THE DECLINE OF BELGIAN FERTILITY, 1800–1970

This book is the fourth in a series on
the decline of fertility in Europe.
A publication of the Office of Population Research
Princeton University.

The Decline of Belgian Fertility, 1800-1970

BY RON J. LESTHAEGHE

PRINCETON UNIVERSITY PRESS
PRINCETON, NEW JERSEY

Published by Princeton University Press, Princeton, New Jersey
In the United Kingdom: Princeton University Press, Guildford, Surrey

Library of Congress Cataloging in Publication Data will
be found on the last printed page of this book

This book has been composed in Linotype Times Roman

Printed in the United States of America
by Princeton University Press, Princeton, New Jersey

To Mams, Paps, and Hi.

Contents

List of Maps and Figures

List of Tables

CHAPTER 1

CHAPTER 2

CHAPTER 3

CHAPTER 5

CHAPTER 6

Foreword

One of the best known generalizations about human populations is that the birth rate tends to fall as a population experiences the set of changes known as industrialization, modernization, or social and economic development. The first statements of this generalization (which describes one-half of the so-called demographic transition) were based on observation of what happened in a few European countries in the nineteenth and early twentieth centuries. By today, the fertility of every national population of Europe is very much lower—in almost every instance at least 50 percent lower—than it was no more than a few generations ago.

About a dozen years ago, the Office of Population Research initiated an ambitious study of the decline in fertility within the provinces of a number of individual European countries. The purpose of the project was a more intensive look at the detailed European statistical records to determine under what conditions the decline in fertility in each province occurred. The project began in 1964 with a "seed" grant from the Rockefeller Foundation, and was subsequently funded by the National Science Foundation and (over most of the project's long life) by the National Institute of Child Health and Human Development. Some of the work has been carried out by members of the Office of Population Research, and some by collaborators at other institutions in Europe and America.

This book is the fourth to be published in a series that includes Livi Bacci's *A Century of Portuguese Fertility* and *The History of Italian Fertility during the Last Two Centuries,* and Knodel's *The Decline of Fertility in Germany, 1871–1939* (van de Walle's *The Female Population of France in the Nineteenth Century* has been published in conjunction with the series).

Belgium is a small country, split both linguistically and economically. To the south are the French-speaking Walloons with their heavy industry and mining; to the north are the Flemish-speaking peoples with a traditional reliance on agriculture and cottage industries. In examining the fertility decline on the basis of the small administrative unit called arrondissement, Lesthaeghe finds the not unexpected result that differences in occupation and language do indeed have an overall effect on fertility patterns. Yet, in a series of statistical analyses, he also shows that a significant portion of the decline remains unrelated to these variables. Lesthaeghe then constructs a variable he calls secularization, and shows that the rejection of traditional values and modes of thinking is equally as important as economic and cultural factors in explaining changes in fertility behavior.

Lesthaeghe's thorough knowledge of the Belgian economy and society, as well as his skill as a demographer and statistical analyst, have produced, in this Belgian study, a solid contribution to the overall project.

Ansley J. Coale
Associate Director
Office of Population Research

Preface

Many books are the result of their author's years of research, teaching, experimenting, and labor. This one is not. It is the result of having spent 18 months with really nice people in one of the most stimulating environments of the demographic profession. I am greatly in debt to all those who have contributed to the European Fertility Project in general, and to the members of the Office of Population Research at Princeton University in particular.

The infectious enthusiasm of Ansley Coale and Etienne van de Walle for reconstructing and interpreting the picture of the European fertility transition has been a major driving force. To this, Hilary Page added substantial improvements and detected numerous inaccuracies and obscurities. She contributed in other ways as well, but there are more adequate means at my disposal to thank her for those.

Guillaume Wunsch, Arthur Campbell, and Luc Danhieux also read the manuscript and offered valuable suggestions. Patricia Taylor took charge of the overall editing and was assisted by Mary Breckenridge, Kirsten Yocom, and Linda Coleman. Anne Ryder (in Princeton) and Gaby Deschepper (in Brussels) typed and retyped the early drafts, while Linda Auerbach prepared the final version.

Behind all this, there is also a financial aspect. Support from the National Institute of Child Health and Human Development (Contract No. NIH-NICHD-70-2077) to the Office of Population Research for the European Fertility Project, and support from the Research Commission of the Vrije Universiteit in Brussels is gratefully acknowledged.

Let me add one afterthought: I thoroughly enjoyed it.

Ron Lesthaeghe
Lagos, Nigeria
October 12, 1976

THE DECLINE OF BELGIAN FERTILITY, 1800–1970

CHAPTER 1: Introduction

In the past two centuries, the population of virtually every European region has experienced an unprecedented reduction in mortality and fertility with the average duration of life substantially increasing, and the average number of children born per woman markedly declining. As a result, changes have also occurred in both the growth rate and age composition of the population. This set of phenomena has often been labeled "the demographic transition." The changes in the vital rates have not provoked much discussion since these are facts that can be documented with little ambiguity by available statistics. However, the reason for the change is not clear and many different viewpoints have been taken to explain the downward trends in mortality and fertility in terms of other demographic, social, economic, or cultural characteristics. Stated differently, the "demographic transition" covers a series of facts, whereas the "demographic transition theory" covers a multitude of possible explanations of these facts.

We restrict ourselves here to discussing that aspect of theory dealing with the fertility decline. We have a double task. First, since data describing the Belgian transition have not been expressed in a way that allows detailed direct comparison with other European experiences, we shall attempt to offer such a description. Second, since a number of different theories have offered specific explanatory hypotheses, we will try to test these hypotheses as fully as possible. This implies that this text is more empirical than theoretical and that a number of hypotheses will remain untested for lack of appropriate data.

1.1 *Why Study the Belgian Fertility Decline?*

The reasons for our interest in the fertility decline occurring in this small country may not be directly obvious. If one were to consider studying population growth in Europe as a whole, the share of the Belgian contingent would be of little significance. The country had only six million inhabitants at the end of the nineteenth century and contributed very little—only three million—to Europe's overall population growth after the turn of the century. However, since we are interested in the decline of fertility and in factors associated with this decline rather than in population growth as such, a closer look at the Belgian situation is worthwhile for two reasons. One is that the decline occurred fairly early; the other is that the country is characterized by a high degree of social, economic, and cultural heterogeneity.

Let us consider the dates of the fertility decline first. In Table 1.1 we present two different indices to measure the date at which fertility started to decline in various European countries. The first list gives the date at which the birth rate fell below 30 live births per 1,000 population, and the second gives the date at which the fertility of married couples declined by 10 percent, never to regain its formal level. The two lists indicate in slightly different ways the national populations that were among the first and last with respect to the fertility decline. The birth

TABLE 1.1

FERTILITY DECLINE, TWO MEASURES OF ONSET, SELECTED EUROPEAN COUNTRIES

Date birth rate falls below 30		Date marital fertility declines 10%	
Decade	Country	Date	Country
1830	France	Pre1830	France
1840	Ireland	1882	Belgium
1880	Belgium, Switzerland	1885	Switzerland
1890	Sweden, Denmark, England and Wales, Scotland, Australia, New Zealand	1890	Germany
1900	Netherlands, Norway, Germany	1892	England and Wales
1910	Canada, Finland, Austria, Hungary, Czechoslovakia	1894	Scotland
1920	Italy, Spain, Portugal	1897	Netherlands
1930	Poland, Bulgaria, Rumania	1900	Denmark
1940	Soviet Union	1904	Norway
1950	Yugoslavia, Japan	1908	Austria
		1910	Finland
		1911	Italy
		1912	Bulgaria
		1918	Spain
		1929	Ireland

SOURCES: N. Ryder, 1967, p. 26; E. van de Walle and J. Knodel, 1967, p. 55.

NOTES: Birth rate is defined as the number of births per 1,000 population. The date of the 10 percent decline in marital fertility is defined as the year in which it declined by that amount, never to return to its former level.

rate indicates roughly the overall level of fertility, combining the effects both of marriage patterns and of fertility levels within marriage; the marital fertility index isolates the fertility level of married couples and is purified of differences in age patterns of marriage. Both lists indicate that the population of France was far ahead of other countries with respect to fertility reduction, preceding them by some 50 years.[1] When we go further down the list based on birth rates, we see that Ireland appears next, followed closely by Switzerland and Belgium. The presence of Ireland high on the list is, however, in some respects accidental, and in the second list based on marital fertility only, Ireland ranks

[1] A systematic presentation of the French data is offered by van de Walle (1974); their interpretation is currently being elaborated by the same author.

fifteenth rather than second. The reason for this discrepancy is that the Irish controlled their overall fertility mainly through a very high mean age at marriage and through high proportions celibate at all ages, rather than through forms of fertility limitation within wedlock. As is shown in the second list, conscious control of fertility within marriage appeared only in the 1920s in Ireland; the birth rate used in the first list is too crude a measure to reflect accurately the fertility level of cohabiting couples.

Belgium, however, ranks as an early decliner on both lists, and if we focus on the marital fertility index, which best captures the onset of fertility control through voluntary and deliberate forms of contraception, we find that Belgium ranks second only to France.

As we indicated previously, the early appearance of marital fertility control is not the only reason why it may be useful to study the Belgian experience. Demographers and historians have also been interested in the relationship between the modernization of fertility behavior and various elements of socioeconomic development such as industrialization and urbanization. In this respect, the examples of France and England are often cited as two poles in Europe's economic and demographic history: France was the first nation to experience the fertility decline and among the last to develop industrial capacity; England, on the other hand, was the pioneer of early industrialization and population concentration, but its first definitive drop in marital fertility occurs 70 years later than in France. The Belgian experience can be situated distinctly between these poles: some areas underwent industrialization as early as 1800–1830 (inaugurating the industrial era on the European continent), while others resembled more closely the French example and shifted away from agriculture and artisanal modes of production only between 1880 and 1910.

In addition, between 1890 and 1900, regional fertility levels in Belgium differed so drastically that a similar heterogeneity within such a small area (11,400 square miles) has remained quite a rare feature in the demographic history of any other European country. For example, the fertility decline in two adjacent Belgian provinces had a time lag of half a century.

Not only do we find a high degree of heterogeneity with respect to the changes in the economic structure and in fertility, but this heterogeneity persists also in many other variables that are of special interest in the study of the fertility transition. Infant mortality rates, for example, varied from about 100 deaths in the first years of life per 1,000 live births in the south to about 350 in some northern coastal areas until 1905. Similarly, life expectancy at birth during the first half of the nineteenth century (i.e., before the breakthrough in mortality control) was only 32 years in a northern province, and at least 46 years in a southern one. Again, these differences occurred in areas only 100 miles apart.

Cultural factors can also be noted for their marked degree of heterogeneity. The process of secularization (more specifically, the gradual shift away from Catholicism) was especially strong in the south and penetrated deeply into most remote villages. In the north, however, adherence to organized religion remained much more intact and only the large urban centers were affected by secularization at the turn of the century. A second cultural feature of great importance in nearly any aspect of Belgian life is the presence of two major linguistic communities. In the north—that is Flanders—Dutch is the local language, and in the south—Wallonia—the vast majority speaks French. Neither language was used originally in its standard form; local dialects were widely used (Flemish and Walloon respectively). Over time the various Flemish dialects survived much longer than the Walloon ones. In the late 1940s there were hardly any Walloons left who could not express themselves in standard French, even in the most remote parts of the countryside; in contrast, a definite majority of the Flemings had trouble shifting to standard Dutch. The Flemish dialect was looked down upon socially, however; in many cases, rather than reveal this dialect in attempting to speak Dutch, the Flemings expressed themselves in French. In fact, the lower degree of secularization and the prolonged attachment to local dialects in Flanders are symptomatic of deeply rooted traditionalism. This higher degree of traditionalism in the north is to a large extent the product of several centuries of economic backwardness and cultural isolation.[2]

To make matters even more complex, both Flanders and Wallonia contain non-negligible linguistic minorities. In Flanders, the cultural and social elite was not Flemish-speaking but Francophone. For example, in 1846 when voting eligibility was a function of wealth, almost

[2] In fact, Flanders was totally cut off from Holland, its linguistic partner, from the middle of the sixteenth century until 1815. Between 1815 and 1830, both countries were unified, but in 1830, following its independence, Belgium was again culturally isolated from Holland. This isolation was only very gradually lifted after 1840, when Belgium and the Netherlands settled their territorial disputes.

three-fourths (14,500 out of a total of 20,000) of the voters in four Flemish provinces were French-speaking. Wallonia contained not only a small German-speaking population (2 percent of the total Walloon population in 1910) but also received a considerable number of Flemish and foreign immigrants as a result of its early industrialization. After World War I, the German-speaking community in Wallonia doubled as a result of the annexation of a previously German area (the "East Cantons"). During the interwar years the industrialized Walloon areas again received the largest share of immigrants from other European countries.

In summary, the Belgian nation in the nineteenth century and in the first half of the twentieth century was a microcosm of European heterogeneity. To a large degree, it shared these economic, demographic, cultural, and linguistic contrasts with Switzerland, its partner on the chronological list of the fertility decline. As a result of its large internal variations, we would expect the Belgian setting to be an interesting laboratory for research on social influences upon such phenomena as fertility levels and fertility decline.

1.2 *Population Growth in the Nineteenth and Twentieth Centuries*

Before turning to a more detailed presentation of the background data and of the fertility variables in the following chapters, it is useful to review briefly the demographic evolution of the Belgian population in general.

During the Napoleonic period, Belgium's population amounted to about 3.2 million and at the time of its independence (1830), there were approximately 3.8 million inhabitants. These grew to 7 million in 1900 and to 9.7 million in 1970 (see Table 1.2). This implies an average annual population growth of 0.8 percent for the period 1830–1900 and a rate of 0.5 percent for 1900–1970. In terms of population density, there were 339 inhabitants per square mile in 1830, 532 in 1900, and 819 in 1970. These general figures cover certain fluctuations over time. To shed more light on these ups and downs, we present Table 1.3, in which we have separated from the total growth rate (balance of births and deaths plus balance of emigration and immigration) the death rate, the birth rate, and the net migration rate for the periods between successive censuses.

Table 1.3 shows first that the total growth rate of the Belgian population exceeded the 1.0 percent level only during a short period (from

TABLE 1.2

POPULATION SIZE AND DENSITY: 1831 TO 1970

Year	Population size (000)	Density per square mile	Density per square kilometer
1831[a]	3,786	332	128
1846	4,337	380	147
1856	4,530	397	153
1866	4,828	423	164
1880	5,520	484	187
1890	6,069	532	206
1900	6,694	587	227
1910	7,424	651	251
1920[b]	7,466	634	244
1930	8,092	687	265
1947	8,512	723	279
1961	9,190	780	301
1970	9,651	819	316

[a]In 1839 Belgium returned a section of the province of Limburg to the Netherlands and ceded the territory which is at present the Grand Duchy of Luxemburg (Treaty of the XXIV Articles). The population figure for 1831 refers to that within the territory of 1840-1919.

[b]As a consequence of the Versailles Treaty, three German cantons (Eupen, Malmedy, Sankt Vith) were placed under Belgian administration in 1919. These cantons joined legally after a plebiscite in 1925. Data from 1920 on incorporate the addition of these cantons.

1901 to 1910) and then only slightly. Similarly, the rate of natural increase (balance of births and deaths) reached the 1.0 percent level only between 1890 and 1910. This moderate growth rate contrasts strikingly with the present rates of increase in most of the developing nations, where levels below 2.0 percent are very rare and levels of

TABLE 1.3

POPULATION GROWTH, SELECTED DEMOGRAPHIC RATES: 1846-1856 TO 1962-1970

Date	Midperiod population (000)	Annual rates per 1,000 population				
		Total increase	Net migration	Natural increase	Birth	Death
1846-1856	4,483	2.0	-3.4	5.4	28.8	23.4
1857-1866	4,679	6.4	-1.8	8.2	32.1	23.9
1867-1880	5,174	9.6	- .3	9.9	32.2	22.3
1881-1890	5,795	9.5	- .3	9.8	30.2	20.4
1891-1900	6,381	9.8	- .3	10.1	29.1	19.0
1901-1910	7,059	10.4	.2	10.2	26.5	16.3
1911-1920	7,413	- .3	-3.1	2.8	18.3	15.5
1921-1930[a]	7,779	8.1	1.8	6.3	19.5	13.2
1931-1947	8,302	3.0	.8	2.2	15.4	13.2
1948-1961	8,851	5.5	.5	5.0	17.0	12.0
1962-1970	9,420	5.4	1.8	3.6	15.9	12.3

[a]Data after 1920 include the population of the annexed German cantons. Their 64,000 inhabitants in 1920 are not counted as migrants and the rates in the table are not distorted by this change in territory.

3.0 percent are often exceeded. The reason for this moderate growth in the Belgian experience is due to the death rate being reduced only gradually and to the control of mortality being fairly well matched by a reduction in the birth rate.

Migration also played a moderating role: there was a negative migration balance (emigration surplus) during the periods of high natural increase and a positive migration balance (immigration surplus) during periods of low natural increase. This dampening effect of migration on population growth was, however, fairly slight since the net migration rate remained in most periods well under the 1.0 per thousand level. In fact, there have only been two times when the Belgian population was affected seriously by emigration: from 1846–1856 (potato blight, crises in textile industry, cholera epidemics); and from 1911–1920 (World War I). Important immigration rates were observed in the period 1921–1930 (return of refugees to the totally devastated province of West Flanders and the import of labor in coal mining areas) and in the period 1962–1970 (import of labor from Mediterranean countries). However, if we take the population of 1846 and add the total surplus stemming from the balance of births and deaths, thereby setting the migration balance to zero and assuming that migrants have the same fertility and mortality conditions as the rest of the population, the 1970 population size would stand at 9.631 million persons compared to the actual 9.651 million. This tiny difference—only 20,000 persons—show very clearly that although migration may have had an effect at particular periods, the overall impact of migration over the last century is virtually negligible. In other words, if the Belgian population would not have been subject to migration since 1830, the growth rates in the nineteenth century would have been slightly higher and those of the twentieth century slightly lower, but by 1970 very much the same population size would have been reached.

1.3 *Administrative and Linguistic Subdivisions*

Most of the statistical material used in subsequent chapters are presented by administrative area. As a result, a short overview of the location of these areas and of the shifts in territory is essential.

During the Napoleonic era, Belgium was an integral part of France; as was customary in post-Revolution France, the territory was also subdivided into départements, most of them named after a river or a geographical feature. Belgium contained nine départements but, as can be seen on Map 1.1, the total area covered by these départements was substantially larger than the present territory. The département Escaut comprised not only the area now called East Flanders, but also most of the modern Dutch province of Zeeland. Similarly, the départements Deux-Nèthes and Meuse Inférieure were made up of a Dutch as well as a

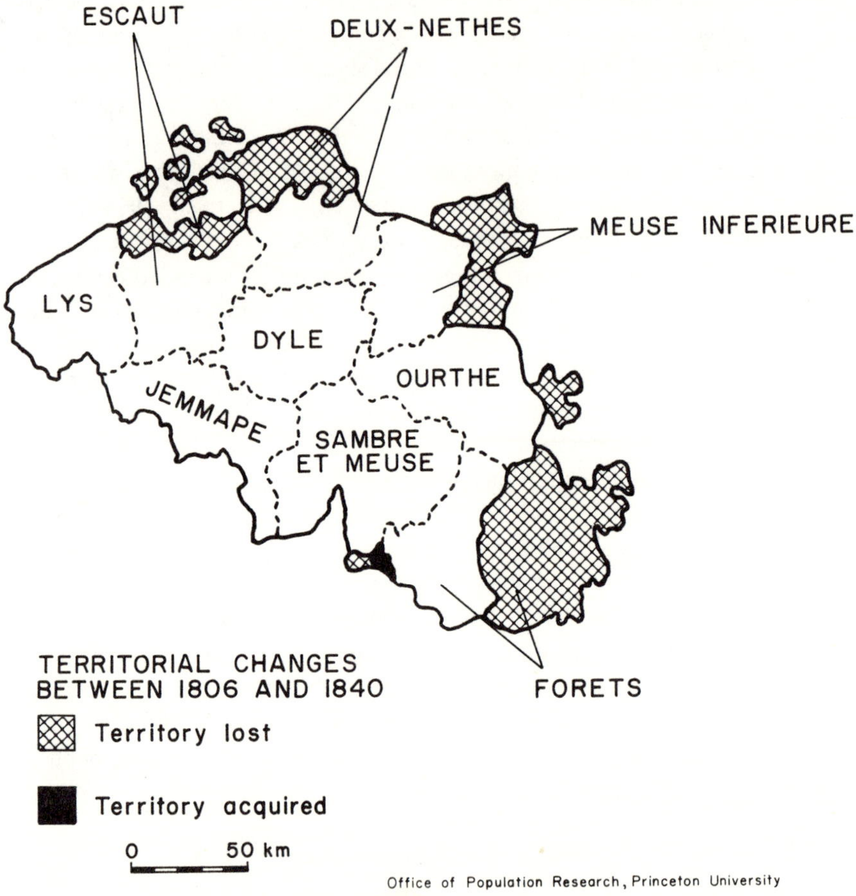

Map 1.1 Boundaries of Belgium and Names of Administrative Units (Départements): 1806–1840.

Belgian part and the département Forêts comprised a portion of the Grand Duchy of Luxemburg, a small part of Germany and a portion of the current Belgian province of Luxemburg. These boundaries were changed by two events: the end of the French Empire in 1815 and Belgium's independence from The Netherlands in 1830. In 1839, a treaty between Belgium and The Netherlands (Treaty of the XXIV Articles) settled territorial disputes between the two countries. Most of the areas shaded on Map 1.1 were either returned to Holland or formed the independent Grand Duchy of Luxemburg. Nearly all of the boundaries of the remainder of the former French départements, however, persist as the boundaries between the nine modern Belgian provinces (see Map 1.2).

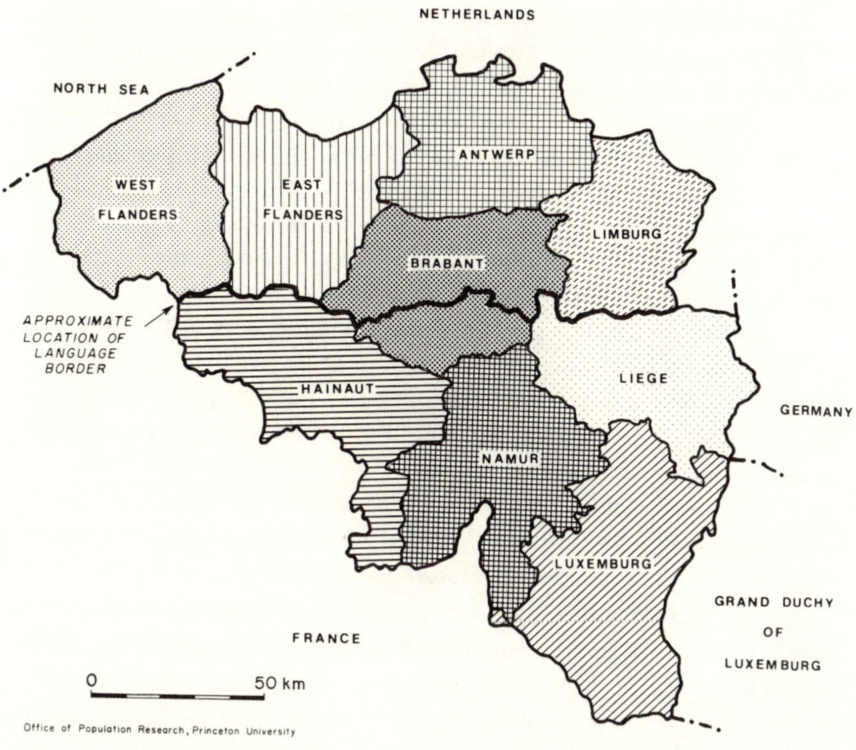

Map 1.2 Boundaries of Belgium and Names of Administrative Units (Provinces): 1840–1919.

From the linguistic point of view, the four northern provinces (West Flanders, East Flanders, Antwerp, and Limburg) speak the Flemish dialect of Dutch and the four southern provinces (Hainaut, Liège, Luxemburg, and Namur) speak French. One province, Brabant, contains not only a Flemish and a French area, but also the bilingual capital of Brussels. When we refer to Flanders, we will have the four Flemish provinces and the Flemish section of Brabant in mind, while the term Wallonia will be used for the four French-speaking provinces plus the Francophone areas of Brabant.[3]

The linguistic situation in Brussels creates a problem of classification. From the sociolinguistic point of view, the area of the capital should definitely not be incorporated with either Flanders or Wallonia. However, administratively, the Brussel's metropolitan area forms one single unit with its Flemish hinterland, and, as such, most social, economic, and demographic data are not only available for that unit as a whole. Under these circumstances, we have occasionally been forced to include the larger Brussels area within Flanders (especially in chapters 5 and 6); wherever possible, however, we have avoided this potential pitfall.

The provinces are further broken down into 41 arrondissements (the names and locations are shown on Map 1.3). These 41 units form the basis of most of the analysis performed in the subsequent chapters. As a rule, the French names are used for Walloon arrondissements and the Dutch names are used for the Flemish arrondissements. However, some areas may be better known to English-speaking readers by their English names and in these instances we have used the English nomenclature instead. To avoid any further confusion, we have prepared Table 1.4, which presents the spelling used in the text, as well as the various linguistic versions of geographical names.

The borders of the 41 arrondissements remained almost completely unchanged from 1840 through 1963. In this period, only the arrondissement of Verviers expanded as a result of the annexation of the German-speaking "East Cantons" following the 1919 Versailles Treaty. After 1963, several arrondissements located along the language border were affected by "linguistic border corrections" and three new arrondissements were created from pieces of others. These alterations after 1920 do not affect the data in our study since detailed analysis of the fertility decline by arrondissement is not taken up after that date.

[3] Until 1963, the metropolitan area of Brussels was administratively joined to a predominantly Flemish section. In 1963, however, this administrative unit was split to reflect more accurately the sociolinguistic composition of the population; the metropolitan area of Brussels became an arrondissement in its own right and the remainder of the territory became a new Flemish arrondissement, Halle-Vilvoorde.

TABLE 1.4

LANGUAGE AND LINGUISTIC NAMES OF BELGIAN ADMINISTRATIVE UNITS

Administrative unit		Name of unit in			
Province	Arrondissement	Dutch	French	English	Language spoken
Antwerp	Antwerp	Antwerpen	Anvers	Antwerp	Dutch (Flemish)
	Mechelen	Mechelen	Malines	Mechlin	"
	Turnhout	Turnhout	--	--	"
Brabant	Brussels	Brussel	Bruxelles	Brussels	Dutch & French
	Leuven	Leuven	Louvain	--	Dutch (Flemish)
	Nivelles	Nijvel	Nivelles	--	French (Walloon)
East Flanders	Aalst	Aalst	Alost	--	Dutch (Flemish)
	Dendermonde	Dendermonde	Termonde	--	"
	Eeklo	Eeklo	--	--	"
	Ghent	Gent	Gand	Ghent	"
	Oudenaarde	Oudenaarde	Audenarde	--	"
	Sint Niklaas	Sint Niklaas	Saint Nicolas	--	"
West Flanders	Bruges	Brugge	Bruges	Bruges	"
	Diksmuide	Diksmuide	Dixmude	--	"
	Kortrijk	Kortrijk	Courtrai	--	"
	Ostend	Oostende	Ostende	Ostend	"
	Roeselare	Roeselare	Roulers	--	"
	Tielt	Tielt	--	--	"
	Veurne	Veurne	Furnes	--	"
	Ypres	Ieperen	Ypres	Ypres	"
Hainaut	Ath	Aat	Ath	--	French (Walloon)
	Charleroi	--	Charleroi	--	"
	Mons	Bergen	Mons	--	"
	Soignies	--	Soignies	--	"
	Thuin	--	Thuin	--	"
	Tournai	Doornik	Tournai	--	"
Liège	Huy	Hoei	Huy	--	"
	Liège	Luik	Liège	--	"
	Verviers	--	Verviers	--	French & German
	Waremme	Borgworm	Waremme	--	French (Walloon)
Limburg	Hasselt	Hasselt	--	--	Dutch (Flemish)
	Masseik	Maaseik	--	--	"
	Tongeren	Tongeren	Tongres	--	"
Luxemburg	Arlon	Aarlen	Arlon	--	French (Walloon)
	Bastogne	Bastenaken	Bastogne	--	"
	Marche	--	Marche	--	"
	Neufchâteau	--	Neufchâteau	--	"
	Virton	--	Virton	--	"
Namur	Dinant	--	Dinant	--	"
	Namur	Namen	Namur	--	"
	Philippe-ville	--	Philippe-ville	--	"

NOTE: Underlined names are those used in this monograph.

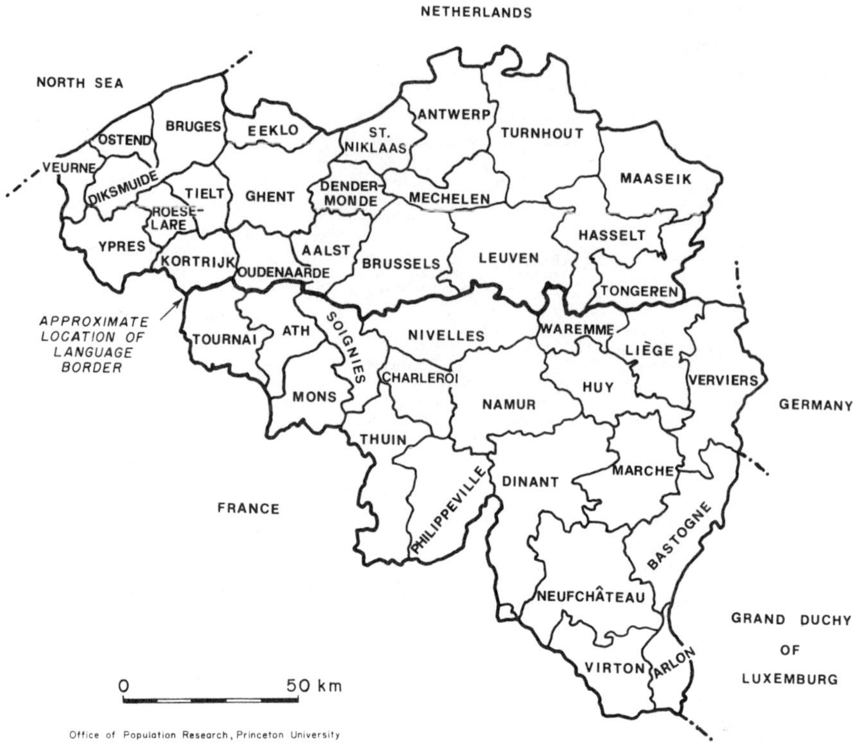

Map 1.3 Arrondissements of Belgium: 1840–1919.

References—Chapter 1

Ryder, N. 1967. The character of modern fertility. *The Annals* (American Academy of Political and Social Sciences) 26:369-374.

Quételet, A., and Smits, E. 1832. *Recherches sur la reproduction et la mortalité de l'homme aux différents âges et sur la population de la Belgique.* Brussels: Louis Hauman et Cie.

van de Walle, E. 1974. *The female population of France in the nineteenth century.* Princeton: Princeton University Press.

van de Walle, E., and Knodel, J. 1967. Demographic transition and fertility decline: the European case. In *Proceedings of the International Population Conference,* pp. 47-55, Sydney: International Union for the Scientific Study of Population.

CHAPTER 2: The Social and Economic Modernization

This chapter on Belgian social and economic development in the nineteenth and early twentieth centuries is meant to give a succinct picture of the background variables that have conditioned the decline in marital fertility and the development of the present marriage pattern. The story of the demographic transition cannot be taken out of its general context in any case and certainly not in this particular one. Hence, a summary of the most important social and economic trends is essential. Their relevance with respect to the demographic change will become apparent in the following chapters.

2.1 *Introduction*

Belgium was the first country on the European continent to adopt the industrial innovations of England and to construct its own industrial revolution. However, the two countries differed socially, politically, and economically, so that the points of departure in industrialization were different in timing and in other ways as well. The market conditions for new industry in Belgium were more limited and unstable. Belgium was governed under four different sovereignties between 1770 and 1840: under the Austrians until the French Revolution; under the French until 1815; under the Dutch until 1830; and, finally, as an independent state from 1830 on. Consequently, the newly developing industry was subject to successive reorientations of its market. Belgium's typical pattern of small-scale, intensive agriculture with a dense rural population was another distinctive feature. In addition, the development of modern financial institutions and apparatus was retarded compared with the English experience, the patterns of social stratification were different from the English ones, and each country had its own cultural traditions.

Within Belgium, the Flemish and Walloon patterns of industrialization should be distinguished. In Wallonia, early full-scale exploitation of coal fields drastically altered the preindustrial structure of the metal industries. Walloon textile mills were independent of locally produced commodities as they operated with imported wool and, later, imported cotton. Consequently, the link between industry and agriculture was to a large extent broken in Wallonia by 1830, so that the former could expand without being hampered by the lagging development of the latter. In Flanders, the tie between industry and agriculture remained very tight: the linen industry was dependent on locally produced flax and when the competition of imported cotton became important, there were severe crises in agriculture. This interdependence found its expression in the prominence of dual labor force participation in subsistence farming and cottage industry. This combination proved to be highly resistant to change during the entire nineteenth century. Only after the two crises of 1841–1845 and 1885 did economic modernization become really evident in Flanders.

Thus, as will be discussed below in more detail, the industrial revolution in Belgium not only differed from the English or any other type (H. van der Wee, 1972), but also led to a dual form of economic development, resulting in major differences between Flanders and Wallonia.

2.2 *Industrialization in Wallonia*

As previously indicated, Wallonia experienced the classic form of industrialization, based on heavy industry and mechanized textile mills. In fact, two poles can be identified: the northern pole was formed by the Liège and Verviers area and the southern pole was located in the central part of the province of Hainaut. Both poles were already well known as industrial centers in the seventeenth and eightheenth centuries.

Until the French Revolution, the northern pole of Liège and Verviers was a principality (that is, an independent political and economic unit). Its industry suffered from protectionism, toll wars, and other trade barriers that separated it from its natural hinterland, the Austrian Netherlands. The first phase of modern industrialization occurred only after the elimination of these barriers under French rule in the first decades of the nineteenth century. The mechanization of the textile industry in the Verviers area, for example, started about 1805–1810, approximately fifteen years after England. The promoters of this early modernization were an English engineering family, the Cockerills, who introduced modern machinery through contracts with local entrepreneurs. The results of their action were evident almost immediately; fully equipped textile mills contributed 50 percent of total production in 1810 (H. van der Wee, 1972, p. 181), thanks to this successful combination of English engineering and local capital. This led not only to a rapid diversification of production, but also, in a short span of only 20 years, to the conversion from partly preindustrial workshops and partly cottage industry to modern textile mills by 1830. The success of the Cockerills did not stop in Verviers. They went on immediately to set up a workshop for machinery and tool construction in Liège and there laid the basis for one of the first integrated industries in the European continent. The Cockerill works introduced the first coke blast-furnace on the mainland and also the puddling method for steel production. They built the first steam locomotive and railway on the continent. Their plant at Seraing (a suburb of Liège) employed 2,000 men in 1840, while Krupp, the German giant of the end of the century, then employed only 70 men (E. A. Wrigley, 1961, p. 14).

The southern pole of industry in Wallonia, located in Hainaut, stretched approximately from Mons to Charleroi; the western part of this area, known as the Borinage and Centre, was an important coal-mining center in the seventeenth century. New infrastructure and technological improvements, together with the opening of the French market after the annexation in 1795, were a boost for Hainaut's coal production. As can be seen in Table 2.1, annual coal production increased from

TABLE 2.1

ANNUAL COAL PRODUCTION, BELGIUM, NORTHERN FRANCE, AND WESTERN GERMANY: 1695 to 1910
(In thousands of metric tons)

	Belgium		Northern France		Western Germany			
Date	Hainaut	Liège	Nord	Pas-de-Calais	Aachen	Düssel-dorf	Arnsberg	Reckling-hausen
1695	ca 24	--	--	--	--	--	--	--
1770-1790	ca 450	--	--	--	--	--	--	--
1807-1811	ca 1,000	--	--	--	--	--	--	--
1829	ca 1,692	--	--	--	--	--	--	--
1850	4,753	1,292	1,000	--	424	1,666		--
1880	12,549	3,824	3,533	4,775	1,175	7,480	13,874	951
1910	16,700	6,500	6,589	19,120	2,636	27,850	43,495	16,972

SOURCES: Hainaut: M. Gillet, 1968 as quoted by H. Van der Wee, 1972, p. 185.
Other areas: E. A. Wrigley, 1961, p. 42.

24,000 metric tons in 1695, to 450,000 metric tons in 1770–1790, and to 1,000,000 metric tons during the Napoleonic period. At the start of the nineteenth century, this area, which formed the French Département de Jemappes, produced 25 to 30 percent of the coal production of the entire European continent (H. van der Wee, 1972, p. 185). The French market for coal remained accessible even after Waterloo, especially since a new network of canals facilitated transportation. However, growth slowed in the years 1815–1835, largely for technological reasons: the pumps of the Newcomen type, which were introduced around 1720, were not replaced by more advanced types until around 1840.

The eastern half of the Hainaut pole, Charleroi, had some metal industries during the eighteenth century, but they were not of great importance. Its industrial boom between 1820 and 1830 was, therefore, all the more spectacular: all the English technological inventions related to metallurgy were introduced almost simultaneously by a few local and English entrepreneurs. The coke-fired blast-furnaces of Charleroi were introduced at a crucial time. The old metal industries located in the nearby Entre Sambre et Meuse area (corresponding to the arrondissements of Thuin and Philippeville), which used charcoal to smelt iron ore, were facing a crisis since they could not boost iron production without endangering the limited supply of local timber. Consequently, the last blast-furnace operating with charcoal in this area was extinguished in 1851 and the new metallurgy of Charleroi became an important customer for the neighboring Borinage coal fields.

The heyday of the Walloon industrialization was reached between 1840 and World War I. As can be seen in Table 2.1, in 1850, the Belgian provinces of Hainaut and Liège produced twice as much coal as the other major coal-mining areas in northern France and western Germany combined, but, after 1870, competition grew at an accelerated pace and the geological features of the Walloon coal layers hampered increased exploitation. Hainaut started to lose its industrial primacy to the more highly diversified economy of the Liège area: iron, steel, and tool and die remained more competitive and such newly mechanized industries as glass and zinc, together with the growing modern chemical industry, consolidated the lead of the northern pole.

2.3 *Industrialization in Flanders*

An industrial structure began in the Flemish provinces of the Austrian Netherlands in the Middle Ages and existed in both the cities and the countryside. It consisted of specialized sectors supplying western Europe with luxury articles. After the Spanish occupation in the second half of the sixteenth century this activity declined, suffering heavily from successive wars and, later, from the protectionist policies of European mercantilism. By the eighteenth century, Flanders mainly produced standardized textiles; this production was concentrated in urban areas and had a weak export position. At the same time, new agricultural techniques brought economic benefits to the countryside of the provinces of East and West Flanders and Brabant; between 1760 and 1780, a century-long import of cereals changed to an annual export. In addition, the production of flax became stimulated by exports to Latin America, and the linen industry developed more fully in the "Sandy Soil" areas of East and West Flanders. This created demand for additional work in the form of rural cottage industry which remained, however, directly linked to the subsistence agriculture in these regions.

The development of rural cottage industry in Flanders, permitting the rural population to stay on their small farms in the second half of the eighteenth century, turned out to be the prime factor of resistance to modernization in the entire nineteenth century. The agricultural sector producing flax and the industrial sector spinning and weaving it into linen were inseparable. A considerable proportion of the very densely settled rural population needed both sectors to survive. At the start of the nineteenth century, a first attempt at modernization occurred in the urban textile mills of Ghent, which processed imported cotton, the main rival of locally produced flax. It was based on advanced equipment, some smuggled from England, including mule jennies, flying shuttles, and progressive techniques for bleaching, dyeing, and printing. However, the Ghent enterprises could thrive only insofar as their market was protected from the merciless competition of English fabrics. Initially, the Continental Blockade of 1806 served this purpose, but the French hinterland was lost in 1815, leading to a first serious crisis. Under the Dutch regime, a new export market was found in Indonesia, but independence in 1830 and the separation from Holland and its colonies brought another crisis in 1831. These years of unstable market and political conditions, combined with the widening of the technological and production gaps between England and Flanders, were economically devastating to the mills of Ghent and resulted in the continued vitality of the rural cottage industry. At the time of the first population and industrial census in 1846, this component made up more than a quarter of the labor force in the provinces of East and West Flanders, employing no less than 120,000 workers (weaving, spinning, lace-making, and embroidery) and 80,000 other artisanal workers. In Brabant and Antwerp another 100,000 workers, or one-fifth of the labor force (B. Verhaegen, 1961, II, 281-285), were engaged in cottage industries. The vast majority of these were in some way directly dependent on the linen industry and earned very low wages compared to other sectors (Figure 2.1). Since cottage weaving and spinning was a family enterprise, a large number of children were employed; this deprived the children of any form of proper education and depressed the wages of

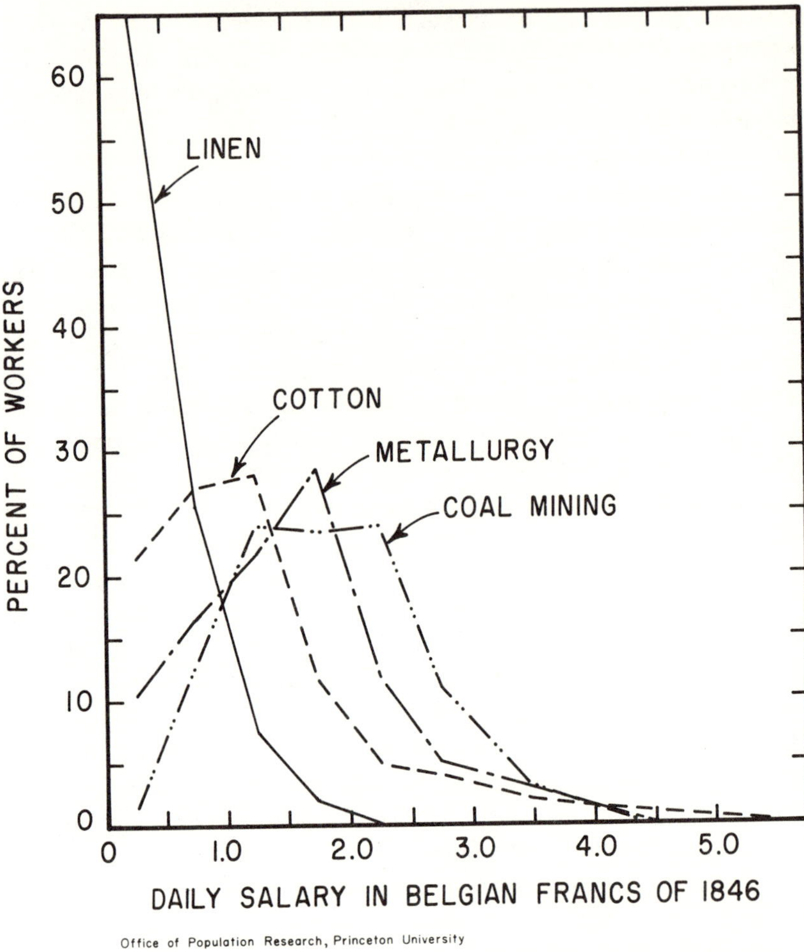

Figure 2.1 Average Daily Salary, Workers in Linen, Cotton, Metallurgy, and Coal Industries: 1846.
SOURCE: B. Verhaegen (1961, p. 201).

adults. This industry, which had provided additional employment in regions with subsistence farming in 1740, became more and more a genuine anachronism in the nineteenth century. This was suddenly revealed in 1841–1845: the stiff competition between domestic linen and foreign cotton and the potato crop failures of the 1840s undermined the economic survival of these two basic sectors. The most serious crisis of the entire century erupted and widespread pauperism in Flanders became a reality. Extensive investment in and expansion of such industrial enterprises as the Cockerill works in Wallonia was in sharp contrast to the poverty and mendicancy in Flanders.

After 1850, the structure of cottage industry changed. As Table 2.2 indicates, the male labor force participation in the sector dropped from 18.0 to 8.7 percent, and this type of work became the preeminent activity for women. Part of the surplus male labor went back into agriculture, causing a rise of 3 to 6 percent in this part of the labor force in the provinces of Brabant, and East and West Flanders. In other

TABLE 2.2

AGRICULTURAL AND SELECTED COTTAGE INDUSTRY WORKERS, BY SEX, COMBINED PROVINCES OF EAST AND WEST FLANDERS: 1846 TO 1910

		Number				Percentage of male labor force			
Sex	Industry	1846	1866	1890	1910	1846	1866	1890	1910
Male workers	Agriculture	159,673	201,633	187,653	166,942	36.0	41.9	34.6	30.6
	Weavers in cottage industry	48,033	41,750	20,273	--	18.0	8.7	3.7	--
	Total	207,706	243,383	207,926	166,942	54.0	50.6	38.3	30.6
						Percentage of female labor force			
Female workers	Agriculture	89,656	90,480	70,603	25,650	24.9	28.5	24.1	8.6
	Lace-making and embroidery	71,921	82,854	48,316	77,157	19.9	26.1	29.0	25.9
	Total	161,577	173,334	118,919	102,807	44.8	54.6	53.1	34.5

SOURCE: Adapted from B. Verhaegen, 1961.

provinces, those without cottage industry, employment in agriculture was reduced by 4 percent between 1846 and 1866. Consequently, provincial changes in agricultural employment differed by some 7 to 10 percent.

With regard to the female labor force, an alternative to spinning linen yarn was sought. The solution was found in lace-making, and between 1846 and 1866 the number of female lace-makers or *dentellières* grew from 49,000 to 62,000. The latter census figure, however, is considered by many authorities to be a serious underenumeration, and alternative figures ranging from 100,000 to 130,000 are commonly quoted. The structure of the lace industry was unusual: 10 to 15 exporters, all located in Brussels, monopolized production. They bought raw materials and distributed them to 1,000 "lace schools" set up by Catholic orders. In these "schools" very little education was offered and all the attention was directed to making different points or stitches. As fashion changed, and this occurred very often, the dentellières had to be retrained repeatedly—to shift now from the *point de Bruges* to the *point de Venise,* then from Irish stitches to the *point d'Armentière*—making them even more dependent on the schools and the entire system. The dentellières received the yarn and returned the small *rosaces* to the nuns who then put them together and returned the finished products to the export firms in Brussels. Contrary to the view of the church and conservative political opinion, this organization of lace-making was not an adequate response to the pauperism arising in the 1840s and 1850s. The small dimension of the enterprises, the concealed structural unemployment, the weak development of the tertiary sector, and, above all, the lack of capital, mobility, drive, and intellectual life meant that lace-making was merely a palliative for Flemish economic and social problems. This was revealed in the crisis of 1880.

2.4 *The Structure of Agriculture and Land Tenure*

Annexation by the French Republic early in the nineteenth century led to the abolishment of all remainders of the feudal system and put an end to all forms of payment other than ordinary rent. The benefits accruing from these moves were wiped out when the confiscated properties of the nobility were subsequently restored to their previous owners by Napoleon. The nationalization of church property had a more important impact, but it cannot be said that the sale of these lands increased the amount of land owned by the farmers themselves or created a class of peasant proprietors. The Catholic peasants remained faithful and it was hard to find purchasers for the *bien noirs* among them. The land of the religious orders was brought primarily by townsmen, foreigners, and speculators, who sought to divide it up and to rent the new plots to tenants.

Contrary to what might have been expected, the effects of the French period constituted a step backward rather than forward in terms of more extensive ownership by small land holders. The peasants even lost the more favorable tenures, since the abolition of church property led to the elimination of the emphyteutic tenures—i.e., long-term leases of some ecclesiastic property (varying from 27 to 99 years) that had given the tenants the possibility of improving the land and the right to erect buildings on it. Short-term leases of 3, 6, or 9 years became the rule, permitting a faster succession of rent increases.

The concentration of land in the hands of fewer landlords developed even further when much of the state land was sold and brought under cultivation between 1815 and 1850, and when the remainder of the commons was abolished after the famines of 1846 and 1847. The careful analysis of E. Vandervelde (1900, 1902) shows repeatedly that the concentration of land ownership also continued into the second half of the nineteenth century. From 1846 to 1895, the number of cultivated hectares (1 ha=2.741 acres) under direct ownership per 100 hectares of arable land decreased from 34 to 31, a remarkably low figure even in European perspective; and, according to Seebohm-Rowntree's representative sample, a third of this land was mortgaged (Seebohm-Rowntree, 1910, p. 42). As shown in Table 2.3, the figure for cultivation

TABLE 2.3

AGRICULTURAL LAND, PERCENTAGE OWNED BY CULTIVATOR, BY PROVINCE: 1846 TO 1895

Province	1846	1856	1866	1895
Antwerp	27.2	27.1	27.4	27.0
Brabant	29.6	30.2	30.9	27.9
West Flanders	15.1	13.7	12.2	11.7
East Flanders	24.1	25.0	24.0	22.2
Hainaut	35.6	35.7	34.9	31.0
Liège	36.8	37.2	35.2	31.0
Limburg	47.6	45.6	42.2	40.8
Luxemburg	74.4	75.9	66.9	66.0
Namur	41.0	41.0	36.4	36.3
Belgium	34.2	34.3	32.7	31.1

SOURCE: E. Vandervelde, 1902, p. 9.

under direct ownership was only 12 percent in the province of West Flanders, leaving 88 percent of the arable land to be cultivated by tenants.

Regional information on the systems of land tenure is given in Table 2.3 and in Map 2.1, where the percentages of rented land are specified by arrondissement in the middle and at the end of the nineteenth century. Only the province of Luxemburg was characterized by fairly widespread cultivation by owner-farmers. However, the concentration of ownership was really a national phenomenon. This strongly capitalistic form of land tenure was directly related to other features: extreme fragmentation of the holdings, a steady rise of rents until 1880, and high rural population densities in certain areas.

In 1846, the census revealed that 56 percent of all agricultural enter-

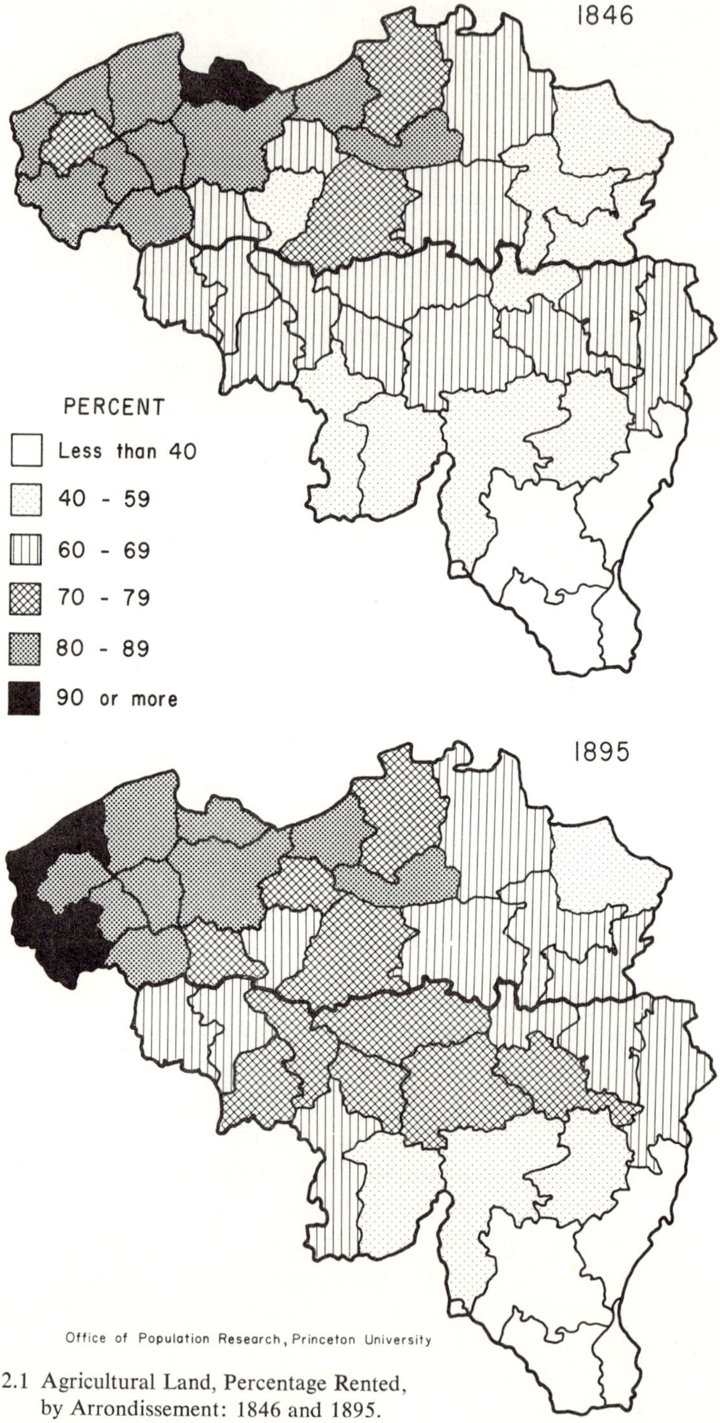

Map 2.1 Agricultural Land, Percentage Rented, by Arrondissement: 1846 and 1895.
SOURCE: Agricultural census of 1895.

prises were smaller than 1 hectare; that these small holdings were often made up of several separate parcels; and that 40 percent were even smaller than 0.5 hectare, constituting merely gardening facilities. To the industrial workers of Hainaut and Liège, this gardening was indicative of a certain prosperity, whereas in Flanders, it was indispensable for the subsistence of small tenants, cottage workers, and farm laborers. Setting the sum of the holdings of more than 1 hectare equal to unity, we still find an extreme concentration of enterprises in the category of 1 to 5 hectares; as shown in Table 2.4, only 11 percent of the holdings are more than 15 hectares. The information in Table 2.4 clearly

TABLE 2.4

AGRICULTURAL ENTERPRISES, PERCENTAGE DISTRIBUTION BY SIZE, BY PROVINCE: 1846

Province	1-5 hectares	5-15 hectares	15-50 hectares	50 or more hectares
Antwerp	56.2	33.0	10.4	0.4
Brabant	74.3	17.5	6.7	1.5
West Flanders	54.5	25.3	18.6	1.6
East Flanders	69.6	23.0	7.1	0.3
Hainaut	69.2	19.9	8.9	1.9
Liège	63.7	24.7	8.7	2.9
Limburg	56.6	32.9	9.4	1.1
Luxemburg	61.3	26.3	10.2	2.2
Namur	69.5	18.3	7.5	4.7
Belgium	65.2	23.6	9.5	1.7

SOURCE: Agricultural census of 1846.

NOTE: 1 hectare = 2.471 acres.

demonstrates that two-thirds of the Belgian agricultural holdings were devoted mainly to subsistence farming and only one-third to regular market farming.

Another, almost unique, feature of the Belgian system of land tenure was that the price or rent of land was not a function of the quality of the soil. E. de Laveleye (1875, p. 445), speaking of some parts of interior Flanders, says: "The soil of Flanders hardly permits the natural growth of heather and furze. It is the worst soil in all Europe. . . . Having been fertilized by ten centuries of laborious husbandry, the soil of Flanders does not yield a single crop without being manured once or twice, a fact unique in Europe." This poor soil to which de Laveleye refers lies entirely within the area of high annual rent, shown on Map 2.2. Of the ten arrondissements having the highest agricultural land

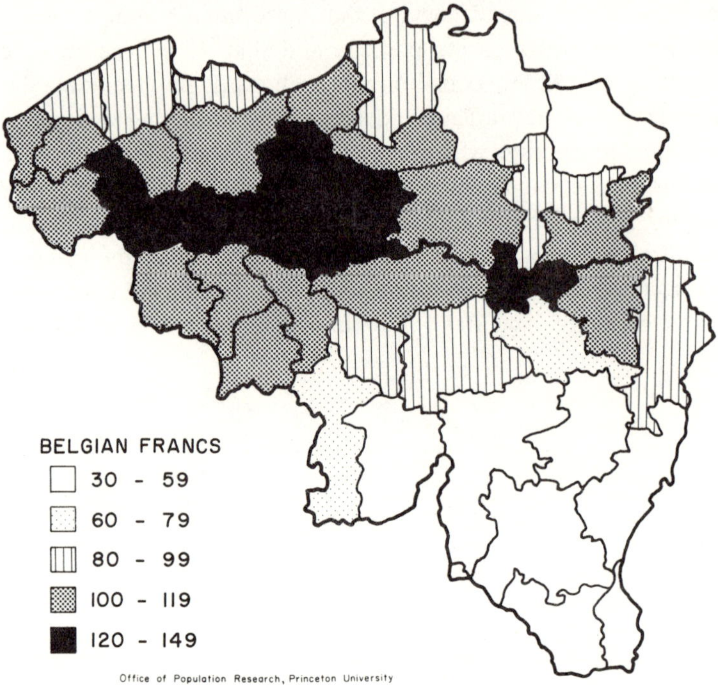

Map 2.2 Agricultural Land, Average Annual Rent per Hectare, by Arrondissement: 1895.
SOURCE: Agricultural census of 1895.
NOTE: Acreage designated as "meadow lands" not included.

values, no less than nine are located, either wholly or in part, within this "Sandy Soil" area of Flanders. Only one is located in Wallonia, the arrondissement of Waremme, where the high land value is due to the spread of industrial crops such as sugar beets.

The explanation for these high land values in Flanders has to be sought in the high rural population densities and the intensive form of agriculture (permitting a high yield despite the condition of the soil) and, in some areas, the growth of flax. The demand for agricultural land in general was not only very large—Seebohm-Rowntree speaks of "land hunger" (1910, p. 151)—but the demand for small farms was also greater than for large ones. Comparatively few people possessed sufficient capital to rent or buy the latter, and there was little demand for large plots when they came onto the market. Competition for the small ones, on the other hand, was keen and prices much in excess of the real worth were frequently paid. As E. Vandervelde (1902, p. 10) notes, the price of land or the rent was low in areas where a large proportion was owned by the farmers, and was double or triple in areas worked by tenants. A comparison of Maps 2.1 and 2.2 illustrates this. In addition, the increase of rent per hectare was considerably larger for small holdings than for the bigger ones. As a consequence, the benefit margins of the small tenants remained compressed.

How could this system have survived for such a long period of time? First, most of the small farmers continued their family enterprise regardless of the marginal productivity of labor and aimed at maximizing the yield per hectare through intensive forms of agriculture (see L. Berkner and F. Mendels, 1972, p. 8). The improvement of fertilization was therefore a crucial issue, and in Belgium more artificial manure per hectare of arable land was used than in any other country of the world. Second, when the marginal productivity fell too low, a supplement of income was earned in rural industry. The large farms, however, operating with wage labor could not afford a dropping marginal productivity of labor. More extensive forms of agriculture had to be used, the output per hectare was lower and so was the rent or the price of land.

Another factor often used as an explanatory variable in connection with the development of these agricultural conditions is the legislation regulating inheritance and succession. Vandervelde (1902, p. 11) suggests that the system of equal division of inheritance among the children was responsible for the fragmentation of the land. This statement cannot be accepted without major qualifications. As early as the eighteenth century, the succession of property was regulated along the lines of partible inheritance and equal division in Belgian Flanders. It is possible that this caused subdivision and fragmentation in the "Sandy Soil" areas. In other regions, such as the *Polders* (a strip along the coast and the upper part of the Scheldt river), subdivision was not the rule and large holdings with regular dairy and market farming were maintained. Although the Walloon areas had a system more along the lines of impartible inheritance in the eighteenth century, many did not escape the tendency of fragmentation. Moreover, even when the *Code Civil* was introduced under the French occupation, making partible inheritance the national rule, those Walloon regions with market farming resisted the consequences of equal sharing and maintained large land holdings. Thus, fragmentation seems to be more a fact of economics than of legislation. Anyway, whatever the system of succession may be, partible or impartible, it can only affect the minority of landowners, not the majority of tenants.

The position of Belgian agriculture on the international market is also of considerable importance. Between 1822 and 1880 this section was heavily protected against foreign competition; under the pretext of assuring the income of the masses, such protection actually served the interests of the landowners and delayed the modernization of rural structures. In the meantime, however, it became more evident that small market farming could not meet the increasing demands of the industrial and urban population, despite the breakthroughs of modern fertilization leading to quality and quantity improvements. The Belgian market had to be opened to foreign products, and when this happened, in the last quarter of the nineteenth century, it was flooded with cheap wheat from the United States. What had been postponed for decades finally occurred: the sale value of land dropped by a third between 1880 and 1895, and 7 percent of the total active male population left agriculture. Once again a growing part of the rural population had to seek employment elsewhere; this time, the cottage industry could not offer an alternative since it had become saturated with underpaid female workers. Many Flemish men moved to the Walloon industrial areas, became seasonal workers in the industries of northern France, or in the large agricultural enterprises of central France. In the same way as Ireland sent its *harvestmen* to England, or Austria its *Wanderarbeiter* to Germany, Flanders exported its *Fransmannen* (Frenchies) to French-speaking areas each summer. Some Belgians, but relatively few in comparison with other European countries, emigrated to America. The largest part of those affected by the agricultural crisis continued to stay on the land and started commuting on a weekly or daily basis to the urban centers. A period characterized by increasing spatial mobility had begun.

2.5 *The Occupational Structure*

It is our intention to use the occupational structure as the principal indicator of economic development, a crucial variable in the study of fertility and nuptiality changes. However, this creates a problem of measurement since the sections in the censuses on occupational distribution are not always directly comparable. Sometimes important differences in the classification of occupations and industries occur in successive censuses, making a systematic comparison over time difficult. For example: (1) agricultural day-laborers are lumped together with other day-laborers in 1846, but are classified with agricultural workers in 1866; and (2) all the censuses of the nineteenth century have a category for nonindustrial laborers, but this category disappears in 1910 and its content is then distributed over the other sections. Problems of under-enumeration arise, particularly for female employment. We have already cited the underenumeration of *dentellières* in 1866; in addition, census figures relative to female labor force participation in agriculture are by no means as trustworthy as the corresponding figures for males. Hence the female employment data in Table 2.2 should be interpreted with care.

A systematic attempt to regroup the various sections of the occupational structure was made by B. Verhaegen in 1961. He put all the original census data on cards and reprocessed this detailed material so as to yield larger and more uniform categories than had been published previously. In this way, he was able to separate out some of the previously entangled material (the number of agricultural day-laborers in 1846 for instance); but his results are still limited by the original questions and classifications used in each census. Verhaegen's main object was to establish a distinction between small, medium, and large industries, based on the ratio of workers to managers. This distinction by size of enterprise led to confusion with regard to self-employed craftsmen, cottage workers, and laborers in other small industries. Other groups, such as agriculture, trade and transportation, or large industries showed more consistent results. Consequently, while his work helps in describing the major trends, the detailed analysis and the construction of specific indices used in the following chapters had to be based on the original tables.

The census takers cannot take the full blame for some of the heterogeneity of their products. The changes in the nineteenth century were not always predictable; classifications used in European censuses varied considerably from country to country; and the occupational structure was complex especially where concealed structural unemployment existed or where the distinction between dominant and secondary occupation remained obscure. A. Quételet, the leading Belgian statistician of the nineteenth century, refused to set up a category of cottage workers in 1846, fearing precisely a double count of those simultaneously engaged in cottage industry and agriculture. It is only from 1910 on that the classification of occupations became more consistent. By then, the occupational structure was already largely modernized and could be captured more easily by fixed categories. The census of 1910 is, therefore, often taken as a starting point in the analysis of professions and industries (F. Pontanus, 1968); the classic authors in this field, such as C. Clark and J. Fourastié, incorporate the Belgian data in their work only from 1910 on.

Rather than ignoring the data prior to 1910 altogether, we prefer to consider them with appropriate reservations. We have represented the apparent evolution in employment in agriculture for the whole country in Figure 2.2, and employment in medium and large industry, trade and

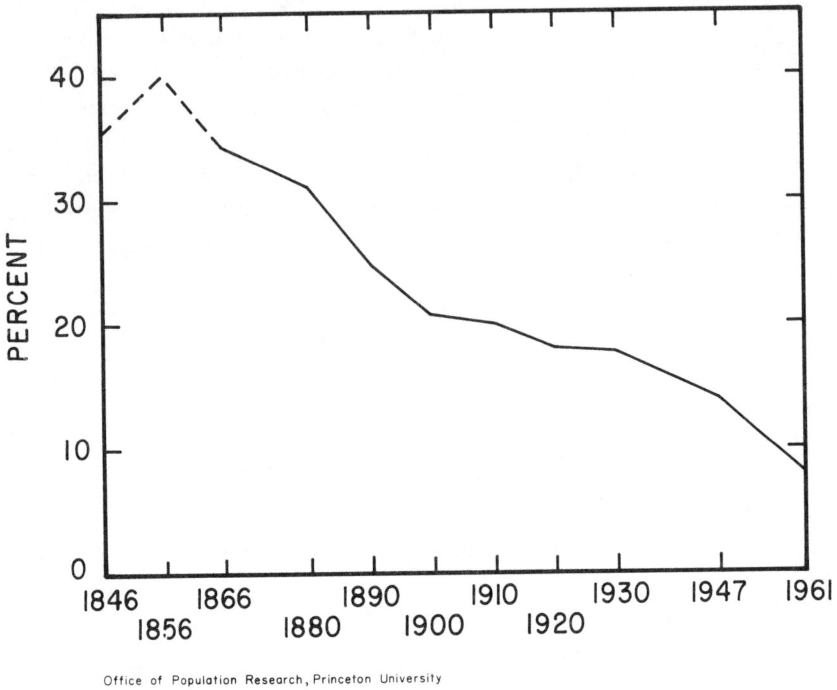

Figure 2.2 Male Labor Force, Percentage in Agriculture: 1846 to 1961.

SOURCES: R. Grooten (1951), B. Verhaegen (1961), and F. Pontanus (1968).

transportation, and agriculture by groups of provinces in Figure 2.3. The percentage of the male labor force engaged in agriculture in Figure 2.2 shows clearly the major trends in this sector. But one must be cautious in interpreting this material. The changes between 1846 and 1866 are represented by dotted lines because these three censuses are not entirely comparable with respect to the figures for agricultural day-laborers and servants. While Verhaegen's corrections were adopted (1961, II, pp. 29-36), we still have to consider the figures for 1846 and 1856 as estimates. However, the initial upward movement of the curve on Figure 2.2 can be accepted as authentic. It corresponds with the temporary drainage back into agriculture (disguised unemployment) following the crisis in the linen sector in the 1840s; the upward movement is most evident in the provinces of Antwerp, Brabant, and East and West Flanders (Figure 2.3). Between 1880 and 1900 the national curve of percentage employed in agriculture registered its steepest downward slope; this corresponds to the crisis of the 1880s. After 1900, the curve becomes more horizontal as the marginal agricultural labor had already found its way into other sectors; it was only after World War II that a new downward acceleration took place (Figure 2.2).

The information in Figure 2.3 shows clearly the main regional trends in occupational structure: in 1910 only the provinces of Antwerp, Brabant, Hainaut, and Liège had less than 20 percent of the male active population in agriculture. In Antwerp and Brabant the sectors of trade

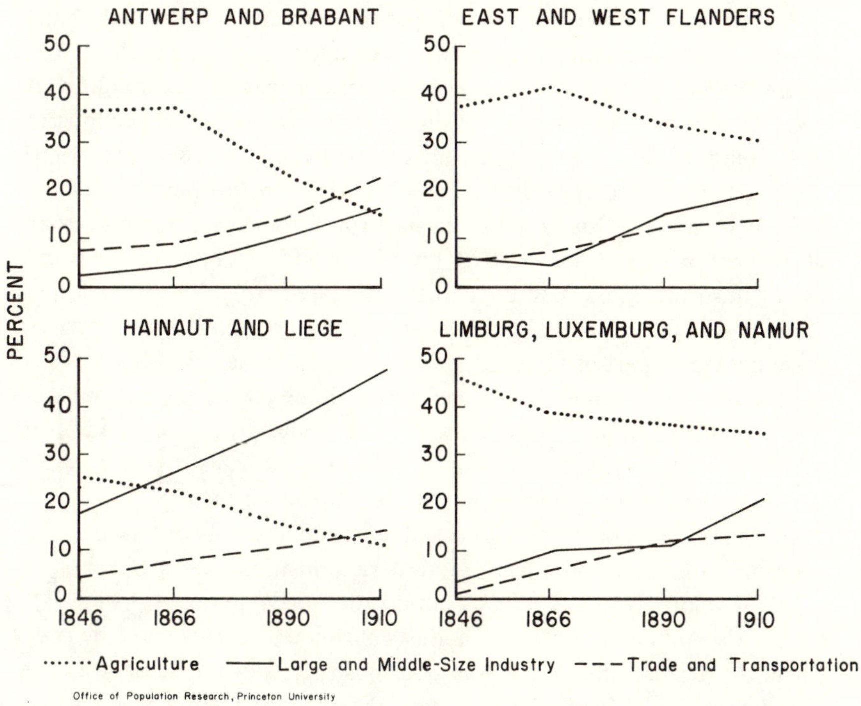

Figure 2.3 Male Labor Force, Percentage in Selected Industries, by Groups of Provinces: 1846 to 1910.

SOURCES: Adapted from B. Verhaegen (1961) and censuses of 1846, 1866, 1890, and 1910.

and transportation became very important as the cities of Antwerp and Brussels developed into large centers of employment in the tertiary sector. Not surprisingly, in Hainaut and Liège, the employment in medium and large industry is considerably more developed than in the rest of the country. Equally important for the two provinces is the fact that the tertiary sector remained very small, given their advanced position with respect to industrialization. The very high concentration in industry alone, already apparent in the nineteenth century, hampered further expansion as well as the economic and social vitality of the Walloon industrial belt throughout the twentieth century. After World War II, modernization was more accurately measured by the development of the tertiary sector than by the extent of industrial employment. The decline of coal mining turned these provinces (Hainaut even more than Liège) into depressed areas lacking a sufficiently diversified economy and occupational structure.

A more detailed view of the occupational structure at the end of the nineteenth and the start of the twentieth centuries is offered on Map 2.3, where the percentage of the male labor force engaged in agriculture is given by arrondissement (the unit used in the demographic sections of this monograph). The comparison of the picture in 1890 and 1910 shows clearly that a considerable shift occurred in this period, particularly in Flanders. Out of 15 Flemish arrondissements with more than 40 percent in agriculture in 1890, only 9 are left by 1910 and the number of those with less than 30 percent increased from 3 to 9. The decline in agriculture in Wallonia was far less spectacular in this period, since the major part of the change had occurred earlier. In fact, there is an increase in the percentage in agriculture in the Ardennes (arrondissements of Bastogne and Neufchâteau); this is due to the dissipation of the effects of the agricultural crisis in 1880 and to the fact that especially the nonagricultural population was affected by out-migration.

A second index of the occupational structure attempts to link through a special ratio the development of modern industrial sectors (Group A) with the more typically nineteenth-century occupations (Group B). Given the different paths to industrialization followed in the two linguistic regions, this index was not constructed in the same way for Flanders as for Wallonia. In Flanders, the male labor force was divided between the following:

Group A: Mining; metallurgy; construction of machinery; other metal industry; modern sectors of textile industry; construction; printing;

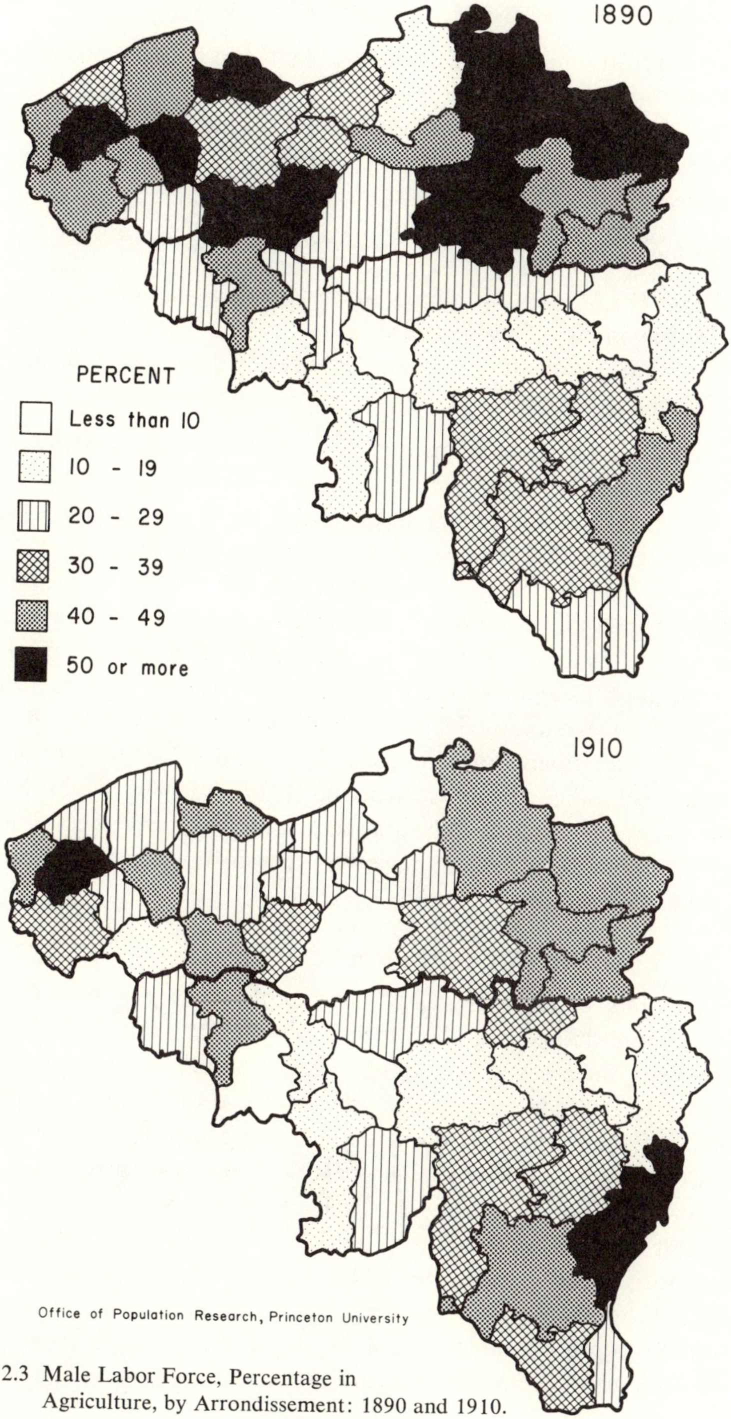

Map 2.3 Male Labor Force, Percentage in Agriculture, by Arrondissement: 1890 and 1910.

SOURCES: Population censuses of 1890 and 1910.

food industry; processing of animal, plant, and mineral materials; and mixed industries.

Group B: Agriculture and horticulture; fishing; cottage weaving and rural textile industry; clothing; servants, and nonindustrial day laborers.

In Wallonia, the male labor force was divided between:

Group A: Mining; metallurgy; quarrying; tool and die; mineral and chemical industry; and textile industry.

Group B: Agriculture and horticulture; clothing; nonindustrial day laborers; and servants.

The ratio for each was defined as the numbers in Group A divided by those in Group B.

Map 2.4 shows the change in the ratios between 1890 and 1910 for Flanders and Map 2.5 shows similar data for Wallonia. The "classic" sectors of the nineteenth century dominated in all of the Flemish arrondissements in 1890 except in Antwerp. By 1910, in 6 arrondissements the "modern" sectors had completely taken over, whereas in 7 more arrondissements an equilibrium was reached. The same trend also holds in Wallonia. The industrial population concentrated in the three arrondissements of Mons, Charleroi, and Liège in 1890 had expanded to 5 other arrondissements in 1910 (Soignies, Thuin, Namur, Huy, and Verviers): the industrial belt was now stretching continuously from Mons in the extreme southwest to Verviers in the extreme northeast of Wallonia.

2.6 *Spatial Mobility and Patterns of Urbanization*

Economic conditions greatly affected the spatial pattern and the volume and kind of migration throughout the nineteenth and twentieth centuries. The areas with a larger emphasis on the "classic" nineteenth-century activities had a negative rate and those with industry and a developed tertiary sectory a positive rate. Consequently, the provinces of East and West Flanders, Limburg, Namur, and Luxemburg were areas of out-migration, while Antwerp, Brabant, Liège, and, to a lesser degree, Hainaut attracted population (Table 2.5). Considering the economic disparities between the regions, the migration rates per thousand inhabitants are not excessively high, even when the information is broken down by arrondissements. In 1901–1910, the average rate of out-migration was nowhere larger than 8.0 per thousand, the rule being that

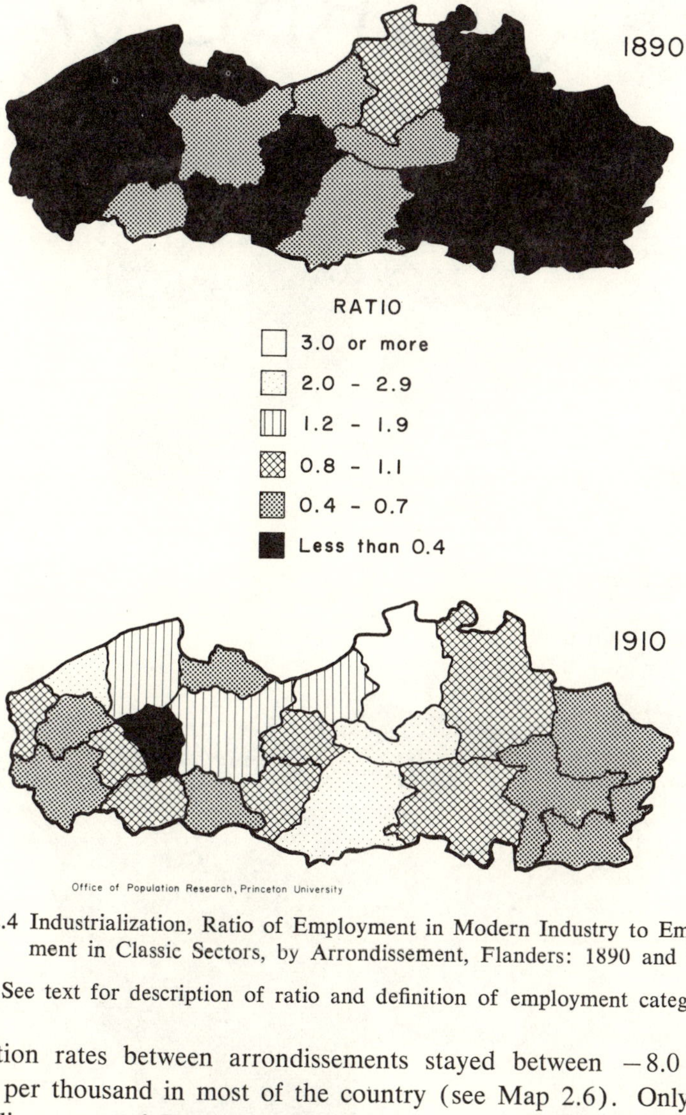

Map 2.4 Industrialization, Ratio of Employment in Modern Industry to Employment in Classic Sectors, by Arrondissement, Flanders: 1890 and 1910.

NOTE: See text for description of ratio and definition of employment categories.

migration rates between arrondissements stayed between −8.0 and +4.0 per thousand in most of the country (see Map 2.6). Only the arrondissements of Brussels and Antwerp were exceptions, with immigration rates above 5.0 per thousand.

Of the four major urban areas, Antwerp, Brussels, Liège, and Ghent, Antwerp was growing fastest (Table 2.6). Antwerp's growth from the middle of the nineteenth century on was closely connected to the development of its Walloon hinterland, and it became an industrial center in the twentieth century. The growth of Brussels was considerable; in

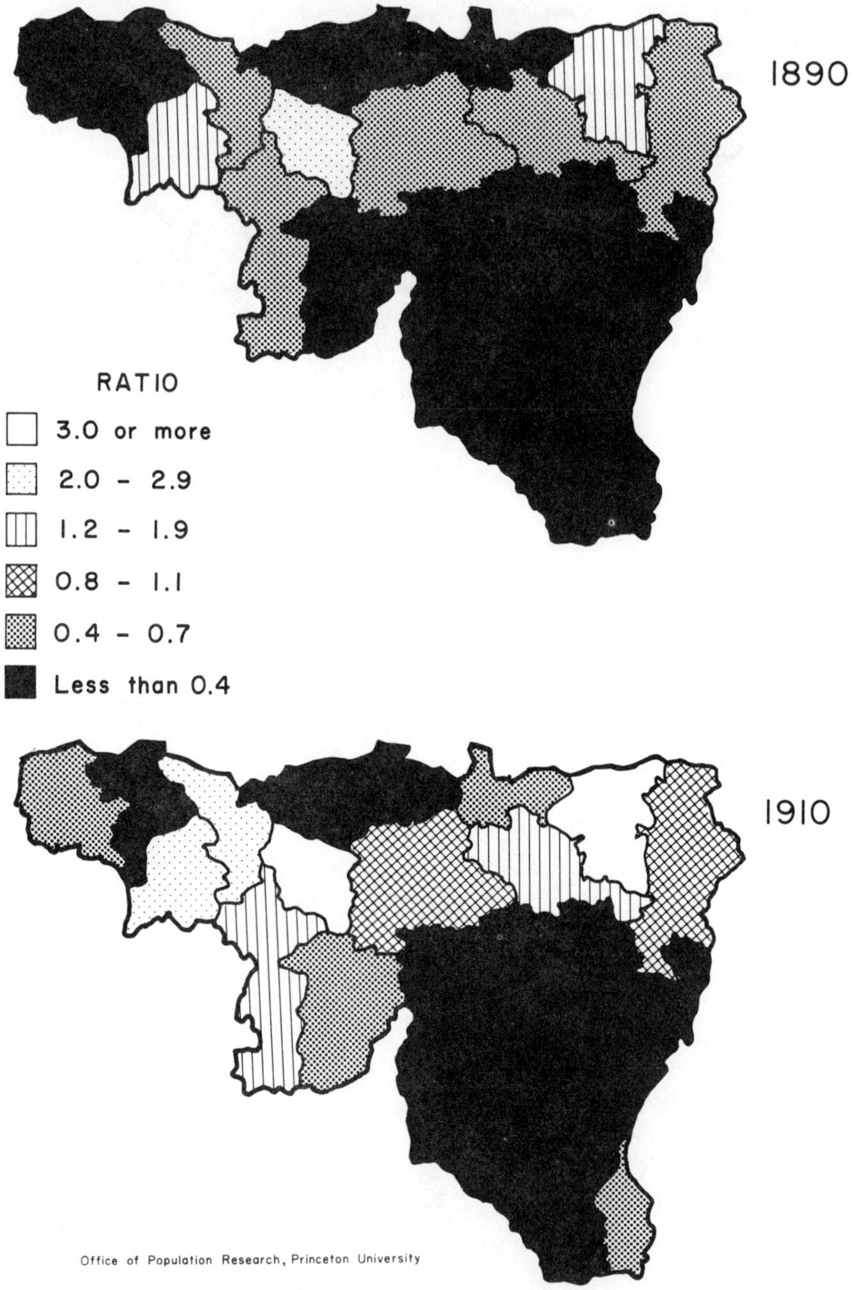

Map 2.5 Industrialization, Ratio of Employment in Modern Industry to Employment in Classic Sectors, by Arrondissement, Wallonia: 1890 and 1910.

NOTE: See text for description of ratio and definition of employment categories.

TABLE 2.5

ANNUAL MIGRATION RATE, BY PROVINCE: 1840-1856 TO 1948-1961

Province	1840-1856	1856-1876	1880-1900	1901-1910	1928-1937	1948-1961
Antwerp	+2.3	+1.3	+3.2	+1.3	+0.7	+0.6
Brabant	+3.5	+2.5	+2.4	+5.7	+5.1	+4.6
West Flanders	-3.7	-3.2	-2.7	-4.2	+1.1	-2.4
East Flanders	-3.3	-2.7	-2.6	-3.5	-1.1	-2.1
Hainaut	+1.0	+0.5	+0.2	+0.1	-0.5	-0.1
Liège	+4.5	+2.2	+1.6	+0.2	+1.6	+1.9
Limburg	+1.7	-3.8	-4.4	-2.9	-0.9	-1.3
Luxemburg	-3.2	-5.3	-4.8	-3.3	-4.7	-4.1
Namur	-0.2	-5.6	-3.2	-1.4	+0.2	-0.5

SOURCE: B. Verhaegen (1961, I, p. 76), H. Damas (1964b, p. 37).

NOTE: The migration rate refers to the annual number of migrants per 1,000 inhabitants.

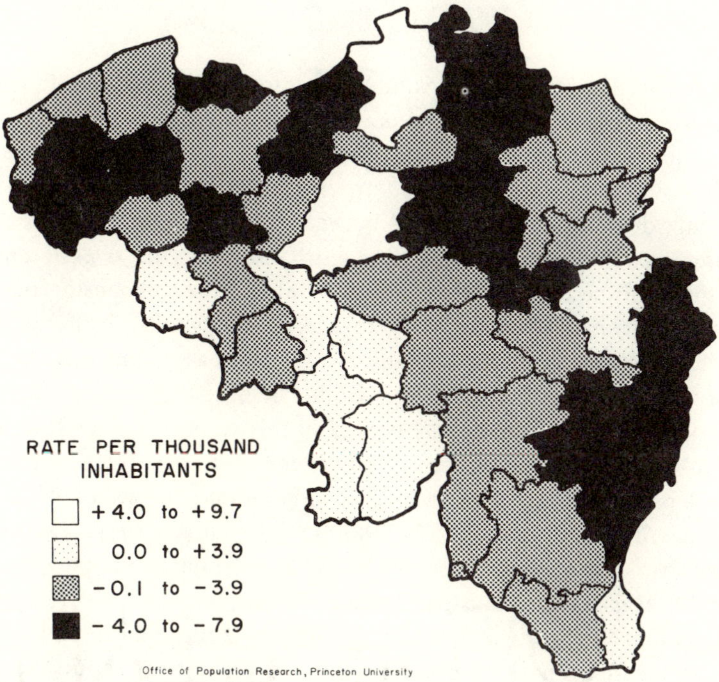

Map 2.6 Annual Migration Rate, by Arrondissement: 1901–1910.

SOURCE: H. Damas (1964, p. 37).

TABLE 2.6

URBANIZATION, POPULATION GROWTH OF ANTWERP, BRUSSELS, GHENT, AND LIEGE: 1856 TO 1930

	ANTWERP		BRUSSELS		GHENT		LIEGE	
Date	Actual population	Relative growth index	Actual population	Relative growth index	Actual population	Relative growth index	Actual population	Relative growth index
1856	117,482	100	250,503	100	118,045	100	109,690	100
1866	136,165	116	298,627	119	127,031	108	122,701	112
1880	202,911	173	421,131	168	153,282	130	156,271	142
1890	275,384	234	500,007	200	180,189	153	190,744	174
1900	340,688	290	599,076	239	198,446	168	214,838	196
1910	398,255	339	720,347	288	210,428	178	242,357	221
1920	408,039	347	756,105	302	211,945	180	240,042	219
1930	484,350	412	825,545	330	218,580	185	297,430	271

SOURCE: Population censuses of 1920 and 1930.

NOTES: Antwerp consisted of 4 communities from 1856 to 1920 and 6 communities thereafter. Brussels consists of 14 communities and Ghent of 4 communities. Liège consisted of 6 communities from 1856 to 1920 and 7 communities thereafter.

addition to its position as a capital, opportunities in medium and small industries grew in step with the development of the tertiary sector. The combined population of the four urban areas accounted for 13.2 percent of the total population of the country in 1856 and 22.6 percent in 1930; the bulk of this growth occurred between 1866 and 1910. While these figures may indicate a considerable urbanization, the overall pattern continued to be dominated by the survival and even expansion of large villages and small towns of 2,000 to 25,000 inhabitants. Not one of the four urban areas developed by any measure into a genuine metropolitan area exceeding 1.0 million inhabitants before 1930. The early industrialization in Hainaut was typical in this respect: rather than leading to the growth of modern urban centers, it spurred the development of a loose conurbation of industrial villages and towns, of which the largest, Charleroi, reached only 29,000 inhabitants in 1930. Ghent and Liège also remained well below 300,000 inhabitants, despite the fact that they were major industrial centers.

This development contrasts with the urbanization experience of England and France, where, especially in the former, entire sections of the countryside depopulated in favor of the far greater growth of metropolitan areas. As can be seen in Figure 2.4, half of the Belgian population remained in small towns and on a semi-urbanized countryside, even during the twentieth century. In fact, the proportion of the population living in communities ranging from 2,000 to 25,000 in-

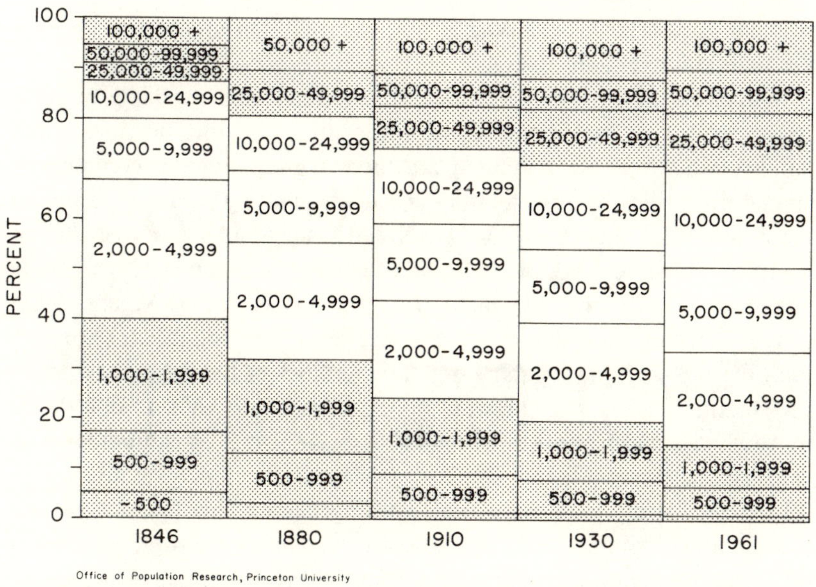

Figure 2.4 Urbanization, Population Distribution by Size of Community: 1846 to 1961.

SOURCE: H. Damas (1964, p. 6).

NOTE: In 1880, data are not reported separately for communities of 100,000 persons or more; rather, the figures were combined with totals for communities with 50,000 to 99,999 inhabitants.

habitants increased during the last century, rising from 48 percent in 1846 to 55 percent in 1961. Only the category of small communities of less than 2,000 inhabitants experienced decreasing proportions of the total population; these communities grew into the next category, became absorbed by larger communities, or lost population through out-migration. Another striking feature is the very comparable degree of urbanization in both language areas, despite their large differentials in industrialization. In addition to Brussels, there were six other arrondissements with more than 50 percent of their population in units larger than 10,000 inhabitants—three in Flanders (Antwerp, Mechelen, and Ghent), and three in Wallonia (Mons, Charleroi, and Liège). Eight Flemish arrondissements had less than 20 percent of their population in units of this size, compared to twelve in Wallonia. Hence, on both sides of the language border, the population remained characterized by moderate rural-urban migration, and by a slow (Hainaut, East and West Flanders) to moderate urbanization (Liège, Antwerp, Brabant). It was not until after World War II that metropolitan areas of more than 1.0 million inhabitants emerged.

This does not imply that work opportunities were available in sufficient quantity in each area. Quite the contrary is true, but in a small country where people remained attached to their original community, spatial disparities in opportunities led to commuting rather than actual migration. The rapid growth of a railroad system and a rural network of tramways, together with the creation of extremely cheap weekly or daily tickets from 1870 on, contributed greatly to this new development. With a weekly ticket, rural laborers were entitled to six round trips for less than the price of one regular fare. The number of these tickets sold by the National Railroad alone went up from 14,000 in 1870 to 6,400,000 in 1908. According to Mahaim (1910, p. 48), the latter number corresponds to the regular movement of 319,000 workmen or more than 20 percent of the male industrial working class. This figure does not include all commuters, such as those on the smaller railroad companies or on the *boerentram* or "peasants' tram"; it also excludes white-collar labor using slightly more expensive season tickets. Vandervelde's notion of *les villes tentaculaires* (1902, p. 103) was as applicable to the urban attraction as expressed in commuting as it was to urban growth by inmigration. From the agricultural crisis in the 1880s onward, the pattern of urbanization became dominated by the development of large semi-urban dormitory areas with a population no longer primarily attached to agriculture or rural industries. This feature curbed the growth of the larger cities to a considerable extent, without, however, stopping it entirely.

2.7 *Sociocultural Change: Secularization*

The change of a society can by no means be described solely in terms of its economic history. While the socioeconomic variables used in the previous sections have had a considerable influence on the sociological differentiation of the areas, ending this chapter with patterns of urbanization and occupational structure would imply that the changes in the social culture were dependent entirely on the changes in the social structures. The connection between structural and cultural modernization is often more contingent than necessary. Socioeconomic changes are only linked, rather than directly related, to phenomena such as the adoption of rational action patterns focusing on maximizing economic returns (M. Weber), the changing patterns of authority and increasing secularization (M. Weber, E. Durkheim), the increase in the division of labor (E. Durkheim), the development of a social stratification based on achieved rather than ascribed status, the accelerating spiral of innovation and imitation processes (G. Tarde), and many other features of the nineteenth- and twentieth-century typologies à la *Gemeinschaft-Gesellschaft*.

Yet, all the elements of cultural change can be related to the demographic transition discussed in the following chapters. Should the fertility decline be viewed as an expression of the Weberian concept of *Zweckrationalität,* the final goal being the prevention of excessive population growth through means other than mortality or migration? Was it a way of endowing a smaller number of descendants with higher chances for promotion in an achieved-status system as A. Dumont suggests in his notion of *capillarité sociale*? Can the spread of modern fertility patterns, occurring throughout most of Western Europe within the very short period of 40 years, be viewed as one of Tarde's imitation processes? Did this become possible as the result of the breakdown of traditional forms of authority? The answer to these questions probably goes in the positive direction, and yet, statistically, it is impossible to ascertain the impact of each of these effects. That statistical measurement of these phenomena is unavailable is no reason for not mentioning the possibilities for a sociocultural explanation. However, as this book deals with *measurable* effects, we are forced, whether we like it or not, to treat these variables in one lumped, residual category, where, in fact, they do not belong. They are indicators of modernization in the same way as industrialization or urbanization, and the fact that we have no precise, concrete statistical way of establishing their impact on demographic changes does not imply that they can be neglected.

One major exception among these unmeasurable sociocultural variables in Belgium is that of secularization. By this concept we refer to the breakdown of traditional religious authority, here of the Catholic Church, and the decrease of adherence to organized forms of religion. The Flemish as well as the Walloon bourgeoisie showed marked signs of anticlericalism, and their refutation of the authority of the church dominated political life in the towns throughout the entire eighteenth and nineteenth centuries. This first form of secularization found a partial expression in the Freemason's lodges, and, after independence, in the Liberal party. A second source of secularization grew in the latter half of the nineteenth century with the spirit of Marxism, particularly in the lower classes. The Belgian form of socialism lost its doctrinal rigor in economic matters very early (the goal of nationalizing industries and resources was abandoned for example). This weakening of its original revolutionary character, plus its emphasis on more feasible political and social reforms within the given economic system and the directly tangible effects of the creation of producer and consumer co-operatives competing freely on the capitalist market, considerably increased its attraction among the working classes. On the matter of religion however, the Workers' party remained inflexible; a softening of its anticlerical views would not appear until after World War II. A third form of secularization was *in se* not inspired by anticlerical feelings or political motivations, but simply grew out of the loss of the functions of organized religion. Whatever the source of the secularization may have been, the movement had spread considerably during the second half of the nineteenth century, leaving no opening for alternative forms of religious authority such as the newly reformed branches of Protestantism growing in the Anglo-Saxon world.

Several historical studies based on Easter records (the parish clergy kept statistical records of the proportion of the population fulfilling its Easter duties) or on Sunday mass attendance (occasional enumerations in church were held) reveal the extent of secularization. The differences between the two language areas were rather striking by 1900. In the whole of West Flanders, for example, few parishes had figures exceeding 10 percent of *nonpascantes* (W. Rombauts, 1971) compared to 30 or 40 percent in certain areas of equally rural Luxemburg and sections of Namur (C. Pourbaix, 1973). The proportion of *nonpascantes* in the industrialized Walloon areas, such as the Liège area, was well above 60 percent (L. De Saint Moulin, 1967). Unfortunately, information based on Easter records is not available for the entire century, so that we have to turn to another, more indirect indicator: the non-Catholic vote in 1919, when the first general elections were held on the basis of the one man, one vote principle. As the non-Catholic vote, we have taken the sum of votes for the Workers' party (socialist), the Communist party and socialist splinter groups (both very small fractions of the total vote), and the Liberal party. This segment of the total vote could almost be labeled as anti-Catholic, since all of these parties had adopted openly a definite position against the social authority of the church. Conversely, voting for one of these parties was anathema for convinced Catholics as they were often reminded of this from the pulpit. The geographical distribution of this non-Catholic vote is pictured on Map 2.7 by election canton. The Walloon industrial belt is once more the spine of the entire movement, a hint that industrialization had greatly fostered the spread of secularization. The arrondissements in the Ardennes (Dinant, Marche, Neufchâteau, and Bastogne) have a smaller proportion of non-

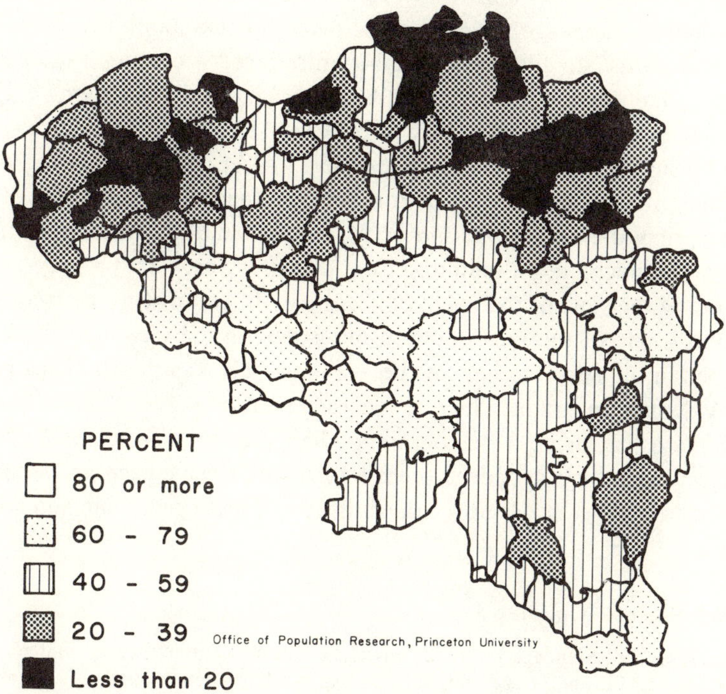

Map 2.7 Secularization, Percentage Votes Non-Catholic, by Election Canton: 1919.

SOURCE: R. De Smet, R. Evalenko, and W. Fraeys (1958).

Catholic vote, rarely exceeding 50 percent. In Flanders, the proportion of the non-Catholic vote is nearly always below 40 percent. The major exceptions to this regional trend were found in the urban areas of Antwerp, Brussels, Ghent, and Ostend. The language border between the two regions runs as a dividing line through the country and only a few nonurban cantons of the Flemish side, with an already linguistically mixed population, contain a more sizeable secularized portion of the population. We do not know the extent to which this trend in secularization is a relevant indicator of sociocultural modernization as a whole, but it is certain that the contingency of this variable with structural changes such as urbanization and industrialization, as well as with demographic changes, cannot be overlooked in Belgium.

2.8 *Summary*

By the middle of the nineteenth century, economic and social development in both language regions was already directed along two critically different paths. In Flanders, changes introduced a century earlier had led to what Mendels (1971) calls a "proto-industrialization." This resulted in some economic growth prior to 1830 but in falling real income per head in the period 1840–1850. After 1860, increasing proportions of the Flemish population became engaged in activities other than agriculture or cottage industry. A slow industrialization started, turning Flanders into a semiurbanized dormitory area with a large labor reserve at the start of the twentieth century. In contrast to the trends in Flanders, one of the most modern industries on the Continent had developed in the northern part of the Wallonia, whereas the southern part, the Ardennes, maintained its rural characteristics.

If there had to be a demographic change in the second half of the nineteenth century, as indeed there was, it would have been an astonishing surprise to see it develop independently of these economic and social trends.

References—Chapter 2

Berkner, L., and Mendels, F. 1972. Legal variables, family structure, and fertility in Western Europe. Paper read at Seminar on Early Industrialization, Fertility, and Family Structure, 1972, at Institute for Advanced Study, Princeton, New Jersey.

Damas, H. 1964a. La concentration de la population en Belgique. *Population et Famille—Bevolking en Gezin* (Brussels) 3:1-24.

———. 1964b. Population de la Belgique: les migrations intérieures. *Population et Famille—Bevolking en Gezin* (Brussels) 4:31–62.

de Laveleye, E. 1875. *Essai sur l'agriculture en Belgique* (Brussels).

De Saint Moulin, L. 1967. Contributions à l'histoire de la déchristianisation; la pratique religieuse à Seraing depuis 1830. *Annuaire d'Histoire Liègeoise* 10:33-127.

De Smet, R., Evalenko, R., and Fraeys, W. 1958. *Atlas des elections belges: 1919–1954.* Brussels: Institut de Sociologie Solvay, Université Libre de Bruxelles.

Grooten, R. 1951. L'évolution de la population agricole et horticole en Belgique depuis 1856. *Revue de l'Agriculture.*

Mahaim, E. 1910. *Les abonnements d'ouvriers sur les lignes de chemins de fer belges et leur effets sociaux.* Brussels–Leipzig.

Mendels, F. 1970. Industry and marriages in Flanders before the industrial revolution. In *Population and economics,* ed. P. Deprez (Proceedings of Section V of the Fourth Congress of the International Economic History Association). Winnipeg: University of Manitoba Press.

———. 1971. Industrialization and population pressure in eighteenth century Flanders. *The Journal of Economic History* 31:269-271.

Pontanus, F. 1968. Un demi-siècle d'évolution de la population active en Belgique: 1910–1961. *Population et Famille—Bevolking en Gezin* (Brussels) 15:39-87 (annex, pp. 3-90).

Pourbaix, C. 1973. La pratique pascale dans le diocèse de Namur. Unpublished thèse de licence, Faculté de Philosophie et Lettres, Université Catholique de Louvain.

Rombauts, W. 1971. *Het paasverzuim in het Bisdom Brugge, 1840–1911.* Leuven: Editions Nauwelaerts.

Seebohm-Rowntree, B. 1910. *Land and labour: lessons from Belgium.* London: Macmillan and Co.

Vandervelde, E. 1900. *La propriété foncière en Belgique.* Paris: Schleicher Frères.

———. 1902. Les villes tentaculaires. *Essais sur la question agraire en Belgique.* Paris: Editions du Mouvement Socialiste.

van der Wee, H. 1972. *Historische aspecten van de economische groei.* Antwerp-Utrecht: De Nederlandsche Boekhandel.

Verhaegen, B. 1961. *Contribution à l'histoire économique des Flandres.* 2 vols. Louvain-Paris: Editions Nauwelaerts.

Wrigley, E. A. 1961. *Industrial growth and population change.* Cambridge, England: Cambridge University Press.

CHAPTER 3: The Evolution of Nuptiality

3.1 *Introduction*

Important demographic changes paralleled the economic and social transformations that occurred within Belgium in the second half of the nineteenth century. One of these demographic changes was a fundamental alteration in marriage patterns. Data from the 1846 and 1856 censuses indicate that the mean age at marriage was 28.6 years for women and 30.5 years for men; in the 1960s figures for both sexes are approximately six years younger. In the middle of the nineteenth century, three-quarters of the men between 25 and 30 years of age were still single; in 1970, more than three-quarters were married. In the 1850s almost as many women married for the first time after age 30 as before age 30; in 1970, the first marriage of a woman older than 30 years was exceptional.

Marriage was not only late, but also far from universal. Using the proportion of singles among those aged 45 to 49 as a measure of definite celibacy (because the chance that a person still single at that age will marry is minimal), we find that in 1846, 15 percent of the women and 18 percent of the men at that age were single. Definitive celibacy grew to 20 percent in the 1850s; by 1970, however, it had fallen to 7 percent.

This fundamental transformation from a schedule of late and non-universal marriage to a pattern of much earlier and more universal nuptiality will be labeled as the modernization of nuptiality.

In this chapter, we will discuss the basic trends in nuptiality, starting with those prior to 1850 and continuing with the changes occurring between 1850 and 1970. The Belgian experience will also be placed in a broader European context. Then, we will present a more theoretical treatment of some of the social and economic reasons underlying (1) the Malthusian patterns of late marriage and (2) the evolution of nuptiality that occurred in the nineteenth and twentieth centuries. Finally, the testing of these theoretical propositions will be made by means of a statistical analysis of empirical material.

3.2 *The Measurement of Nuptiality and Fertility*

As a first step in assessing the important demographic changes, it is necessary to introduce as accurate measures as possible. Since the proportion of women remaining single influences overall fertility as well as nuptiality, we will introduce measures of both marriage and fertility here. The indices used are those developed by Coale (1965b, 2, p. 207) specifically for use in the European Fertility Project of which this monograph is a part. These indices utilize the statistical data that were most readily available in nineteenth-century Europe.

A measure of nuptiality, called the index of proportion married and labelled I_m, was computed from the proportions of women reported currently married in the census. This index summarizes the nuptiality pattern within the childbearing span and its effect on overall fertility by comparing the number of children *married* women would bear if they were subject to natural fertility to the number of children *all* women, married or not, would bear under the same circumstances. Natural fertility was represented by the Hutterite schedule from 1921–1930, since this population had one of the highest fertility schedules on record.[1] Hence,

$$I_m = \frac{\Sigma\, m_i F_i}{\Sigma\, w_i F_i}$$

where, for a given age group i, m_i is the number of married women, w_i is the total number of women, and F_i the marital fertility rate from the Hutterite schedule. Consequently, I_m can be interpreted as a weighted index of the proportion currently married, giving a larger weight to the proportion of married women in the younger and, hence, more fecund ages. The advantage of this fertility-weighted aggregate index of nuptiality among women of childbearing age, over the simple calculation of proportion married in the age interval 15-50 years, is that it incorporates an indirect standardization for age distribution. The index I_m has a value of unity if all women in the fecund ages are married; thus, the later and less universal marriage is, the lower the value of I_m.

The intuitive meaning of this index becomes more apparent if we state its relationship to overall and marital fertility. Overall fertility is measured by an index I_f, defined as:

$$I_f = \frac{B}{\Sigma\, w_i F_i}$$

where B is the annual number of live births, observed in a five-year period centered around a census, and where F_i and w_i are already de-

[1] The marital fertility rates by five-year age group for the Hutterite population are .300, .550, .502, .447, .406, .222, .061, starting at the age group of 15-19 years and ending with 45-49 years.

fined quantities. The index of marital fertility (I_g) relates the annual number of legitimate live births (B_L) to the number of legitimate births that would occur to married women in each age group of the childbearing span (m_i), if they were subject to natural fertility. Hence, this index is

$$I_g = \frac{B_L}{\Sigma\, m_i F_i}$$

In the same way, an index of illegitimate fertility can be constructed as

$$I_h = \frac{B_I}{\Sigma\, u_i F_i}$$

where B_I is the number of illegitimate live births and u_i the number of unmarried (i.e., widowed and single) women in a given age group. The three indices of fertility measure the relative fertility experience of all three categories of women (married, unmarried, and all women) compared with that of the Hutterites.

These four indices can furthermore be related in a simple way:

$$I_f = I_g \cdot I_m + I_h(1 - I_m)$$

or in the case of negligible illegitimate fertility, this relationship becomes

$$I_f = I_g \cdot I_m$$

Since the level of I_f is determined by various combinations of levels of marital fertility and nuptiality, breaking it into the product of I_m and I_g enables us to trace the evolution from a Malthusian pattern of reproduction (high marital fertility curbed by a late age at marriage and extensive life-long celibacy) to a neo-Malthusian pattern (reduced marital fertility and widespread nuptiality).

The calculation of these four indices for the nineteenth century requires the complete registration of live births and the exact enumeration of the female population by age and marital status. In Belgium, the basic data were checked by various techniques; it appears that the indices err by only a few percent. The reader interested in the more detailed description of these checks will find a full report in the Appendix.

Now that the basic demographic measures are defined, we will return to the subject of nuptiality, and more precisely to the situation prior to 1850.

3.3 *Nuptiality Patterns before 1850*

In the middle of the nineteenth century, Belgium recorded close to the lowest levels of I_m ever observed. In 1846 the value of the index of proportion married was .375 and in 1856 only .366. In the province of East Flanders, a record low of .303 was registered in 1856; the highest value of I_m at that time, found in the already highly industrialized province of Hainaut, was only .424.

There is, however, a possibility that these levels were not typical of the beginning of the century. In the Netherlands, for example, nuptiality reached its lowest level in the 1840s and 1850s. Hofstee (1972, p. 52) notes a decline in the percentage of married among men aged 25-29 from 42.5 in 1830 to 34.0 in 1849. After this sharp decline, it took another 25 years for the proportion married in this group to regain its 1830 level. The explanation for the unusual figures in the 1840s and 1850s is to be found in the economic and agricultural crises of this period that plagued Belgium, the Netherlands, and many other western European countries.

The first piece of evidence indicating a downward trend in the proportion married from early to mid-century is the curve of the proportion single in the age group 45-49 years. This proportion, taken as an approximate measure of definitive celibacy, was lower in the 1846 census than in the three later ones of 1856, 1866, and 1880. In fact, the percentage of single women in that age group was 18.0 percent in 1846, compared with 20.0 percent in 1856. For the male population, the increase in definitive celibacy was larger: from 16.5 percent in 1846 to 20.5 percent in 1856 and 1866. Moreover, some other age groups also show this tendency (see Figure 3.1). Hence, the cohorts susceptible to marriage prior to 1835 may have had slightly higher probabilities of first marriage than the cohorts entering the marriage market in the late 1830s, the 1840s, and 1850s.

Additional evidence of earlier marriage in the last quarter of the eighteenth century and the first decades of the nineteenth century can be found in several areas. First, the distribution of the female population by age and marital status is available for the canton of Lede and for several villages of East Flanders in 1796 (J. de Brouwer, 1968, p. 130). In these areas, the value of I_m was .434 in the canton of Lede, and .431 in the other four rural communities. In 1846, half a century later, the rural part of East Flanders had a value of I_m of .319, considerably lower than the value in the selected East Flanders areas in 1796.

A reconstruction of the female population by age and marital status

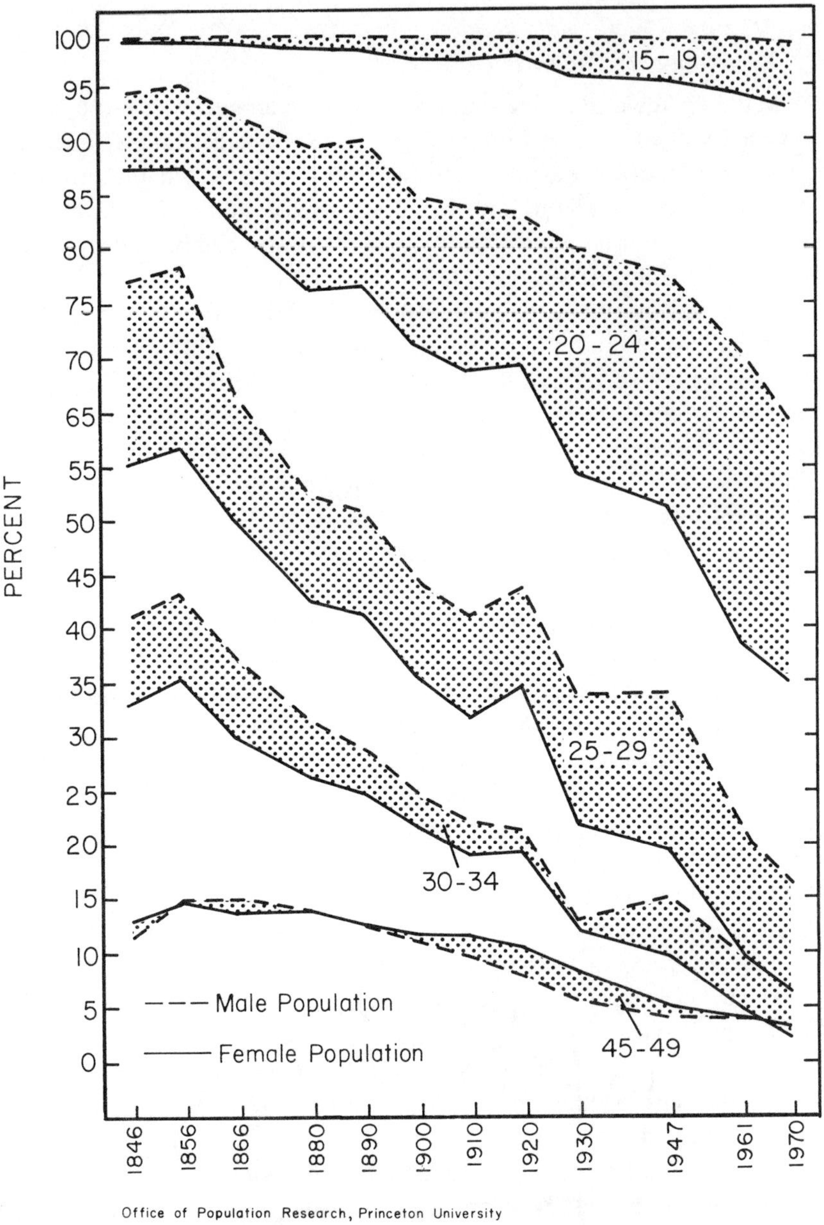

Figure 3.1 Percentage Single, by Sex and Age Group: 1846 to 1970.

is possible for eight of the nine Belgian départements in 1806 (J. Duchène and R. Lesthaeghe, 1975). (The data for the département Meuse Inferieure were considered to be too unreliable to attempt that reconstitution.) The values of I_m were considerably larger in 1806 than in 1846 in all the Flemish regions, while no significant difference appeared in the Walloon areas. The lowest and highest estimates of I_m in 1806 are compared with those observed in 1846 in Table 3.1.

TABLE 3.1

PROPORTION MARRIED (I_m), BY FRENCH DEPARTEMENT/BELGIAN PROVINCE: 1806 AND 1846

Département/Province	Area	1806 Lowest estimate	1806 Highest estimate	1846
Deux-Nèthes/Antwerp	Flanders	.400	.446	.365
Dyle/Brabant	Flanders and Wallonia	.419	.420	.384
Escaut/East Flanders	Flanders	.389	.445	.345
Lys/West Flanders	Flanders	.400	.414	.347
Jemmape/Hainaut	Wallonia	.385	.410	.411
Ourthe/Liège	Wallonia	.403	.416	.404
Meuse Inférieure[a]/ Limburg	Flanders	--	--	--
Forêts/Luxemburg	Wallonia	.453		.421
Sambre et Meuse/Namur	Wallonia	.407	.419	.415

SOURCE: J. Duchène and R. Lesthaeghe, 1975.

NOTE: The first name is that of the département during the Napoleonic period; the second name refers to the post-independence division of the territory into provinces. The later provinces overlap substantially with the French départements, but it should be noted that the département Deux-Nèthes included the Dutch province of Noordbrabant, that Escaut included the islands of the Dutch province of Zeeland, and that Forêts covered the Grand Duchy of Luxemburg together with a small section of German territory as well.

[a]Data for the département Meuse Inférieure are considered unreliable.

The next piece of information available on marital status compositions has been compiled by A. Quételet and E. Smits (1832, pp. 16-17) from the census of 1829, taken in the last year of the Dutch occupation. Again, these data are not equal in reliability to those of 1846: the census results for several areas were not returned and in other areas they were collected only partially. From these 1829 data, a mean age at marriage of 28.9 years for women and 29.8 years for men can be obtained. These values differ only by a fraction of a year from those calculated by E. van de Walle (1965, p. 45) for 1851–1856.

On the basis of this information, we accept that I_m for the whole of Belgium declined from 1800 to 1829 and 1846. This decline occurred solely in Flanders, however, whereas a horizontal trend seems to characterize the Walloon experience during the first half of the nineteenth century; by 1866, I_m had returned to the level of .403 and increased steadily afterwards.

3.4 *The Belgian Nuptiality Evolution after 1850 and Its Place in European Perspective*

Marriage patterns following the middle of the nineteenth century can be traced in three ways. First, data are available on the percentage of persons single in selected age categories. These are reported in Figure 3.1 for both sexes and show that a change in nuptiality started between 1856 and 1866 and continued until the 1960s. The trend was interrupted by several events: the agricultural crises of the 1880s, World War I, and, to a lesser degree, World War II. Second, the values of the index of proportion married (I_m) portray the same picture. These are reported in Table 3.2 for the period 1846 to 1970. The low level of

TABLE 3.2

PROPORTION MARRIED (I_m): 1846 TO 1970

Date	I_m	Date	I_m
1846	.375	1910	.517
1856	.366	1920	.501
1866	.403	1930	.602
1880	.435	1947	.617
1890	.436	1961	.705
1900	.479	1970	.703

nuptiality suppressed overall fertility in 1846 and 1856. Later on, in the second half of the nineteenth century, the relative impact of marital fertility on overall fertility increased, as the value of I_m started its upward movement for a period of more than a century. In 1866, only 40 percent of the value of I_g was translated into I_f. At the turn of the century the figure was 50 percent; in 1930, it increased to 60 percent; and, in 1970, it reached the unprecedented level of 70 percent. The old Malthusian function of nuptiality, of restraining overall fertility and consequently also population growth, had virtually disappeared.

A third, and perhaps more classic, way of summarizing nuptiality trends consists of following the mean age at marriage. This is reported in Table 3.3 and has been calculated from the proportion singe reported in two successive censuses. It represents the central tendency of the age pattern of marriage in a hypothetical cohort during the intercensal period (E. van de Walle, 1965, p. 46; C. Wattelar and G. Wunsch, 1967,

TABLE 3.3

MEAN AGE AT MARRIAGE, BY SEX: 1852-1856 TO 1961

Date	Females	Males
1852-1856	28.6	30.5
1862-1866	28.0	30.0
1886-1890	26.7	28.6
1896-1900	25.7	27.6
1906-1910	25.2	27.3
1916-1920	25.6	27.5
1926-1930	24.2	26.6
1947	23.4	26.3
1961	22.4	24.9

SOURCE: E. van de Walle, 1965, p.46; C. Wattelar and G. Wunsch, 1967, p. 48.

p. 48). In 1846, the mean age at marriage was at very high levels: more than 28 years for women and over 30 years for men. In 1961, when the rising trend of nuptiality was essentially completed, these mean ages stood respectively at 22.4 and 24.9 years.

At the middle of the nineteenth century, Belgium was by no means the only country characterized by tardy and nonuniversal marriage. In fact, if one divided Europe by an imaginary line stretching from Trieste on the Adriatic Sea to Leningrad on the Baltic, one would find this Malthusian pattern in nearly all populations to the west of the line. The index of proportion married (I_m) varied in these regions between .300 and .600. In the eastern half of Europe, however, the mean age at marriage and the incidence of definitive celibacy were considerably lower; values of I_m smaller than .550 were exceptional.

There were several gradations of marriage patterns within this broad western-European picture. First, France had a more modern nuptiality behavior developed by 1850. There, I_m had reached the value of .526 (E. van de Walle, 1974, Appendix), and a few areas even had values of I_m around .650. Other French areas, however, continued to exhibit substantially lower levels of I_m, i.e., between .400 and .500. On the whole, the rest of western Europe was behind France with respect to the nuptiality change.

A second pattern is found in Belgium, the Netherlands, and, to a lesser degree, Germany. This pattern is characterized by a gradual rising trend, starting sometime around 1860 and continuing at least until the 1960s. This gradual change is described in Table 3.4. The table also includes the highest and lowest levels of I_m recorded by administrative unit. These sets, describing the range and the central tendency of the movement, reveal that the change in the national averages was not caused by changes in a few areas. In Germany and the Netherlands, the relative change of I_m in the provinces with the lowest levels of I_m is as large as in the provinces with the highest levels.

A third pattern existed in most of the remaining western-European countries: the change in I_m was insignificant during the nineteenth century and the first decades of the twentieth. After 1930, and especially after World War II, these countries exhibited a nuptiality revolution and reached I_m levels of .700 in only a few decades.

Now that we have an idea of the overall European pattern of marriage, we will turn our attention to the regional differences within Belgium.

3.5 *Nuptiality Patterns after 1850*

According to Quételet and Smits (1832, p. 63), the highest relative marriage frequencies in the period 1803–1829 were found in the province of Luxemburg and the lowest in the provinces of East and West Flanders. These levels still held in 1846. However, I_m values decreased in those provinces affected by the agricultural and industrial crisis in the linen sector. The most industrialized province, Hainaut, was barely affected by these economic factors and developed the least restrictive pattern in 1856.

From the middle of the nineteenth century on, very little changed in the ranking of the provinces with respect to I_m. Hainaut maintained its advanced position and was followed by Namur (1856–1947). This is shown on Figure 3.2 and in Table 3.5. In 1856, the intermediate provinces were Liège, Antwerp, and Brabant; until 1961, the values of I_m for these provinces remained clustered around the national average. The lowest indices of proportion married were found in Limburg East Flanders, and West Flanders. They still had the lowest values of I_m in 1961. As can be seen in Figure 3.2, only the province of Luxemburg was somewhat exceptional: between 1846 and 1890, I_m varied little;

TABLE 3.4

PROPORTION MARRIED (I_m), NATIONAL AVERAGES AND ADMINISTRATIVE UNIT EXTREME LEVELS, BELGIUM GERMANY, FRANCE, AND THE NETHERLANDS: 1840 TO 1910

Approx. date	National averages				Highest levels				Lowest levels			
	Belg.	Fr.	Ger.	Neth.	Belg.	Fr.	Ger.	Neth.	Belg.	Fr.	Ger.	Neth.
1840	--	.516	--	--	--	.634	--	--	--	.385	--	--
1845	.375	.520	--	--	.421	.648	--	--	.345	.394	--	--
1850	--	.526	--	.389	--	.657	--	.437	--	.400	--	.321
1855	.366	.530	--	--	.424	.670	--	--	.303	.402	--	--
1860	--	.531	--	.406	--	.683	--	.444	--	.400	--	.319
1865		.530	.454	--	.464	.701	.537	--	.361	.388	.334	--
1870		.529	.472	.438	--	.705	.549	.481	--	.385	.388	.366
1875	--	.533	.495	--	--	.710	--	--	--	.396	--	--
1880	.435	.538	.501	.469	.489	.713	.583	.514	.384	.404	.422	.410
1885	--	.541	.494	--	--	.714	.575	--	--	.410	.413	--
1890	.436	.540	.497	.450	.502	.705	.584	.502	.395	.409	.412	.379
1895	--	.541	--	--	--	.695	.585	--	--	.411	.411	--
1900	.479	.543	.513	.450	.572	.700	.595	.524	.411	.406	.418	.382
1905	--	--	--	--	--	--	--	--	--	--	.429	--
1910	.517	--	.524	.469	.617	--	.647	.545	.448	--	.433	.418

SOURCES: France: E. van de Walle, 1974; Germany: J. Knodel, 1974; The Netherlands: E. van de Walle, unpublished.

NOTES: To facilitate comparison, only administrative units of comparable population size were used; these included 9 provinces in Belgium, 86 départements in France, 55 to 71 administrative areas in Germany, and 11 provinces in The Netherlands.

Areas which recorded the highest levels were the Belgian province of Hainaut, the French départements of Oise and Lot-et-Garonne, the German administrative areas of Anhalt and Arnsberg, and the Dutch provinces of Friesland and Drente.

Areas which recorded the lowest levels were the Belgian provinces of East Flanders and Limburg, the French département of Ille-et-Vilaine, the German administrative areas of Aachen and Niederbayern, and the Dutch provinces of Noordbrabant and Limburg.

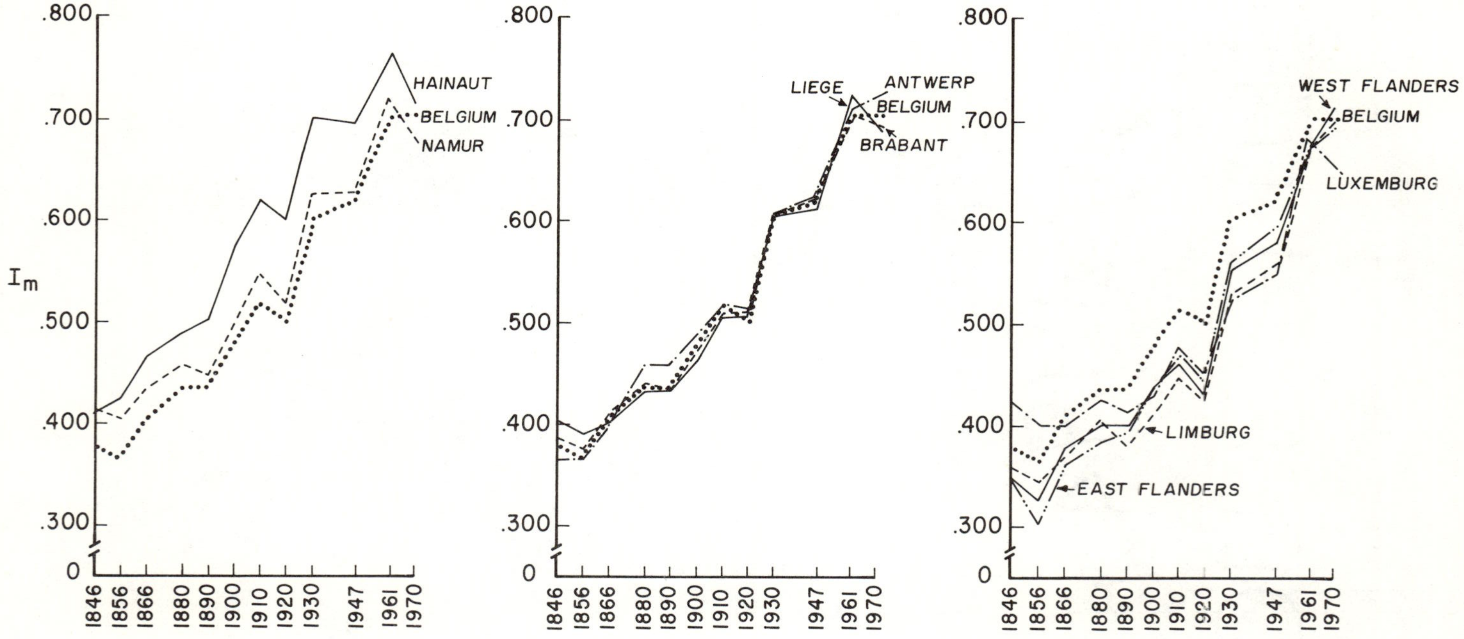

Office of Population Research, Princeton University

Figure 3.2 Proportion Married (I_m), by Province: 1846 to 1970.

TABLE 3.5

PROPORTION MARRIED (I_m), BY PROVINCE: 1846 TO 1970

Date	Antwerp	Brabant	East Flanders	West Flanders	Hainaut	Liège	Limburg	Luxemburg	Namur
1846	.365	.384	.345	.347	.411	.404	.359	.421	.415
1856	.365	.374	.303	.326	.424	.390	.347	.400	.405
1866	.395	.408	.361	.375	<u>.464</u>	.401	.370	.398	.432
1880	<u>.457</u>	<u>.440</u>	<u>.384</u>	<u>.400</u>	.489	.434	.406	.424	<u>.457</u>
1890	.457	.431	.395	.401	.502	.433	.380	.412	.444
1900	.482	.470	.439	.437	.572	<u>.468</u>	<u>.411</u>	.432	.497
1910	.518	.509	.473	.463	.617	.509	.448	<u>.476</u>	.546
1920	.512	.507	.446	.432	.597	.503	.427	.449	.520
1930	.604	.602	.561	.551	.699	.605	.529	.524	.621
1947	.623	.622	.596	.579	.694	.612	.558	.547	.625
1961	.709	.703	.676	.672	.766	.720	.671	.682	.717
1970	.721	.691	.696	.710	.715	.689	.700	.653	.679

NOTE: Underlined values of I_m represent initial 10 percent increase over 1846 values.

after 1890, I_m followed very closely that of the other provinces with more restricted patterns of nuptiality.

In the twentieth century, the upward trend of the index of proportion married was interrupted by both World Wars. The civilian population was especially affected by World War I. The front lines cut through the southern part of West Flanders, and there, any form of activity, other than military, came to a complete halt for a period of four years from 1914 to 1918.

On the whole, provincial levels of I_m were remarkably parallel for more than a century: the differences in nuptiality existing at the start of the upward trend persisted during the entire movement.[2] Only very recently has a major reordering of the provinces according to I_m level occurred: between 1961 and 1970, all the Walloon areas have undergone a decrease, whereas all the Flemish areas have continued the upward trend.

After 1880, basic data for the calculation of I_m became available for the arrondissement as well as for the four major metropolitan areas of Antwerp, Brussels, Ghent, and Liège. These data are reported in Table 3.6 and Map 3.1 for the dates 1880, 1890, 1900, and 1910. These

[2] Exactly the same phenomenon was observed by A. C. de Vooys (1964, p. 229) in the Netherlands: the Dutch provinces of Friesland and Drente developed an earlier age at marriage in the 1850s and maintained it during the century thereafter, whereas the provinces of Noord Brabant and (Dutch) Limburg have had the most restrictive nuptiality schedule throughout the entire period between 1860 and 1960.

TABLE 3.6

PROPORTION MARRIED (I_m) AND PROPORTION EVER-MARRIED AGED 20-24 (EM), BY ARRONDISSEMENT: 1880 TO 1910

	I_m				EM			
Flanders	1880	1890	1900	1910	1880	1890	1900	1910
Aalst	.377	.385	.443	.469	.172	.186	.244	.252
Antwerp	.463	.466	.485	.519	.252	.264	.308	.319
Bruges	.383	.379	.414	.456	.195	.191	.219	.260
Brussels	.442	.431	.467	.505	.302	.229	.282	.303
Dendermonde	.379	.389	.441	.482	.191	.185	.242	.259
Diksmuide	.412	.408	.426	.444	.205	.201	.207	.231
Eeklo	.378	.367	.409	.459	.161	.170	.231	.258
Ghent	.394	.410	.449	.480	.195	.209	.250	.272
Hasselt	.418	.398	.410	.449	.200	.156	.199	.225
Kortrijk	.397	.410	.452	.467	.188	.218	.248	.257
Leuven	.432	.433	.464	.495	.218	.228	.253	.283
Maaseik	.395	.381	.429	.467	.168	.136	.179	.229
Mechelen	.459	.456	.480	.521	.262	.261	.297	.317
Ostend	.481	.465	.502	.517	.297	.258	.322	.316
Oudenaarde	.349	.371	.407	.431	.136	.169	.189	.210
Roeselare	.370	.378	.415	.445	.155	.192	.214	.251
St. Niklaas	.395	.396	.437	.486	.180	.214	.261	.277
Tielt	.348	.349	.383	.406	.130	.161	.168	.164
Tongeren	.400	.376	.402	.434	.155	.133	.175	.186
Turnhout	.439	.422	.469	.507	.215	.218	.270	.297
Veurne	.481	.451	.472	.506	.247	.246	.266	.303
Ypres	.407	.411	.446	.471	.200	.214	.248	.264
Wallonia								
Arlon	.450	.460	.482	.535.	.211	.232	.268	.339
Ath	.444	.440	.499	.548	.241	.212	.282	.331
Bastogne	.402	.381	.401	.443	.178	.169	.179	.188
Charleroi	.534	.536	.611	.660	.342	.353	.471	.514
Dinant	.437	.434	.462	.490	.221	.195	.229	.268
Huy	.420	.414	.455	.504	.190	.192	.232	.272
Liège	.448	.454	.494	.526	.228	.246	.297	.305
Marche	.414	.391	.392	.425	.199	.165	.177	.177
Mons	.504	.520	.582	.617	.309	.324	.411	.461
Namur	.450	.432	.495	.552	.267	.229	.294	.349
Neufchâteau	.430	.416	.449	.479	.201	.187	.218	.231
Nivelles	.441	.434	.497	.556	.269	.207	.289	.352
Philippeville	.503	.499	.560	.611	.290	.273	.384	.428
Soignies	.473	.507	.573	.625	.308	.332	.410	.463
Thuin	.510	.523	.607	.645	.295	.327	.454	.490
Tournai	.402	.414	.462	.500	.193	.201	.266	.304
Verviers	.415	.404	.418	.466	.188	.178	.187	.206
Virton	.424	.419	.435	.498	.186	.170	.221	.280
Waremme	.417	.402	.433	.489	.193	.181	.222	.246

SOURCE: Population censuses of 1880, 1890, 1900, and 1910, Institut National de Statistique - Nationaal Instituut voor de Statistiek, Brussels.

maps show clearly the existence of three areas with particularly low values of I_m:

1. All the arrondissements in the province of East Flanders, and their neighboring arrondissements in West Flanders (the arrondissements of Bruges, Tielt, Roeselare).
2. All the arrondissements of the province of Limburg.
3. The arrondissements of Marche and Bastogne, located on the Ardennes plateau.

Areas with earlier marriage and higher values of I_m coincide with the industrial basin of Hainaut (arrondissements of Charleroi, Mons, Soignies) and with the adjacent Entre Sambre et Meuse region (arrondissements of Thuin and Philippeville). Several other arrondissements such as Arlon in the southeast and the rural part of Liège in the east, also had higher than average values, but they did not cover large areas. In Flanders, the least restrictive nuptiality patterns were found along the North Sea coast in the arrondissements of Ostend and Veurne, and in the arrondissements of Mechelen and Antwerp in the northern part of the country.

Not only the levels of I_m can be studied by arrondissement from 1880 on, but also the pace at which nuptiality was changing. A slightly different measure than I_m was adopted as a basis for measuring this change.

The index I_m is basically a period measure of nuptiality, and it reflects the experience of cohorts who contracted their marriages in periods prior to the one under observation as well as more recent experiences. At this point, we introduce a second index of nuptiality to help us measure the pace at which nuptiality was changing. This index is the proportion ever-married among women aged 20-24 (*EM*). It reflects the behavior of a particular cohort at the start of the nuptiality process, and is not affected by the behavior of cohorts that went through this phase several decades earlier. The index of proportion married (I_m) measures the combined effect of age at marriage and the ultimate proportion ever marrying in a hypothetical cohort, whereas the proportion ever-married aged 20-24 (*EM*) reflects more specifically the tempo of nuptiality in a specific cohort. The two indices correlate very highly: the proportion ever-married among women in the age group 20-24 carries the highest weight in the calculation of I_m, and in Belgium, at least, the behavior of the cohort at older ages can be predicted accurately from their performance in the age group of 20-24 years. The correlation coefficients between these two measures of nuptiality are calculated for the arrondissements of both language areas and are reported in Table 3.7. As can be verified there, they never fall below the .876 level for the period on which we are focusing our attention.

Hence, rather than defining a measure of change on the basis of I_m, we will base it on the proportion ever-married in the age group 20-24. We refer to this index as ΔEM and define it as

$$\Delta EM = \frac{EM_{t+x} - EM_t}{.800 - EM_t}$$

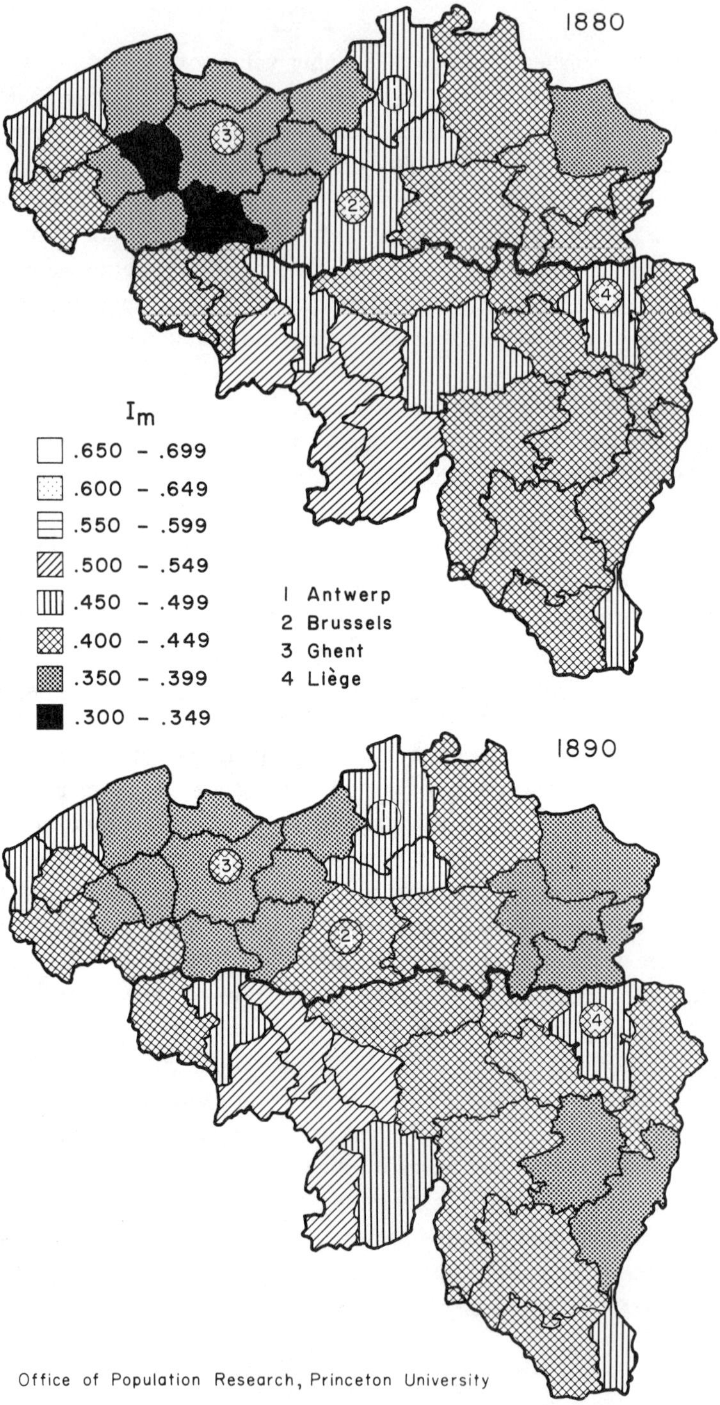

Office of Population Research, Princeton University

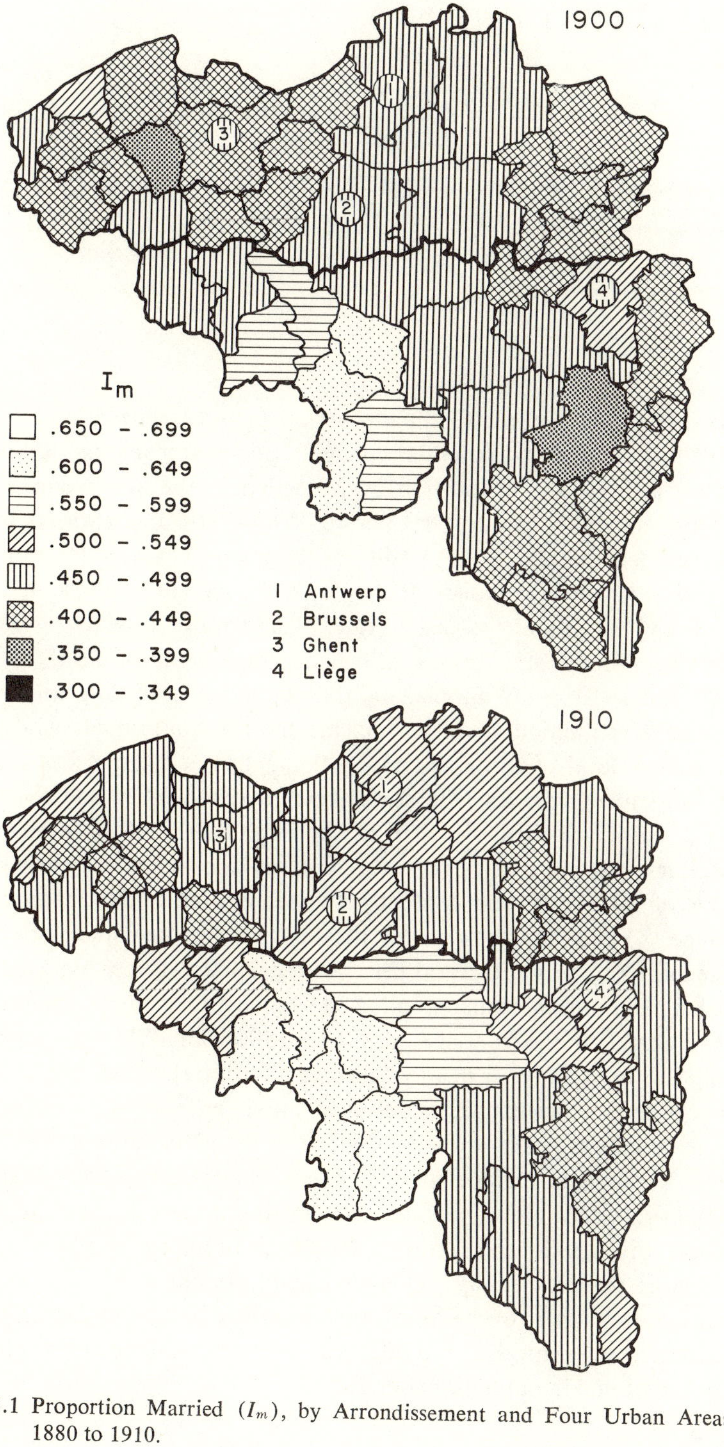

Map 3.1 Proportion Married (I_m), by Arrondissement and Four Urban Areas: 1880 to 1910.

TABLE 3.7

PROPORTION MARRIED (I_m), CORRELATION WITH PROPORTION EVER-MARRIED AGED 20-24 (EM), FLANDERS AND WALLONIA: 1880 TO 1910

Date	Flanders (N=22)	Wallonia (N=19)
1880	.876	.928
1890	.890	.967
1900	.928	.991
1910	.956	.993

where the observed change in the period between times t and $t+x$ is related to the possible potential change at moment t, taking .800 as the highest level of the proportion ever-married in the age group 20-24.

The values of ΔEM for the period 1880–1910 are reported by arrondissement in Map 3.2. Again, the entire province of Hainaut and several adjacent arrondissements in Wallonia were changing their nuptiality patterns at the fastest rate. The arrondissements of Belgian Lorraine (Virton and Arlon) also had a high value of ΔEM between 1880 and 1910. In Wallonia, the differentiation according to the rate of change in nuptiality was very clear: the arrondissements which had the highest level of I_m or EM in 1880 changed at the quickest pace in the subsequent decades (the correlations between ΔEM and the levels of I_m or EM are all above .836 as shown in Table 3.8). In Flanders, such high positive correlations were entirely absent: on the basis of the levels of EM or I_m one could by no means predict the speed of the change. One of the reasons for the instability of regional patterns in Flanders was the agricultural crisis of the 1880s. In certain areas this caused an important setback, followed by recovery of varying magnitude. If one correlates the level of I_m or EM in 1890 with ΔEM measured from that date until 1910, instead of measured from 1880 on, the resulting correlation coefficients are larger than those reported in Table 3.8 and fluctuate between .234 and .597. Never in Flanders, however, has there been such a clear regional pattern of nuptiality change as in Wallonia.

With this description we have concluded our review of the nuptiality trends. In the following sections, the subject of nuptiality will be treated in a more theoretical way. There, we shall present some economic and social consequences of the Malthusian marriage pattern in the eighteenth and nineteenth centuries, and offer theoretical possibilities for explaining the rising trend in nuptiality after 1850.

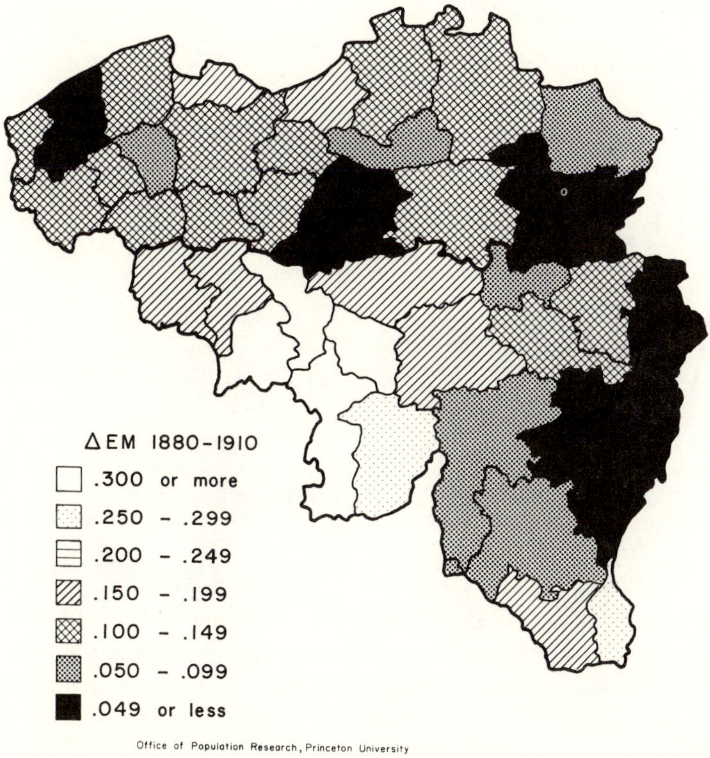

Map 3.2 Change in Proportion Ever-Married Aged 20-24 (ΔEM), by Arrondissement: 1880 to 1910.

3.6 *Nuptiality in Preindustrial Societies of Western Europe*

Before studying modern marriage patterns, it is necessary to understand the role played by restricted nuptiality in the economic and demographic setting of preindustrial western European countries. When we know more precisely the functions of the Malthusian marriage pattern, we may gain a better insight in exploring the possible explanations for its disappearance in the nineteenth and twentieth centuries.

In the preindustrial western European societies of the seventeenth and eighteenth centuries, the rate of marriage was a major factor in determining the rate of population growth. With an essentially uncontrolled marital fertility, population losses suffered during the frequent and often severe mortality crises could only be restored through an increase in nuptiality. The literature of the time shows that the demographic importance of nuptiality was fully understood, at least in a gen-

TABLE 3.8

CHANGE IN PROPORTION EVER-MARRIED AGED 20-24 (ΔEM) 1880-1910, CORRELATION WITH PROPORTION MARRIED (I_m) AND PROPORTION EVER-MARRIED AGED 20-24 (EM), FLANDERS AND WALLONIA: 1880 TO 1910

Measure and date	Correlation with ΔEM 1880-1910 Flanders (N=22)	Wallonia (N=19)
EM 1880	-.371	.836
EM 1890	.084	.919
EM 1900	.117	.955
EM 1910	.213	.977
I_m 1880	-.260	.871
I_m 1890	-.135	.919
I_m 1900	.016	.952
I_m 1910	.123	.963

eral policy oriented context. Malthus' reference of 1803 to the role of nuptiality was by no means new; before him an extensive literature had developed, linking nuptiality to population growth and population policies. Mercantilists such as Colbert (1666), and a group of French "populationists" such as Plumard de Danguel (1754), Abbé Joubert (1767), and Poncet de la Grave (1801) all attributed a key role to nuptiality. While the French advocated a decrease in celibacy to provoke an acceleration of population growth and to prevent a "depopulation" of France, (see J. J. Spengler, 1942, pp. 77-110), English authors, such as Young and Malthus, desired an increase in the mean age at marriage to curb the growth of a jobless and landless class of paupers.

Modern historical and demographic research has confirmed the importance of nuptiality and provides a more detailed picture of the situation. Drawing on French village studies, J. Dupâquier (1972, pp. 177-211) finds that the seventeenth- and eighteenth-century system of marriage, fertility, and household formation was based on the following three principles:

1. No conceptions outside wedlock.
2. No sharing of the same dwelling by more than one married couple.
3. No marriage without "establishment" (i.e., the availability of an independent means of living).

The first principle was generally well observed and fairly widespread in Western Europe. It was certainly applicable to Belgium; even in the nineteenth century, illegitimate fertility in the rural areas was remarkably low. As a result, procreation was almost wholly confined within wedlock, and nuptiality thus played a major role in determining overall fertility. The second and third principles made marriage (and hence also overall fertility) dependent on the economic system. In an agrarian and artisanal economy, marriage had to be delayed until a business, a farm, a workshop, a cottage, or at least a dwelling became available (E. W. Hofstee, 1954, p. 77).[3] In most cases, this occurred only at the death of the father. Mortality crises in the seventeenth and eighteenth centuries eliminated the older "established" generations, and the younger ones took over. As Dupâquier notes (1972, p. 202), the longer such mortality crises were postponed, the higher rose the mean age at marriage and the more numerous became the group of older candidates on the waiting list. As soon as the climax of a mortality crisis was over, the older bachelors, spinsters, and widowed persons had their immediate chance for a "good match," and generally shortly thereafter, an increase in marriage frequencies among the younger people occurred.

In such a structure, the inheritance system may have played an important role. According to H. Habakkuk's hypothesis (1955, pp. 1-12), when property is passed along the lines of a system with impartible inheritance (either primogeniture or strong testamentary preference), control is exerted mainly through marriage. Thus siblings who do not share their father's property have to postpone marriage, and in many cases they seek work in rural or urban industries or become employed as day laborers, seasonal workers, farmhands, or servants. In a system with partible inheritance and equal sharing, the check lies more in marital fertility, as parents want to limit further division of property through limitation of family size.

According to E. W. Hofstee (1954, p. 78), a late and nonuniversal marriage pattern results in the formation of extended households. In such a household other relatives are present in addition to a conjugal family (parents plus single children) (P. Laslett, 1972, p. 29). In Hofstee's description, only one son would marry upon the death of the

[3] In some instances a dowry was also required. Convinced that the French population was decreasing in the eighteenth century, Plumard de Danguel advocated the diversion of funds, originally destined to the organization of community fetes, to the dowering of poor adolescents (Plumard de Danguel, 1754, p. 322).

father, and rather than dividing the heritage, the other siblings would continue to live within this new household. According to this hypothesis, the modernization of nuptiality is not only the change from a pattern of late and nonuniversal marriage to a pattern of earlier marriage and reduced definitive celibacy, but also the change from an extended to a nuclear family system. These interrelations between the agricultural and artisanal economy, late marriage, and the prevalence of extended households form the core of what Hofstee has labeled "the agrarian-artisanal phase" (Hofstee, 1954, p. 77).

In the Malthusian framework, late age at marriage fulfilled an important economic role. As the formation of a new household implied additional births and the prospect of population increase, the age at marriage had to remain high to prevent a further fragmentation of the land, the division or overexploitation of the commons, the possibility of a decrease in real wages, and above all the formation of a class of paupers who would rely solely on community poor relief and charity. In Young's and Malthus' opinion, poor relief tended to waste capital and to facilitate "imprudent" marriage and natural increase, which then aggravated further the situation that the poor relief was supposed to alleviate. Even in France, where the "populationist" voice was traditionally very strong, the *Comité de Mendicité,* established in 1790, rejected the idea that population growth was necessarily advantageous to the state and blamed the French laws for encouraging marriage and hence the growth of indigence (J. J. Spengler, 1942, p. 312). In Germany and Switzerland, several states had adopted rigid marriage laws, explicitly forbidding marriage to anyone who could not prove the adequacy of his means of subsistence. Such legal prohibtions remained fully in force in several areas in Germany until as late as the second half of the nineteenth century (J. Knodel, 1967, p. 280).

A clear example showing the relation between economic conditions and late marriage has been described by R. Braun (1972, p. 9). He reports the existence of a closed village settlement in the lowlands of the canton of Zurich in eighteenth-century Switzerland. These farming areas had a traditional three-field system of cultivation that was based on a comprehensive and binding interdependence of the villagers. The field servitudes, crop rotation, and common pasture use were strictly regulated. Population growth, either through in-migration or through natural increase, was undesirable in these closely knit socioeconomic units, where the division of land and labor had to be so firmly organized.

Consequently, a settlement fee for newcomers (*Einzugsgeld*) was claimed, and a rigid *numerus clausus* of chimneys existed. This prevented the erection of any new dwelling, except upon the demolishing of an older one. Given this tight economic structure, family formation was not a simple matter and age at marriage was high. Together with the legal system, nuptiality fulfilled very clearly its function as a "preventive check" in that part of the Swiss lowlands.

The nuptiality valve worked consequently in two directions: by restricting marriage, a relative demographic and economic "equilibrium" could be maintained; by encouraging marriage, a substantial "reproductive reserve" could make up for the population loss suffered during years of hardship. In this way, nuptiality was a key element in a larger "self-regulating mechanism" (J. Dupâquier, 1972, pp. 177-211) or "homeostatic adjustment process" (E. A. Wrigley, 1969, p. 113) where at least a long-term "equilibrium" was sought between population size and economic conditions.[4]

This system might have been a valid model for picturing long-term trends in specific areas. In the short run, however, there are several examples showing that portions of the population tried to break away from it. R. Braun gives an example for the canton of Zurich. In the seventeenth and eighteenth centuries, a "proletarization" occurred in the more mountainous parts of this canton. In these areas, which were previously sparsely settled and characterized by very poor soil and the near absence of agriculture, industrial villages grew and attracted some of the surplus population from the lowlands. These landless classes, whose opportunities had been limited in the close village settlements of the plains, could now engage as cottage workers in the cotton industry. One of the striking phenomena in this development is the decline of the age at marriage. In fact, bundling became practiced as the chances for a young girl of being wed by her "seducer" had increased. There is no sign, however, that these sections of the population became more affluent. Quite the contrary was true: the cottage workers remained

[4] There is a possibility that the Malthusian marriage pattern did not exist in Western Europe prior to the sixteenth century (J. Hajnal, 1965, p. 131). We have no precise idea about marriage and family formation in a demographic, social, and economic context at that time. Hence, the three principles on which Dupâquier's model is based may not have been valid in the late Middle Ages. It is also interesting to note that both Dupâquier and Wrigley take their notion of "self-regulating mechanism" and "homeostatic adjustment process" from biologists' studies in animal populations.

paupers, only the economic *raison d'être* of the Malthusian nuptiality check did not apply to them any longer to the same degree. Their income was solely determined as a wage for their labor, and they did not have to wait to get married until capital became available in the form of a farm or an artisanal enterprise.

In Belgium, and more particularly in Flanders, such a "proletarization" occurred in the eighteenth century. When exports of linen to Latin America increased after 1740, the number of cottage spinners and weavers proliferated rapidly. P. Deprez has described this movement in the rural areas near Ghent (Castellany of Oudburg) (1965, p. 64), and F. Mendels has directly linked the periodic fluctuations in marriage frequencies to the expansion of this linen sector. He attributes the acceleration of population growth in the eighteenth century in these areas of interior Flanders to increasing marriage rates (1970c, p. 83).[5] Again, the decrease in the mean age at marriage was not the result of increased affluence. It was a consequence of the fact that there was no reason to postpone marriage: there was no land to divide, no property to inherit, no commons to protect.

In the Netherlands the phenomenon of "proletarization" occurred as well, and in more than one region. The case of the province of Overijssel in the eighteenth century has been described by B. M. Slicher van Bath (1968, p. 616): there, the proportion of landless labor, made up of cottage workers, day laborers, and peat diggers, increased substantially. A continuous population growth was observed during this period, and a mean age at marriage lower than in the nineteenth century may have been among the causes of this expansion in Overijssel.

Hence, the "agrarian-artisanal" pattern of which Hofstee speaks and the "self-regulating mechanisms" of Dupâquier did not necessarily exist everywhere before the nineteenth century. The landless proletariat that grew in many areas of Western Europe tried to escape from the Malthusian rules: they married earlier and had a higher overall fertility. Only mortality remained an important check, and the living conditions of these lower classes often led to very high levels of infant as well as adult mortality. Despite their high death rates, the development of

[5] The statistical links between the revival of the linen industry in Flanders and the nuptiality trends were studied by F. Mendels, but, since better measures of nuptiality were lacking, Mendels had to rely on the periodic fluctuations in overall marriage frequencies. The key issue in the argument, age at marriage, is in our view insufficiently documented in historical research so far conducted in Belgium to accept Mendel's theory without precaution.

landless classes was often associated with the acceleration of population growth in the eighteenth century. Consequently, they were living very close to what Wrigley (1969, p. 113) calls "the verge of the Malthusian precipice."

3.7 *Modern Nuptiality Patterns: Explanatory Hypotheses*

In eighteenth-century Flanders, Overijssel, and the canton of Zurich, the emergence of sharp breaks from the old Malthusian setting were caused by far-reaching economic alterations. In all three examples, the shift away from the restrictive nuptiality pattern occurred as the result of what could be called the "proletarization" of a large section of the rural population. New groups of wage-earning persons were growing and were engaged in different rural industries (cottage spinning and weaving in Flanders and the canton of Zurich, peat digging in Overijssel). As cottage industry developed, there was no longer a need for boys to engage in long apprenticeships during which they could not marry. Nor did they have to wait to establish themselves until an entire artisanal workshop became available; only a hand-loom had to be procured. Where there was a combined activity in cottage industry and agriculture, as in Flanders, the young adults did not have to wait to inherit land: most of the small plots were rented rather than owned. The basis of the subsistence of these classes was their labor, not their property; as a consequence of the increasing separation between these two elements of production, tardy and nonuniversal marriage started losing its capacity to maintain an "equilibrium" between population and the classic agricultural artisanal economy.

What Deprez, Mendels, Braun, and Slicher van Bath tried to find in the eighteenth century, Hofstee (1954, p. 90) placed in the nineteenth: with the accelerated growth of employment outside the family-related artisanal workshops or agricultural enterprises during the Industrial Revolution, an even larger section of the population became both economically independent and capable of establishing a household at an earlier age. The precariousness of the wage-earners' sustenance ceased to be related to their age, and they had no more grounds for postponing their marriages. Hence, the "agrarian-artisanal phase" is followed by the "intermediary proletarian phase." While we are introducing more of Hofstee's terminology here, we should note that the qualification "intermediary" is not given with respect to nuptiality; rather, it relates to the lack of any attempt to control marital fertility. The control of marital fertility occurs in Hofstee's third phase with the development of "modern reproductive behavior."

Both the economic and demographic functions of the Malthusian pattern disappeared with the arrival of the Industrial Revolution and the unprecedented growth of wage-earning classes. First, mortality crises played an important role in the Malthusian marriage system by occasionally creating a large number of vacancies with respect to occupational posts. The filling of these posts by survivors implied generally a temporary increase in nuptiality rates and a decrease in the mean age at marriage. In this way, the Malthusian marriage pattern filled the role of a "reproductive reserve," which was occasionally released after a mortality upswing. When mortality crises became scarcer and less severe, however, there was a diminishing need to maintain such a "reproductive reserve" and this particular function of the classic marriage pattern grew less important. Second, the old marriage pattern was the most important factor preventing largely uncontrolled marital fertility from becoming translated into excessive population growth. Subsequently, when marital fertility was gradually brought under control, this corrective function became obsolete as well, and the more natural tendency to marry earlier could be released.

Most hypotheses explaining the increase in nuptiality in the nineteenth century point to the disappearance of factors that had maintained the mean age at marriage at its Malthusian level. There were at least four reasons for a rising trend in nuptiality: (1) the "agrarian-artisanal" phase was succeeded by the "proletarian" one; (2) the extended family structure was no longer a social necessity in a changing economic structure; (3) mortality declined; and (4) marital fertility was gradually brought under control.

3.8 *Some Research Topics*

On the basis of the hypotheses formulated in the preceding section, we will retain several topics for analysis. Given the size of the subject of the nuptiality evolution, the choice of these topics is, of course, largely arbitrary, and in this instance is also the result of a particular interest and the availability of certain data.

The first topic to be examined more carefully is the link between the Malthusian marriage pattern and the extended household structure. which existed during Hofstee's "agrarian-artisanal phase." In our view, one could just as well expect that the prevalence of extended households would lead to early rather than late marriage, as was the case in Eastern Europe.[6] We hypothesize that there is no necessary association between late marriage and extended household structure.

The second research topic is also related to Hofstee's three-phase theory. More precisely, the explanation of increasing nuptiality as a function of the growth of wage-earning classes (i.e., the explanatory power of Hofstee's "proletarian intermediary phase") seems to be an attractive subject for further investigation. Of course, Hofstee has never pretended that his three-stage evolution would be applicable to Belgian demographic trends; his theory was only constructed to explain Dutch data. The testing of several of his claims on the basis of the Belgian materials may, however, lead to some clarifications and add interesting amendments.

As a third area of investigation, we will test the claim that the increase in nuptiality started only when the demographic effect of late marriage ceased to exist, i.e., when marital fertility was reduced. According to this hypothesis, the marital fertility transition must have preceded or at most occurred simultaneously with the increase in nuptiality. Putting the relationship in the other direction (i.e., considering nuptiality change as a factor triggering the marital fertility decline) would be unacceptable given the classic function of nuptiality in Western Europe. In the pre-industrial setting, the age at marriage went down without alterations in marital fertility, when the population had to draw on the so-called "reproductive reserve" to make up for losses suffered during epidemics and famines. Now, as a result of rapidly modernizing economic structures, the old economic functions of late marriage were gradually disappearing and the combination of earlier marriage and natural fertility would lead to higher overall fertility and increased population growth, which, at least temporarily, could easily be absorbed in a situation of accelerated economic growth.

The first and second topics will be discussed in the sections immediately following. The third subject involves the prior description of the decline of marital fertility. The discussion of the link between marital fertility and nuptiality will consequently be treated in chapter 5.

[6] In Eastern Europe, economic independence was not a major prerequisite for marriage. A newly married couple found more frequently a place in the household of the parents or of another married relative. As a result, the formation of extended households was not incompatible with early marriage.

Let us now turn our attention to the relationship between household structure and late marriage in preindustrial Belgium.

3.9 *Average Household Size Before 1850*

Given the overall late age at marriage and the importance of definitive celibacy and widowhood, one can readily pose the question of what happened to the large numbers of unmarried people. As we know, Hofstee has suggested that extended family households were, of necessity, very common as these individuals joined the families of relatives (1954, p. 78).

More recently, however, evidence has been collected in several western European countries, and most clearly in the Netherlands (A. M. van der Woude, 1972, pp. 300-318), indicating that extended family households were the exception rather than the rule, and that the presence of unmarried persons in the population, either single or widowed, did not necessarily lead to the formation of extended families. Consequently, what is possible for certain Dutch provinces with economic and social characteristics relatively similar to the Belgian ones, seems a priori possible in our case also.

To clarify the issue, we have constructed a few elementary models of household formation that take into account the demographic conditions prevailing in Belgium for the period 1750–1830. As a first input, six different stable age structures are used. They correspond to growth rates of 0.0 percent (stationary model), 0.5 percent, and 1.0 percent, and to the mortality conditions bracketing the life table computed by Quételet and Smits (1832, p. 32) for the 1820s. These mortality conditions correspond to the North life tables of the Princeton set with life expectancies at birth of 30.0 and 35.0 years. In addition, three hypotheses concerning the mean age at marriage are adopted: 25.0, 27.5, and 30.0 years, bracketing what has been found in the canton of Lede in 1796 and in the 1829 census for the whole of the country. On the basis of the model life tables for both sexes, the proportion widowed, by age, was approximated. From this and the proportion ever-married by age, the proportion currently married could be obtained. These approximations were the direct inputs in our calculations of household sizes. All calculations were performed on the female population only.[7]

[7] These values of the mean age at marriage were converted into a proportion ever-married by age group. Following Coale's standard nuptiality schedule

With respect to the hypotheses regarding household formation, we have adopted methods different from those developed by A. J. Coale (1965a, pp. 64-69) and T. K. Burch (1972, pp. 92-95). These authors followed a typology of household structures and tried to picture the conditions necessary to obtain an extended, stem, or nuclear household system. Rather than making a clear distinction between these various types, we have made assumptions regarding the destiny of widows and single adults. It is our purpose to find out whether or not unmarried individuals joined other households, rather than to describe precisely the types of household that would result.

In Model A, we have assumed that neither single women (children or adults) nor widows above the age of 45 years would set up a separate household.[8] Hence, these unmarried persons continue to live with married children, married siblings, or other married relatives, or become servants in the household of an unrelated family. In Model B, single adults above the age of 30 form a separate household and widows over the age of 45 either join in a household with a single daughter or return to a household of a married child or any other couple. In Model C, this combination has been reversed: widows form a separate household, but single women above age 30 do not. To a considerable degree, Models B and C lead to the same household type, since in both cases single adults form a common household with widowed mothers. Differences in average household size between Models B and C stem from the differences between the number of widows and single women. In Model D, everyone goes their own way: married women form a household with their husbands and children (conjugal family), widows over 45 and single persons over 30 years of age form separate household units.

The resulting average household sizes for A through D are given in

---

(explained in full detail in the technical appendix), the mean age at marriage was translated into the value of parameter k through the following equation

$$k = (\overline{x}_m - a_o)/11.36$$

In this formula, 11.36 is the standard deviation of Coale's model curve, $\overline{x}_m$ is the mean age at marriage, and a_o the lowest age at which first marriges occur (set at 17.0 years). The value for C, or the final proportion ever-married, was taken as 0.85. The formula for translating x_m into k was kindly made available by D. Ewbank.

[8] It was assumed that remarriage probabilities for widows younger than 45 years were so high that they formed another conjugal household immediately upon the dissolution of their first union.

Table 3.9. Certain values are presented in parentheses and are to be viewed as theoretical rather than actual possibilities, given certain demographic constraints. A female mean age at marriage of 30.0 years was probably rare and so were birth rates below 30.0 per thousand. From Table 3.9 it is clear that the impact of the demographic parameters

TABLE 3.9

AVERAGE HOUSEHOLD SIZE, FOUR STABLE POPULATION MODELS INCORPORATING SPINSTERS AND WIDOWS: DEMOGRAPHIC CONDITIONS OF 1750-1830

Model	Intrinsic growth rate (%)	Life expectancy at birth=30.0 years: Mean age at marriage 25.0	27.5	30.0	Birth rate	Death rate	Life expectancy at birth=35.0 years: Mean age at marriage 25.0	27.5	30.0	Birth rate	Death rate
A. Widows and single adults do not form separate households	0.0	6.00	6.65	(7.39)	33.3	33.3	(5.66)	(6.47)	(7.16)	28.6	28.6
	0.5	6.36	7.08	(7.91)	38.4	33.4	6.09	6.76	(7.50)	33.1	28.1
	1.0	6.77	7.56	(8.32)	43.8	33.8	6.56	7.33	(8.20)	38.0	28.0
B. Single adults over age 30 form separate households, widows over age 45 join other households	0.0	5.13	5.55	(5.89)	33.3	33.3	(4.99)	(5.34)	(5.67)	28.6	28.6
	0.5	5.47	5.85	(6.35)	38.4	33.4	5.35	5.77	(6.16)	33.1	28.1
	1.0	5.87	6.40	(6.89)	43.8	33.8	5.66	6.14	(6.59)	38.0	28.0
C. Single adults over age 30 join other households, widows over age 45 form separate households	0.0	4.50	4.87	(5.25)	33.3	33.3	(4.30)	(4.62)	(4.96)	28.6	28.6
	0.5	4.89	5.31	(5.77)	38.4	33.4	4.66	5.04	(5.44)	33.1	28.1
	1.0	5.33	5.83	(6.27)	43.8	33.8	5.07	5.51	(6.00)	38.0	28.0
D. Single adults over age 30 and widows over age 45 form separate households	0.0	4.00	4.22	(4.44)	33.3	33.3	(3.80)	(4.01)	(4.20)	28.6	28.6
	0.5	4.35	4.63	(4.89)	38.4	33.4	4.21	4.47	(4.71	33.1	28.1
	1.0	4.76	5.10	(5.41)	43.8	33.8	4.51	4.81	(5.09)	38.0	28.0

Note: Figures are average number of females per household multiplied by 2 (female dominant model)

is considerable; but the variation introduced by the four different assumptions regarding the destiny of widows and single adults is as large. In Model A, the acceptable average household sizes vary between 6.00 and 7.56, whereas in Model D, household sizes of 4.00 to 5.10 are found. Not surprisingly, Models B and C give intermediate results.

These theoretical values of average family size can be compared with the actual ones reported in Table 3.10. On the basis of the census of 1829, values are available for urban and rural regions in the majority of the provinces that made up the territory of Belgium after 1830. Values are also reported for the major cities in 1829, and they can be compared

TABLE 3.10

AVERAGE HOUSEHOLD SIZE, SELECTED PROVINCES, CITIES, AND VILLAGES: 18TH AND EARLY 19TH CENTURIES

Area	Prior to 1739 Size	N	1740-1779 Size	N	1780-1810 Size	N	1829 Urban Size	1829 Rural Size
Provinces:								
Antwerp	--	--	--	--	--	--	4.53	5.22
Brabant	--	--	--	--	--	--	4.61	5.20
East Flanders	--	--	--	--	--	--	4.67	5.16
West Flanders	--	--	--	--	--	--	5.00	5.31
Hainaut	--	--	--	--	--	--	4.42	4.80
Liege	--	--	--	--	--	--	4.52	4.78
Namur	--	--	--	--	--	--	4.79	4.77
Cities:								
Antwerp	--	--	3.10	--	--	--	4.65	N.A.
Brussels	--	--	3.20	--	3.80	--	4.49	N.A.
Ghent	--	--	--	--	--	--	5.09	N.A.
Liege	--	--	--	--	3.70	--	4.50	N.A.
Villages:								
Aalst area	5.03	9	5.14	2	4.98	5	N.A.	5.43
Eeklo area	5.09	3	--	--	5.19	1	N.A.	5.06
Oudenaarde area	4.71	4	5.02	3	4.84	2	N.A.	5.30

SOURCES: Data through 1810: J. de Brouwer, 1968, pp. 117-127; G. van Laere, 1961, p. 54; C. Rammelaere, 1959, p. 54; and E. Hélin, 1972, p. 319.
Data for 1829: Quételet and Smits, 1832, p. 60.

NOTE: Data for villages in 1829 are for complete rural districts, corresponding closely to arrondissements without urban units.

with those found in earlier periods. It should be noted, however, that the values for 1829 are overestimated since collective households (e.g., convents, hospitals) were incorporated in the calculations. Finally, information is given for 29 villages in the province of East Flanders for the entire eighteenth century. Their levels of average household size were remarkably homogeneous and stable over time (median: 4.98; interquartile interval: 0.48).

Clearly, nowhere are average household sizes obtained comparable to those in Model A: the extended family household could not have been the dominant type, and many other alternatives were open to the unmarried. In Model B and C, the formation of a simple but nonconjugal family unit (e.g., widow[er]s with single offspring) becomes possible. The average household size drops considerably, and the observed values for the rural areas now fit better the theoretical ones. In the major cities, however, the observed values are much closer to—or even smaller than—the theoretical averages of Model D: a considerable number of households must have been made up of widowed or single adults living alone.

Even where the extended family household was not the rule, the difference between urban and rural areas was important. Very few single adults were found in the countryside but a great many more in the cities. In eight East Flanders villages combined, (1786–1792) only 4.5 percent of all households consisted of one person, compared with 18.0 percent in Liège and 14.6 percent in the Liège suburbs (1801) (E. Hélin, 1972, p. 324). Obviously, the very low figures for average household size in the cities can only be explained by the in-migration of single adults, probably those who did not want or were unable to find a place in a rural society as a member of another household.

The large numbers of unmarried individuals typical for the demographic conditions in the late 1700s and early 1800s did not necessarily lead to extended family households. Simple family households on a conjugal or nonconjugal basis were present in the countryside and dominated in urban settings.

3.10 *Nuptiality Patterns*

On the basis of E. W. Hofstee's "proletarian phase" one should find the breakdown of the Malthusian marriage pattern occurring first in areas with a growing labor force participation outside of agricultural and artisanal activities. In studying the Dutch case, Hofstee (1972, p. 59) makes no distinction between the marriage behavior of the urban industrial working classes and the landless rural proletariat. In his view, there is no need for such a distinction as both groups became independent of the "agrarian-artisanal" pattern.

Failure to distinguish between a rural proletariat and the urban or industrial working classes in the Belgian experience would be difficult to defend. As we shall prove in the subsequent paragraphs, the newly growing wage-earning classes were not homogeneous with respect to their nuptiality behavior. The urban (especially the industrial group) developed earlier marriage, whereas the rural proletariat continued to follow a more Malthusian pattern.

In chapter 2, two indices documented the modernization of the occupational structure. The first was the percentage of the male labor force engaged in agriculture and the second was the ratio of those employed in modern industry over those engaged in more typical nineteenth-century activities (see chapter 2, Section 2.5). The second index was not constructed entirely in the same way for Flanders as for Wallonia, because of the different economic structures of the two areas.

To obtain more nearly linear relations with the dependent variable proportion ever-married aged 20-24 (*EM*), the second index was calculated in logarithmic form and will be referred to in subsequent tables as "log. occupational structure."

The results of a multiple regression analysis between the nuptiality variable *EM* and the characteristics of the occupational structure are given in Table 3.11. The analysis is performed in three steps, as follows:

TABLE 3.11

TWO INDICES OF MARRIAGE, PROPORTION OF VARIANCE (R^2) EXPLAINED BY TWO INDICES OF OCCUPATIONAL STRUCTURE, FLANDERS AND WALLONIA: 1880 TO 1910

		Flanders (N=22)						Wallonia (N=19)					
		Percentage males in agriculture and log. occupational structure			Δ percentage males in agriculture and Δ log. occupational structure			Percentage males in agriculture and log. occupational structure			Δ percentage males in agriculture and Δ log. occupational structure		
Marriage index	Date	1890	1900	1910	1890-1910	1890-1900	1900-1910	1890	1900	1910	1890-1910	1890-1900	1900-1910
Proportion women ever-married aged 20-24 (EM)	1890	.472	--	--	--	--	--	.567	--	--	--	--	--
	1900	--	.641	--	--	--	--	--	.553	--	--	--	--
	1910	--	--	.653	--	--	--	--	--	.525	--	--	--
Change in proportion women ever-married aged 20-24 (ΔEM)	1880-1910	.040	--	--	.005	--	--	.400	--	--	.588	--	--
	1880-1900	.001	--	--	--	.042	--	.455	--	--	--	.489	--
	1890-1910	.077	--	--	.232	--	--	.321	--	--	.396	--	--
	1890-1900	.102	--	--	--	.366	--	.382	--	--	--	.315	--
	1900-1910	--	.208	--	--	--	.007	--	.202	--	--	--	.208

1. The levels of industrialization as measured through the occupational structure are related to the regional levels of the proportion ever-married aged 20-24 years (*EM*).
2. The levels of industrialization at time *t* are used to predict the change in the rate of nuptiality (Δ*EM*) in the years following time *t*.[9]
3. The relative changes in the occupational structure (the pace at which industrialization proceeded) are used as predictors for the regional change in rates of nuptiality (Δ*EM*).

In the first purely static analysis, the regional differences in proportions ever-married at ages 20-24 (*EM*) are found to be clearly related to industrialization: in each linguistic region, 45 to 65 percent of the

[9] The values of Δ*EM* 1880–1900 and Δ*EM* 1880–1910 are predicted from the variables of occupational structure measured in 1890 instead of 1880. No observations by arrondissement were available for 1880.

variance of *EM* is explained by differences in occupational structure. In the second and third forms of analysis relating ΔEM to occupational structure and changes in this structure, strong relationships are still found for Wallonia: roughly half of the variance of ΔEM for the entire period 1880–1910 is explained by either the level or the pace of industrialization in the different arrondissements. In other words, in this part of Belgium, clear and undeniable associations are found between the levels and rates of change of nuptiality on the one hand, and the extent or rates of change in industrial occupation on the other hand.

In Flanders, however, the relationship breaks down when the rates of change in nuptiality (ΔEM) are introduced. In Table 3.8 we had found a weak relationship in Flanders between the levels of nuptiality, as measured by I_m or *EM,* and the change in their rates (ΔEM). This phenomenon appears again in the form of a negligible correlation between ΔEM and the occupational structure. Once more, a partial explanation is offered by the effects of the agricultural crisis: in some arrondissements the values of ΔEM may have responded to the pace of industrial growth, whereas in others nuptiality may have changed primarily as part of the recovery from the setback between 1880 and 1890.

The multiple regression analysis that yielded the values of R^2 in Table 3.11 gives us an opportunity to search for regional patterns of nuptiality not accounted for by regional differences in occupational patterns. We predicted the values of *EM* by means of the regression equations and compared the results to the actual values; in this manner a residual was obtained that is the difference between the observed and the predicted values. To adjust for arbitrary units of measurement, these residuals can be standardized by their own standard deviation. For each value of R^2 in Table 3.11 we have obtained a set of such standardized residuals. Upon inspection of these series of residuals, a very stable regional pattern was found in which some areas were more advanced (positive residuals) and some areas were lagging behind (negative residuals) in the rise in nuptiality (relative to their degree of industrialization). On Map 3.3, the average of the standardized residuals is given for the following regressions:

Flanders: -*EM* 1890, 1900, and 1910 regressed on the levels of the indices of occupational structure at these dates.

Wallonia: -*EM* 1890, 1900, and 1910 regressed on the levels of the indices of occupational structure at these dates.

-ΔEM 1880–1910, 1880–1900, 1890–1910, and 1890–1900 regressed on the levels of the indices of occupational structure.

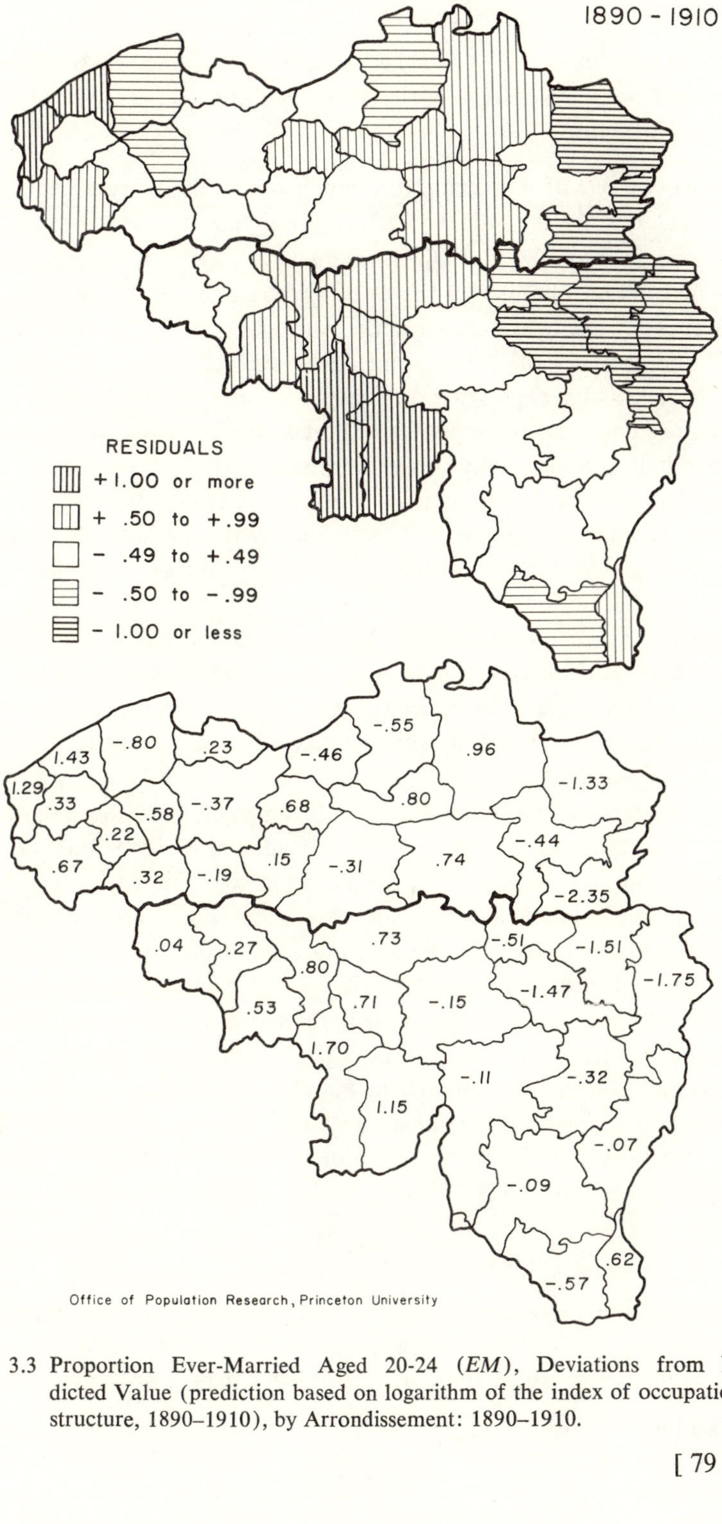

Map 3.3 Proportion Ever-Married Aged 20-24 (*EM*), Deviations from Predicted Value (prediction based on logarithm of the index of occupational structure, 1890–1910), by Arrondissement: 1890–1910.

-ΔEM 1890–1910, 1880–1900, 1890–1910, and 1890–1900 regressed on Δ Percentage Males in Agriculture and Δ Log. Occupational Structure.

The last two sets of standardized residuals for Wallonia were not plotted for Flanders since the values of R^2 were insignificant (see Table 3.11).

The regional pattern of these residuals is especially interesting for Wallonia. After eliminating the overall impact of industrialization and differences in occupational structure, the areas located in the western half—the province of Hainaut and the arrondissements of Philippeville and Nivelles—have persistently positive residuals, indicating a more modernized pattern of nuptiality, whereas the arrondissements in the eastern half and especially in the northeast corner of Wallonia—Huy, Liège, Verviers, and Waremme—have negative residuals and are consequently behind in the nuptiality transition. While the index of "occupational structure" explains about 40 to 50 percent of the variation in nuptiality (either EM or ΔEM in Wallonia), there is still a distinct regional pattern, independent of this measure. The arrondissements in the west of Wallonia, which were in direct contact economically and socially with France, had higher values of EM than the arrondissements in the northeast of Wallonia, which had economically and socially closer ties to Flanders and Germany.

In Flanders, a more confused picture emerges from the analysis of standardized residuals. The arrondissements of Ostend and Veurne, located along the coast and in the Polder area, seem to have a systematically more modern pattern of nuptiality, whereas the arrondissements of Maaseik and Tongeren in the eastern part of Flanders share their negative residuals with the adjacent Liège area in Wallonia. The arrondissements with the large metropolitan areas of Antwerp, Brussels, and Ghent all have negative residuals. An additional explanation for the overall pattern of nuptiality in Flanders is taken up in subsequent paragraphs through an examination of the rural areas. The feature of later marriage and higher frequency of celibacy in large urban areas is discussed in Section 3.12.

3.11 *Nuptiality in Rural Areas*

The analysis in Wallonia suggests that wherever a large group of industrial laborers could be found, a high value of EM would also exist. Where the active population was primarily made up of farmers and artisanal workers, or of rural laborers such as cottagers, farmhands, day laborers, and servants, a lower nuptiality intensity would be expected.

In rural Flanders, the working class did not follow the trend set by urban and inustrial workers. Using the census of 1890, we have calculated the values of I_m and *EM* for the rural parts of arrondissements (obtained by eliminating urban units of 10,000 or more inhabitants). In the census of professions and industries of 1896, more detailed information was found on the occupational structure of these rural parts, and this allowed us to correlate the values of *EM* with three indices of the rural occupational structure. The first measure relates the number of agricultural laborers and cottage weavers to the nonagricultural male population aged 15 to 55. The second utilizes the percentage of the active male population in agriculture. The third deals with the female labor force: agricultural laborers and servants together with lace-makers and women employed in other sectors of the cottage industries are compared to the nonagricultural female labor force between the ages of 15 and 55. The results of the correlation analysis are shown in Table 3.12 for each language region. In Wallonia, the percentage in agriculture explains most of the relationship with the degree of nuptiality in the age group 20-24 (*EM*). In Flanders, however, the relative numbers of day laborers, farmhands, servants, and cottagers of either sex are responsible for the strong negative relationship with the measure of nuptiality (*EM*). This is definitely a clear indication that the rural proletariat did not follow the pattern of the industrial workers. In other words, Hofstee's concept of "proletarization" is too general and does not allow for the major difference in nuptiality patterns among the rural and the strictly industrial wage earners.

3.12 *Nuptiality in Urban Areas*

The degree of urbanization can be expected to have two opposing effects on nuptiality. First, according to the "proletarization theory," a large concentration of wage earners in industrial towns and city suburbs should lead to an earlier pattern of marriage in these communities. Second, given the attraction that cities traditionally have exercised on the labor force of the countryside, and especially on single persons who did not fit well into the agricultural setting, the value of I_m should be low in urban areas (see Section 3.7). In view of this, the socioeconomic background of the migrants and the economic function or specialization of urban units may be two factors of great importance

TABLE 3.12

PROPORTION WOMEN EVER-MARRIED AGED 20-24 (EM), CORRELATION WITH THREE MEASURES OF OCCUPATIONAL STRUCTURE, RURAL PARTS OF ARRONDISSEMENTS, FLANDERS AND WALLONIA: 1900

	Correlation with occupational structure ratios					
	Flanders (N=19)			Wallonia (N=19)		
Measure	Ratio 1	Ratio 2	Ratio 3	Ratio 1	Ratio 2	Ratio 3
Proportion women ever-married aged 20-24 (EM)	-.91	-.35	-.76	-.43	-.63	-.39
Ratio 1: Farm laborers/cottage weavers to non-agric. male pop. aged 15-55	--	+.47	+.79	--	+.92	+.64
Ratio 2: Male pop. active in agric. to male pop. aged 15-55	+.47	--	+.39	+.92	--	+.59
Ratio 3: Female agric. workers to non agric. female pop. aged 15-55	+.79	+.39	--	+.64	+.59	--
Proportion of variance in EM explained by three occupational ratios ($R^2_{4.123}$)		+.84			+.57	

NOTES: The three arrondissements of Limburg province in Flanders are omitted.
Female agricultural workers include farm laborers, servants, and lace makers and other cottage workers.
In explaining the porportion of variance in EM, the value of R^2 was corrected for the effect of the number (3) of independent variables approaching the number (19) of observations.

in explaining both the urban-rural differentiation and the heterogeneity among urban areas with respect to nuptiality.

Testing these assumptions with the Belgian data,[10] we cannot deny the existence of a very clear-cut differentiation in Wallonia between two categories of urban units: (1) the industrial towns of the province of Hainaut, with their specialization in heavy industries, and the industrial suburbs of Liège and (2) the city of Liège itself and the provincial towns. The industrial towns had values of I_m that far surpassed the national or even the Walloon average. Hence, when a pronounced degree of industrialization was coupled with the dominant presence of a

[10] The information necessary to calculate the value of I_m is available only for urban units with a population larger than 10,000. This explains why the number of units for which I_m is calculated increases with time.

wage-earning class, a much more modern nuptiality pattern prevailed, and few women remained single. On the other hand, the provincial towns and the city of Liège itself had a high concentration of single persons, which is translated into substantially lower values of I_m. These places had a much more balanced occupational structure corresponding to their more diversified economic function.

In-migration played a key role in the mechanism linking nuptiality to economic specialization. It is hard to imagine, for example, that coal-mining towns and other industrial centers of metallurgy or machinery construction would attract a labor force of women. Only men were requested, and they came, either single or married. The two classical statistical characteristics of these towns were a low female employment rate and a sex ratio indicating a surplus of men.

In contrast, provincial towns and larger cities were attracting significant numbers of women. Light industries—above all the textile and clothing industry—recruiting cheaper labor, turned typically to the female labor reserve. In addition, jobs in education, small trade, and domestic service were open to women, and, as a consequence, the sex ratios of large cities and provincial towns indicated a deficit of men. This is documented for Wallonia in Table 3.13 where we have contrasted several characteristics of the Liège industrial suburbs with those of other Walloon provincial towns. The industrial suburbs of Liège had a small female active population (not exceeding 30 percent of all women between 15 and 55 years of age), a smaller concentration in the classic women-oriented sectors (education, textiles and clothing, and domestic service), a considerable surplus of males in the age group of 20 to 30 years, and a much higher I_m than the national or the Walloon average. The picture is completely reversed in the Walloon provincial towns. The central city of Liège has, as expected, all the characteristics of the provincial towns, while the more mixed industrial and commercial center of Charleroi has the characteristics of the industrial suburbs. Compared with the urban areas of Hainaut, however, the value of I_m in Charleroi lies midway between that of the Hainaut provincial towns of Mons and Tournai and that of the typical industrial towns [11] (see Figure 3.3).

[11] Only the occupational structure of a few urban communities was published in the 1910 census. In this way, no information on female labor force participation was available for the Hainaut industrial towns. The sex ratio in these 15 communities in 1910 showed again a considerable surplus of males and ranged

TABLE 3.13

LABOR FORCE PARTICIPATION OF FEMALES, SEX RATIO, AND PROPORTION MARRIED (I_m), SELECTED URBAN UNITS, WALLONIA: 1910

Urban unit	Female workers as percentage of female pop. aged 15-55	Female workers in education, textiles, and domestic service as percentage of total female workers	Sex ratio, ages 20-30, of males to females	Proportion married (I_m)
Industrial suburbs of Liège:				
Angleur	14	71	1.16	.619
Bressoux	19	62	1.07	.596
Grivegnée	24	73	1.10	.567
Herstal	26	38	1.01	.580
Ougrée	15	64	1.17	.619
Seraing	19	44	1.16	.612
Provincial towns:				
Mons	46	82	.94	.482
Namur	41	80	.90	.455
Tournai	54	83	.90	.454
Verviers	50	86	.90	.460
Larger cities:				
Charleroi	25	66	1.07	.581
Liège	46	68	.89	.450

Among the urban units that form the large urban areas of Antwerp, Brussels, and Ghent, those with the smallest surplus of women and the smallest female active population had values of I_m substantially larger than central cities or suburbs with an important female labor force and a considerable surplus of women. These associations are shown in Table 3.14 for 13 communities belonging to the three urban areas. For 10 other communities, only the sex ratio for the age group 20 to 30 is available. Including these 10 with the 13 just mentioned, one finds a correlation coefficient between this sex ratio and I_m of .826 in 1910.

A similar analysis can be made for the Flemish provincial towns (the fourth group in Figure 3.3). The range of I_m values in 1910 is substantial, from .604 in the industrial town of Boom (clay-digging and brickyards) to .412 in Bruges, the center of lace-making, an activity per-

between 1.04 (Marcinelle) and 1.17 (Marchienne-au-Pont). The median stood at 1.11.

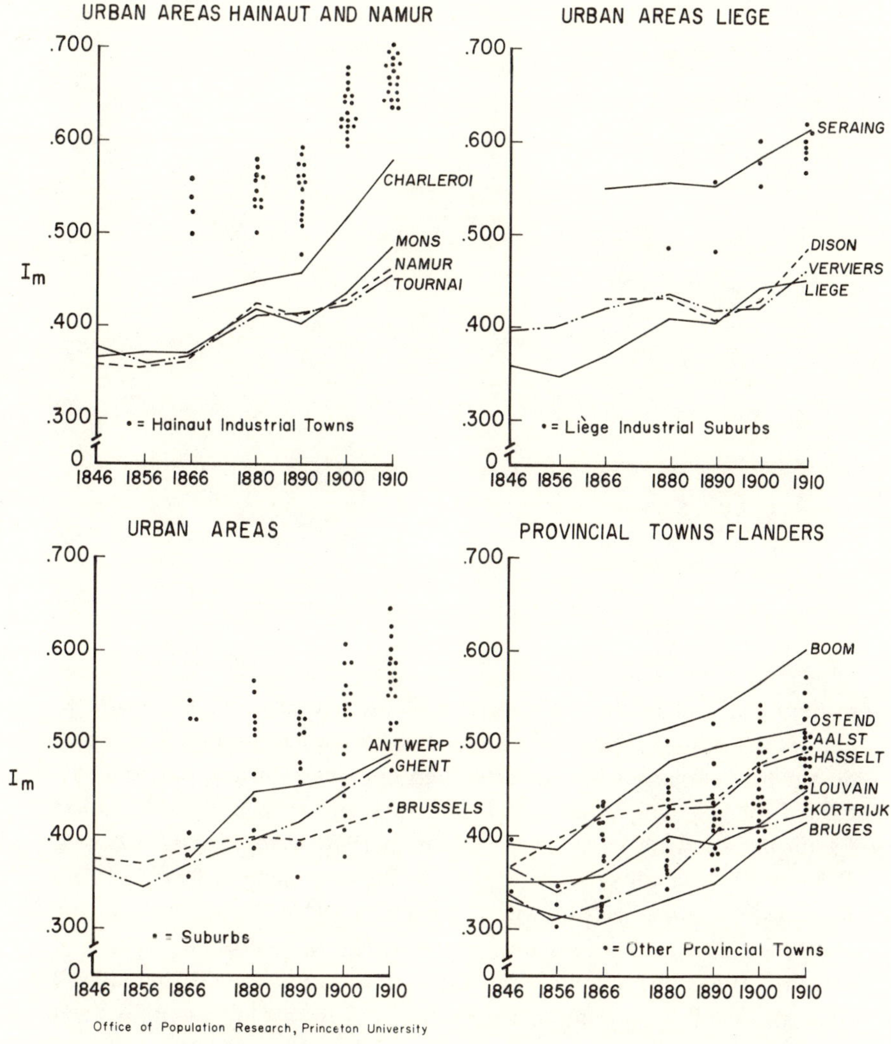

Figure 3.3 Proportion Married (I_m), by Selected Urban Areas: 1846 to 1970.

formed only by women. High values of I_m were recorded for Willebroek (.600) and Vilvoorde (.571), two fast-growing industrial centers along a canal linking Brussels to the Scheldt river. The town of Moeskroen, an industrial center on the French border and actually the Belgian part of the French industrial complex near Lille and Roubaix, had an I_m of .566. The center of sugar refineries, Tienen, had an I_m of .525. Together, these towns had the highest values of I_m and sex ratios above

TABLE 3.14

LABOR FORCE PARTICIPATION OF FEMALES, SEX RATIO, AND PROPORTION MARRIED (I_m), CITIES AND SUBURBS OF ANTWERP, BRUSSELS, AND GHENT: 1910

Suburb	City	Female workers as percentage of female pop. aged 15-55	Female workers in education, textiles, and domestic service as percentage of total female workers	Sex ratio, ages 20-30, of males to females	Proportion married (I_m)
Berchem	Antwerp	22	83	1.10	.564
Borgerhout	Antwerp	29	69	.98	.573
Gentbrugge	Ghent	35	77	1.02	.599
Hoboken	Antwerp	22	72	1.09	.646
Koekelberg	Brussels	36	71	.96	.616
Laken	Brussels	32	80	.96	.576
St. Jans-Molenbeek	Brussels	37	76	.96	.587
--	ANTWERP	35	71	.86	.486
--	BRUSSELS	56	74	.81	.426
Elsene	Brussels	44	86	.71	.429
--	GHENT	58	80	.86	.484
St. Gillis	Brussels	41	78	.74	.429
St. Joost-ten-Node	Brussels	45	77	.74	.406

unity, indicating a male surplus in the age group 20 to 30. I_m values at the other end of the scale were .412 for Bruges, .421 for Kortrijk, and .456 for St. Niklaas. The latter two towns had a labor force predominantly employed in the textile and clothing industry, and thus attracted many young women from the surrounding countryside. Other Flemish towns with very low I_m values in 1910 were Tielt (.430) and Eeklo (.448), small provincial places with some light industry. In all five towns characterized by low I_m values in 1910, the sex ratio in the age group 20 to 30 was below .90, showing an important surplus of women. When the number of observations was expanded to all 32 Flemish towns, a correlation coefficient of .756 was obtained between this sex ratio and I_m. Stated in a different way, 58 percent of the variance of I_m in Flemish urban areas outside of major cities was explained by the sex ratio. When the values of I_m in the surrounding rural parts of each arrondissement were used as a second set of predictors of the value of I_m in the urban units, the explained variance increased to 62 percent, which is hardly larger than the percentage explained by the factor "sex ratio" alone.[12] The value of I_m in the provincial Flemish towns was far

[12] The partial correlation between I_m in the urban units and the urban sex ratio in the age group 20 to 30 years, controlling for the value of I_m in the rural

more a result of sex differentials in employment, migration, and population composition than of the nuptiality patterns prevailing in the adjacent countryside.

Hence, in both Wallonia and Flanders there was largely a chain of associations between the following variables: economic function of the urban units, the occupational structure, sex differentials in migration, the sex ratio in the age group 20 to 30, and I_m. Consequently, an explanation based solely on the "proletarization theory" is inadequate and disregards some important variables involved in a more complex network of relationships.

3.13 *The Problem of Ecological Correlation*

In most of the analysis conducted so far, we have measured the degree of association between nuptiality and industrialization on the basis of indices calculated for aggregate populations of entire arrondissements or communities. In general, the label of "ecological measurement" is attached to statistical procedures that operate with characteristics of aggregate units rather than with characteristics of individual persons. The problem with ecological measurement is that the variance of the characteristics of the individuals constituting an aggregate unit is not taken into account.

In our analysis, for example, two arrondissements may have a similar value of I_m, but in the first it reflects the nuptiality pattern of the vast majority of the population, while in the second it is the average of individuals exhibiting either a much earlier or much later age at marriage. If this second arrondissement was split into two subunits, one consisting of those who marry early and the other of those who marry late, an entirely different picture would result. Hence, if the boundaries of arrondissements in Belgium were shifted around, different values of I_m could arise and the value of the correlation coefficients between I_m and other characteristics could increase or decrease.

Similarly, if heterogeneous arrondissements were broken down into more homogeneous communities, different values of the correlation coefficients might result. Furthermore, these coefficients might change again if heterogeneous communities were in turn broken down, and if measurements were performed on the basis of individuals. In this way,

area adjacent to each urban unit, was .702. The partial correlation between urban and rural I_m, controlling for the sex ratios of the urban units, was only .336 ($N = 32$).

the shift from measurement on an individual level to a level involving small aggregates, and the shift from small aggregates to larger ones may cause a substantial inflation of the values of the correlation coefficients.

Consequently, whenever relationships are measured on an ecological level one should be very careful about interpreting these in terms of individual behavior. The negative correlation between *EM* and the percentage of the male active population in agriculture observed in Table 3.12, for instance, does not ipso facto mean that farmers married late in life. It means that areas characterized by a late marriage pattern were those with large agricultural populations; but, it may well be that persons employed in sectors other than farming married equally late in life in those rural areas. Hence, ecological correlations should be checked against those compiled from data on an individual basis. In the early Belgian censuses, such information is scarce. Nevertheless, we were able to find a few tables that allowed us to control some of the relationships found between nuptiality and occupational structure.

First, the group of cottage workers, the core of the rural proletariat, definitely married much later than the regular industrial workers. The census of industries and professions of 1896 reported substantially higher percentages of single men among the cottage workers than among the industrial workers employed outside their homes. In the age group 21 to 29, 58.1 percent of the cottagers were single compared to 52.2 percent of the industrial workers. In the next age group, 30 to 49, these percentages were respectively 20.9 and 14.8. Definitive celibacy for cottagers was found to be 13.2 percent, but only 8.4 percent for the regular industrial workers.

Non-ecological information on the intensity of nuptiality could also be obtained for other groups of industries or occupations in the 1910 census. There, the age distribution by five-year intervals is given for each occupation or industrial branch, together with the total number of single persons. On the basis of this age distribution, weighted by the national schedule of proportions single by age group, an expected number of single men was obtained. The reported total number single divided by the expected number yielded a ratio that gives an idea of the relative frequency of celibacy. The resulting celibacy ratios are plotted in Figure 3.4. Public transportation shows the smallest proportion of single men relative to the national schedule. People in this category, along with those in the civil service, held municipal or government jobs, which were renowned for their job security and for more advanced

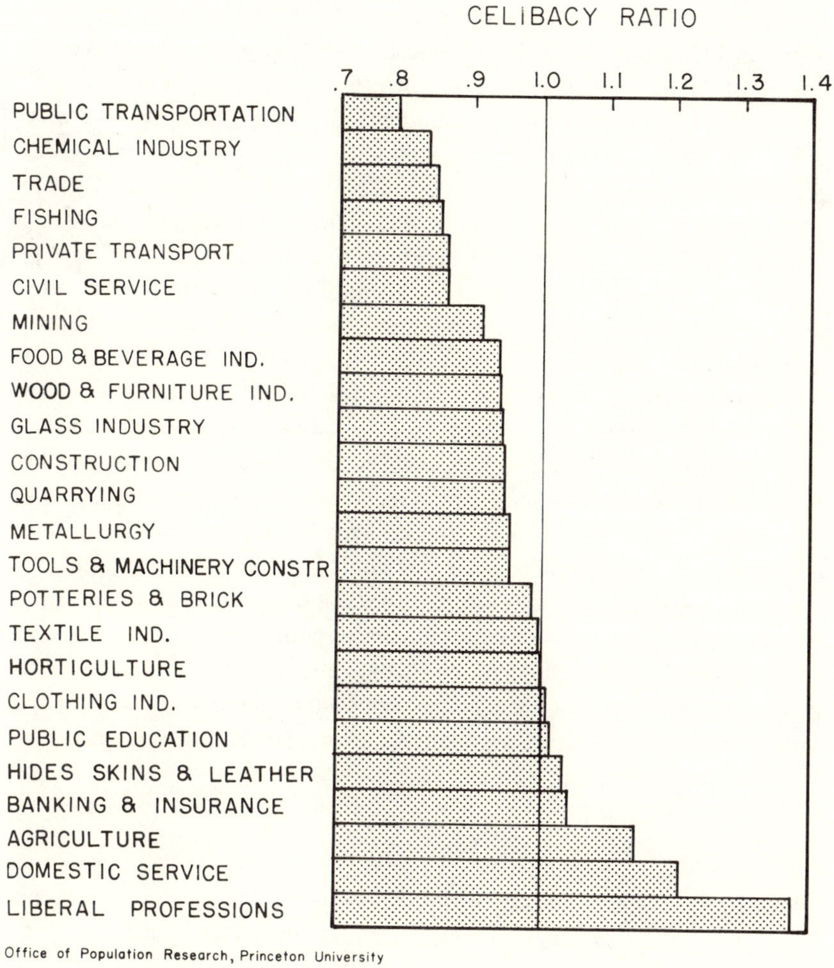

Figure 3.4 Celibacy (Males Not Married) Ratios, Selected Industries and Professions: 1910.

NOTE: See text for definition of ratio.

social and labor conditions.[13] Other occupations with low celibacy ratios are fishing, private transportation, chemical industries, and, more surprisingly, trade. This last category contained a large number of small-

[13] The vast majority of persons included under "public transportation" were employed by the national railroad system. As the railroads were a public enterprise, the railroad workers benefitted from equally favorable labor conditions as civil servants.

shopkeepers, who, in general, did not exhibit patterns of early marriage. Most probably, the low ratio for this group is the result of a negligible degree of definitive celibacy [14] and not of early marriage. Often, future shopkeepers did not engage independently in a new business at a very young age; they had to gather at least a part of the initial starting capital or await the inheritance or vacancy of a parental enterprise. By the same token, however, there was a deeply rooted belief that no shopkeeper could run his business efficiently without the assistance of his wife behind the counter. Consequently, the nature of this occupation may have led to this less-common combination of later but nearly universal marriage.

More intermediate celibacy ratios are found among industrial branches. Not surprisingly, those in lower-wage or more-artisanal industries (textiles, clothing, hides, skins, and leather industries) have higher ratios than those in better paid heavy industry (mining, quarrying, metallurgy, and chemical industries). Finally, the branches requiring a prolonged education (liberal professions, teaching, banking, and insurance), together with agriculture and domestic service, contain larger proportions of single men relative to the national schedule.

On the basis of the calculations of the celibacy ratios by industry or profession, we can also obtain a corresponding ecological measure by arrondissement. This measure, called C for each arrondissement j, is a weighted average and defined as

$$C_j = \frac{\Sigma P_{ij} r_i}{\Sigma P_{ij}}$$

where r_i, the original celibacy ratio of profession i, is weighted by P_{ij} or the number of persons in arrondissement j employed in profession i. If the regional variation in nuptiality were entirely the result of the regional variation in occupational structure, one would expect the ecological celibacy ratios C to be good correlates of—

1. the other previously introduced measures of occupational structure by arrondissement; and
2. the measures of nuptiality EM or I_m by arrondissement.

As can be seen in Table 3.15, this holds in practice to a large degree,

[14] The expected and reported numbers of single persons used in the calculation of the celibacy ratio contain the frequencies not only in the younger age groups, but also in all age groups above age 50. Consequently, the celibacy ratios reflect the size of definitive celibacy to a large degree.

TABLE 3.15

ECOLOGICAL CELIBACY RATIO (C), CORRELATION WITH PROPORTION WOMEN EVER-MARRIED AGED 20-24 (EM) AND TWO INDICES OF OCCUPATIONAL STRUCTURE, ARRONDISSEMENTS OF FLANDERS AND WALLONIA: 1910

Measure	Correlation with ecological celibacy ratio (C) Flanders (N=22)	Correlation with ecological celibacy ratio (C) Wallonia (N=19)
Percentage males in agriculture	+.863	+.977
Log. occupational structure	-.953	-.951
Proportion women ever-married aged 20-24 (EM)	-.755	-.727

which means that our conclusions from sections 3.10, 3.11, and 3.12 are justified and that the magnitude of the correlation coefficients reported in these sections is not inflated.

3.14 *Conclusions*

The clearest fact produced by this analysis is that the considerable but gradual change in nuptiality which took place in Belgium over a period of slightly more than a century cannot be explained by an mono-causal theory. In this view, Hofstee's "proletarization" phenomenon has an explanatory power that cannot be overlooked, but it remains largely inadequate and incomplete on more than one point.

Very generally speaking, it is true in Belgium that the nuptiality schedule of the wage-earning classes tended to depart earlier and more strongly from the Malthusian pattern prevailing before 1860, and that, as a result, a "proletarization" movement linked to increasing industrialization provoked the collapse of the "agrarian-artisanal" pattern. This generalization may be too sweeping, however, and overlooks important features.

First, Hofstee's departure point, the link between late and nonuniversal marriage and the dominance of the extended family household is questionable. In the seventeenth and early eighteenth centuries we do not find any value of average family size that, given the demographic conditions or mortality and fertility at that time, justifies the acceptance of this feature. In the countryside there must have existed a rather heterogeneous mixture of simple family households on a conjugal basis and more extended versions, but by no means a predominance of the latter type. In urban areas the prevalence of extended family households was probably very rare. There, simple family households and solitary units (single or widowed persons alone) must have formed a vast majority. A system where the urban areas attracted a substantial number of single persons, where the family structure was relatively modern, and where the mean age at marriage was occasionally able to go below the Malthusian level (either as a result of a mortality increase or as the consequence of a temporary growth of an industrial sector) seems to correspond better to the pretransitional Belgian scene than the picture presented by Hofstee in the "agrarian-artisanal" phase.

A second element that adds to the complexity of the matter is the marked heterogeneity of the wage-earning classes with respect to their nuptiality behavior. The Flemish rural proletariat in particular, made up primarily of female lace-makers and farm laborers of both sexes, did not follow the leading role of the typical industrial workers in the nuptiality change. The fact that many persons in the former group were employed part time in small-scale subsistence farming may be a possible explanation for their discordant behavior. At any rate, the term "proletarization" proves to be too general and overlooks this heterogeneity with respect to nuptiality.

A third feature concerns the impact of the type of industrialization on nuptiality in urban areas. Towns or suburbs specializing in sectors of the heavy industries attracted primarily men, single or married; there, the sex ratio shows an important deficit of women, and a large proportion of the female population is married. In provincial towns, suburbs with light industries, and central parts of metropolitan areas, a high inmigration of single women took place, responding to employment opportunities in the textile and clothing industry, domestic service, small trade, education, and other branches of the tertiary sector. Again, not only do we have to allow for large differentials within the group of wage earners with respect to nuptiality, but also for a heterogeneity within the types of industrialization and urban growth, leading to considerably diverging patterns of marital status and sex composition of the population.

Finally, even after the elimination of effects of differences in industrialization and occupational structure, strong regional residuals persist. The arrondissements in the province of Hainaut and in the southern part of the province of Namur developed a leading position in 1860 and kept it till 1960, whereas the provinces of East Flanders and Limburg remained behind throughout most of the entire period. This may indicate that a certain life style, with more favorable attitudes toward earlier marriage, came into existence in the western half of Wallonia and that the impact of it was felt for an entire century. In this way, several arrondissements (Thuin and Philippeville, for example) kept their advanced place in the nuptiality evolution, even when other areas reached considerably higher levels of industrialization or economic development and had a much faster expansion of the industrial working class.

So far we have treated the increase in nuptiality only in relation to social and economic development. The third research topic, linking nuptiality to marital fertility, has not been explored. There, we hypothesized that the transition in marriage patterns would be explained by increasing control of marital fertility. This additional analysis is performed in chapter 5, where the characteristics of the marital fertility decline are presented.

References—Chapter 3

Braun, R. 1972. Early industrialization and demographic change in the canton of Zurich (Switzerland) in comparison with English and German cases. In *Seminar on Early Industrialization, Fertility and Family Structure* pp. 1-34. Princeton: Institute for Advanced Study.

Burch, T. K. 1972. Some demographic determinants of average household size: an analytic approach. In *Household and family in past time,* ed. P. Laslett, pp. 91-102. Cambridge, England: University Printing House.

Coale, A. J. 1965a. Estimates of average size of household. In *Aspects of the analysis of family structure,* ed. A. J. Coale et al, pp. 64-69. Princeton: Princeton University Press.

———. 1965b. Factors associated with the development of low fertility: an historic summary. In *World Population Conference,* vol. 2, p. 207. New York: United Nations.

de Brouwer, J. 1968. *Demografische evolutie van het Land van Aalst.* Brussels: Pro Civitate, Historische Uitgaven.

Deprez, P. 1965. The demographic development of Flanders in the eighteenth century. In *Population in history,* eds. D. V. Glass and D. E. C. Eversley, pp. 608-630. Chicago and London: Aldine Publishing Co.

de Vooys, A. C. 1964. De regionale verscheidenheid in de geboorte-frekwentie in de tweede helft der 19e eeuw. *Tijdschrift van het Koninklijk Nederlandsch Aardrijkskundig Genootschap* 81:220-232.

Duchène, J., and Lesthaeghe, R. 1975. Essai de reconstitution de la population belge sous le régime francais: quelques chatactéristiques démographiques de la population féminine. *Population et Famille* (Brussels).

Dupâquier, J. 1972. De l'animal à l'homme; le mécanisme auto-régulateur des populations traditionnelles. *Revue de l'Institut de Sociologie* (Université Libre de Bruxelles) 2:177-211.

Habakkuk, H. J. 1955. Family structure and economic change in nineteenth-century Europe. *Journal of Economic History* 15:1-12.

Hajnal, H. 1965. European marriage patterns in perspective. In *Population in history,* eds. D. V. Glass and D. E. C. Eversley, pp. 101-143. Chicago and London: Aldine Publishing Co.

Hélin, E. 1972. Size of household before the industrial revolution: the case of Liège in 1801. In *Household and family in past time,* ed. P. Laslett, pp. 299-318. Cambridge, England: University Printing House.

Hofstee, E. W. 1954. Regionale verscheidenheid in de ontwikkeling van het aantal geboorten in Nederland in de tweede helft der 19e eeuw. *Akademiedagen Koninklijke Nederlandse Akademie van Wetenschappen.*

———. 1962. De groei der Nederlandse bevolking. *Drift en Koers,* pp. 16-64.

———. 1972. Enkele opmerkingen over de ontwikkeling van de huwelijks-vruchtbaarheid in Nederland. *Mens en Maatschappij* ("Onderzocht en Overdacht") pp. 43-91.

Knodel, J. 1967. Law, marriage, and illegitimacy in nineteenth century Germany. *Population Studies.* 20:279-294.

———. 1974. *The decline of fertility in Germany, 1871–1939.* Princeton: Princeton University Press.

Laslett, P. 1972. Introduction. In *Household and family in past time,* ed. P. Laslett. Cambridge, England: University Printing House.

Mendels, F. 1970. Industry and marriage in Flanders before the industrial revolution. In *Population and economics,* ed. P. Deprez (Proceedings of section v of the Fourth Congress of the International Economic History Association) pp. 81-89. Winnipeg: University of Manitoba Press.

Plumard de Danguel, N. 1754. *Remarques sur les avantages et les désavantages de la France et de la Grande Bretagne.* Leiden.

Quételet, A., and Smits, E. 1832. *Recherches sur la reproduction et la mortalité de l'homme.* Brussels.

Slicher van Bath, B. 1968. Historical demography and the social and economic Development of the Netherlands. *Daedalus* 97:604-621.

Spengler, J. J. 1942. *French predecessors of Malthus—a study in eighteenth century wage and population theory.* Durham, N. C.: Duke University Press.

van de Walle, E. 1965. La nuptialité en Belgique de 1846 à 1930 et sa relation avec la déclin de la fécondité. *Population et Famille—Bevolking en Gezin* (Brussels) 6-7:37-56.

———. 1974. *The female population of France in the nineteenth century.* Princeton: Princeton University Press.

van der Woude, A. M. 1972. Variations in the size and structure of the household in the United Provinces of the Netherlands in the seventeenth and eighteenth centuries. In *Household and family in past time,* ed. P. Laslett, pp. 299-318. Cambridge, England: University Printing House.

van Laere, G. 1961. De demografische evolutie in Assenede, Bassevelde, Boekhoute, Ertvelde, Oost-Eeklo en Watervliet gedurende de 18e en 19e eeuw. In *Handelingen der maatschappij voor geschiedenis en oudheidkunde te Gent,* p. 54.

Wattelar, C., and Wunsch, G. 1967. *Etude démographique de la nuptialité en Belgique.* Louvain: Université Catholique de Louvain.

Wrigley, E. A. 1969. *Population and history.* New York: McGraw-Hill Book Co.

CHAPTER 4: The Transition of Marital, Illegitimate, and General Fertility

Changes in marriage patterns were by no means the only demographic transformation occurring in the second half of the nineteenth century. Shortly after 1850, we find the first indications that couples were beginning to control their fertility within marriage.

This evolution will be studied in this chapter. We will examine marital fertility characteristics when fertility control is not a widespread phenomenon. This leads us to the concept of "natural fertility" and to the extent and nature of contraceptive practice in the eighteenth and nineteenth centuries. Then, a short comparison of the marital fertility transition in Belgium and its neighboring countries will follow. Next, we shall turn our attention to the regional pattern of the decline in Belgium. Since the transition of fertility within wedlock was accompanied by a similar decline in fertility outside wedlock, we shall seize the opportunity to have a closer look at the regional variation in the decline of illegitimate fertility. Finally, taking advantage of the relation between the three indices, I_g, I_m, and I_h (defined in the previous chapter), the evolution of general fertility (I_f) will be followed over a period of slightly more than a century.

4.1 *Natural Fertility and the Index of Marital Fertility* (I_g)

When demographers refer to a situation in which marital fertility is not controlled directly through any conscious method of contraception, they adopt the term "natural" or "uncontrolled fertility." This concept of natural fertility has been defined by L. Henry (1961, p. 81). According to this definition, natural fertility does not refer solely to the physiological level of fertility. It also includes the indirect effect of those social factors that may reduce fertility to a large degree, but which cannot be considered as a form of direct and *conscious* action aimed specifically at preventing births.

Hence, the level of natural fertility is influenced by a series of biological and social factors. We should mention among these factors the incidence of sterility. In strictly biological terms, this factor is mainly a function of age. Adolescent sterility is quite common in the first months or years following menarche. The incidence of female sterility reaches a minimum around age 20 (2 to 3 percent) and then increases gradually to complete sterility at menopause. The level of sterility may vary considerably, however, from society to society, as a function of the incidence of venereal diseases, infections, and poor health conditions in general. In this context, social factors can be important. For example, in some African societies (Southern Sudan, and Uele province in Zaire), unstable marriage patterns have contributed to the spread of venereal diseases among some ethnic groups; these diseases, in their turn, lower the level of natural fertility substantially (A. Romaniuk, 1967, pp. 297-322; A. Retel-Laurentin, 1967, p. 841).

A second factor influencing natural fertility levels is the frequency of intercourse, which also varies from population to population. In this context, it is often observed that women living in a polygamous union have lower fertility (in the absence of any form of contraception) than women living in a monogamous union. One possible explanation for this is that women in polygamous unions probably have, on the average, less-frequent sexual relations.[1] Abstinence, too, falls within this framework, provided that it is practiced for reasons other than that of deliberately controlling the number of offspring. Here, we have the example of seasonal migrants in nineteenth-century Europe, who left their wives and families behind for a substantial period of time each year. Flemish farmhands left early in May and returned home from France only after they had finished the sugar-beet harvest in November. Except possibly for an occasional extramarital excursion, their wives were unexposed to the risk of conception for a period of six months. When such seasonal migrations affected the majority of the population, as was the case in the Swiss canton of Ticino, the level of natural fertility was automatically lowered.

Yet a third factor affecting the level of uncontrolled fertility is the duration of lactation and the existence of sexual taboos related to lactation. Prolonged lactation leads, not necessarily individually but in the aggregate, to a longer postpartum sterile period, and hence, other things being equal, to lower levels of natural fertility (E. van de Walle and J. Knodel, 1967, pp. 109-131; A. Jain et al., 1970, p. 255; H. Léridon, 1973, pp. 81-90). The impact of lactation on the fertility level is even further increased when certain taboos, such as those existing in many African societies, prohibit intercourse during the period of breastfeeding. It should be understood, however, that one stops using the notion of

[1] A more plausible explanation for the lower fertility of polygamous unions can be offered by pointing out that older and less-fecund women are considerably overrepresented in such unions.

natural fertility when lactation is prolonged specifically to reduce the chance of a conception, i.e., when this act is inspired by the couple's judgment that the desired number of children has been reached, either definitely or temporarily.

In addition to sterility, coital frequency, lactation, and postpartum sterility, many other factors affect natural fertility. There is the effect of fetal wastage and intrauterine mortality, the possibility that not all cycles may be equally fertile, and that not all sexual behavior necessarily results in coitus.

On the basis of the above, one can expect that natural fertility will result in very different fertility levels under different biological and social conditions. If we were to base the calculation of I_g on the theoretical combination of different incidences of sterility, various frequency distributions of intercourse, alternative magnitudes of fetal wastage, and different lengths of postpartum sterility, as done by J. Bourgeois-Pichat (1965, p. 383), then we would obtain values of I_g ranging between 1.928 and .670. This means that, assuming that the various fertility-maximizing conditions are not mutually incompatible, strictly biologically conditioned fertility could be almost twice as high as the fertility found among the Hutterites (who have the highest marital fertility on record).

Looking at the other side of Bourgeois-Pichat's results, we find that a value of I_g equal to .670 still falls within the range of natural fertility. In real populations not practicing conscious and manifest forms of birth control, I_g values as low as .620 have been recorded (marriages of 1946–1947 in selected Hindu villages of Bengal). If data were available, the value of I_g in Uele (Zaire) and among the Azande people in central Africa would probably be much lower still, despite the fact that contraception is virtually unknown in these communities.

From this evidence, it is clear that the notion of natural fertility covers a wide range of possible overall fertility levels. Hence, we have no yardstick for the level of marital fertility from which we could infer directly whether or not fertility is natural or controlled. The only way demographers can unequivocally confirm the presence of voluntary control is by inspecting the shape (and not the general level) of marital fertility, specific by age, marriage duration, or parity. Control generally appears first among couples who have reached a desired number of offspring (either temporarily or definitively). Consequently, with fertility control, the fertility of women with longer marriage durations and higher parities ceases to be in line with the uncontrolled fertility of women of the same ages. For our study, detailed data of this kind are virtually nonexistent, and we have to rely on the aggregate level of fertility rather than on the distribution of the marital fertility function. Hence, we are forced to make an arbitrary decision: in the following sections we assume that any value of I_g larger than .700 indicates uncontrolled fertility. Also, absence of a trend is indicative of no control.

4.2 *Contraceptive Practice before 1850*

Though the distribution of marital fertility by age, marriage duration, or parity has a form typical for natural fertility, this does not ipso facto mean that couples did not try to limit their childbearing. One can find the demographic appearance of natural fertility in two situations. In the first, one is indeed dealing with a situation in which no effort is made to control family size. In the second, contraception is practiced, but in such an ineffective way as to have no significant consequences demographically.

There are several elements indicating that reality was somewhere between these alternatives before the present century. A vast literature is available concerning contraceptive practice before 1900, and although the bulk of it is made up of interesting but statistically inconclusive anecdotes, it gives the impression that efforts to limit fertility are as old as human culture itself.

Let us group the types of contraceptive techniques known before the twentieth century. The first category is made up of mechanical devices. An abundant literature, either medical, ethical, or erotic in nature, mentions the use of sheaths, condoms, sponges, and primitive cervical caps. All these methods had a certain effectiveness, but they were probably not widespread. Indeed, one has the impression that each of their advocates had to reinvent his or her own particular type of sponge or condom. The same holds true for douching. There are almost as many recipes for concocting douching liquid as there are mentions of the method.

The second category is made up of folk beliefs. These were probably far more widespread than mechanical devices, but in most instances nearly always totally ineffective. Some of them were strictly ritualistic and bore more relation to witchcraft than to contraception. Others, equally bizarre, were savage and dangerous in addition. Among the non-ritualistic folk beliefs, a large place is occupied by potions and plant or mineral extractions that were believed to have some contraceptive or abortive power. Many of them were taken orally after intercourse, so that their effectiveness was negligible indeed. Those that were not taken orally were generally aimed at provoking abortion or miscarriage, but then the increased effectiveness was dearly paid for by a high risk of infection, impairment, or death.

From this discussion, it seems reasonable to conclude that the most widespread forms of contraception were those with little or no effectiveness, and that the better methods were either too dangerous or insufficiently known to have any effect on the fertility level of an entire population (see N. E. Himes 1936, p. 184).

There is, however, another method, which can be invented in principle by any couple and in any society: coitus interruptus. Physiologically speaking, it is not harmful, and theoretically it could be practiced by large segments of the population. Despite the fact that the method is not a sure means of preventing conception on an individual level, it is a powerful means of reducing fertility in the aggregate. Hence, coitus interruptus cannot be treated in the same way as the other premodern forms of contraception, since it is neither ineffective nor unknown.

Outside Europe, coitus interruptus seems to have been relatively popular in the Islamic world, and no religious or ethical condemnation of the method was raised. In Western Europe, however, the "crime of Onan" or "conjugal Onanism" [2] was condemned by Catholic and Protestant authorities alike. As early as 1557, Calvin gave a very clear description of what was understood by coitus interruptus and labeled it an "act of monstrosity." [3] Despite the condemnation, certain theologians of great influence started amending the church's official teaching on it. The first was Sanchez; in 1614, in Antwerp, he published the thesis that impregnation of a women during extramarital relations was an additional sin committed by the man, over and above the sin of adultery. Hence, retreat before ejaculation should not be condemned, at least not in adulterous relations. His followers in the "Probabilist School" went

[2] Outside ecclesiastic literature, onanism is synonymous with masturbation. In the ecclesiastic texts, however, masturbation is referred to as "polution," whereas onanism generally stands for coitus interruptus. At the end of the nineteenth century the term "onanism" denoted more and more the use of contraception in general (see J. Stengers, 1971, p. 423, note).

[3] Calvin's original description in French is as follows: "Et de se retirer tout exprès de la femme afin que la semance tombe en terre, c'est un double monstre car c'est estreindre l'espérance du lignage, et meurtrir l'enfant qu'on esperoit avoir avant qu'il soy nay" (J. Calvin, *Commentaire sur le premier livre de Moyse, dit Genèse,* Geneva, 1554, p. 418; quoted by J. Stengers, 1971, p. 427).

even further and advocated that, "in "copula fornicaria," the male partner had an actual moral obligation to retreat "ante seminationem" (J. Stengers, 1971, p. 407).

A second breach in the classic teaching was made by Alphonso de Liguori (1696–1787), who defended the idea that the confessor had no right to interrogate confessants on sins committed during the conjugal act. Later, the notion that coitus interruptus constituted a sin on the part of both partners was challenged; in 1827, Monseignor Bouvier, bishop of Le Mans, claimed that no woman could be blamed if her husband committed the "crime of Onan."

Not only in theological writings, but also in everyday experience, the clergy were exposed to the question of whether or not coitus interruptus was a sin. This is clear from the repeated questions directed at their superiors by French clergymen. No clear directions were forthcoming, however, and the local parish priests remained badly in need of practical guidelines along which they could pattern their attitude toward confessants. In this climate, there emerged in French theological writings and practice an outlook that we call "laxist." Monseignor Bouvier fully accepted, for example, that "conjugal Onanism" could be practiced in good faith, i.e., not knowing that it was a sin. The local priests were advised not to preach on the matter nor to scare the faithful away (their number was probably rapidly diminishing in early nineteenth century France) by interrogations on these subjects in the confessional. At this time—the first half of the nineteenth century—a substantial proportion of the French population must have practiced coitus interruptus. This is evident not only from the concern of the clergy, but also from demographic data. By 1830, I_g in Normandy and the area around Bordeaux had dropped to levels that, beyond any doubt, no longer corresponded to uncontrolled fertility.

In Belgium marital fertility levels remained stable and high up to 1860. In Table 4.1 we have gathered various measurements of I_g prior to that date. The figures of 1846 and 1856 come directly from census and vital registration data and are fully reliable (see the reliability test in the Appendix). For other dates prior to 1860 we have little information. The only age-specific marital fertility schedule available is that for the Brabant village of Walem from 1715 to 1755 (G. Tack, 1973, p. 68). As can be expected, the schedule shows no traces of fertility control. Levels of I_g calculated from a reconstitution of the East Flanders rural population, 1750–1800, were approximately .828 (R.

TABLE 4.1

MARITAL FERTILITY (I_g), SELECTED AREAS: 1715-1755 TO 1856

Area	1715-1755	1750-1800	1802-1809	1846	1856
Village of Walem	.943	--	--	--	--
Rural East Flanders	--	.828	--	.824	--
Département/Province:					
Deux-Nèthes/Antwerp	--	--	.744	.786	.799
Dyle/Brabant	--	--	.787	.737	.765
Escaut/East Flanders	--	--	.836	.793	.923
Lys/West Flanders	--	--	.892	.810	.897
Jemmape/Hainaut	--	--	.829	.717	.722
Ourthe/Liège	--	--	.798	.765	.790
Meuse Inférieure/ Limburg	--	--	--	.773	.839
Forêts/Luxemburg	--	--	.854	.774	.768
Sambre et Meuse/Namur	--	--	.756	.743	.745
Belgium	--	--	--	.757	.827

NOTES: For 1846 and 1856 the values of I_g are calculated on the average number of births during the five-year period centered around the census at each date.

Under Département/Province, the first name is that of the département during the Napoleonic period; the second name refers to the post-independence division of the territory into provinces. The later provinces overlap substantially with the French départements, but it should be noted that the département Deux-Nèthes included the Dutch province of Noordbrabant, that Escaut included the islands of the Dutch province of Zeeland, and that Forêts covered the Grand Duchy of Luxemburg together with a small section of German territory as well.

Lesthaeghe, 1974, p. 4). Finally, figures are available for the Napoleonic period on the basis of a reconstitution of the population of eight of the nine Belgian departments (J. Duchène and R. Lesthaeghe, 1975). In all cases I_g is well above the .700 level, and we have to acknowledge that contraception was either not widespread or was largely ineffective. We cannot rule out that coitus interruptus might have been known, but it is likely, judging from the levels of marital fertility, that it was not in general use in Belgium prior to 1860.

4.3 *The Decline of Marital Fertility in Belgium and Adjacent Countries*

There is no sign of a significant fertility decline in Belgium in the first half of the nineteenth century. We may assume that marital fertility was very near natural fertility and that it probably fluctuated between .700 and .950. The same could also be said of two neighboring countries, Germany and the Netherlands. In 1865 every province of the

Netherlands and nearly all the administrative units in Germany (with the exception of Lüneburg and Berlin) had a value of I_g greater than .700. Levels above .800 were observed in parts of all three countries up until World War I (see Table 4.2). In France, the situation was

TABLE 4.2

MARITAL FERTILITY (I_g), NATIONAL LEVELS AND ADMINISTRATIVE UNIT EXTREME LEVELS, BELGIUM, FRANCE, GERMANY, AND THE NETHERLANDS: 1840 TO 1910

Approx. date.	National levels				Highest levels				Lowest levels			
	Belg.	Fr.	Ger.	Neth.	Belg.	Fr.	Ger.	Neth.	Bel.	Fr.	Ger.	Neth.
1840	--	.579	--	--	--	.760	--	--	--	.313	--	--
1845	.757	.531	--	--	.810	.727	--	--	.717	.315	--	--
1850	--	.503	--	--	--	.686	--	--	--	.298	--	--
1855	.827	.481	--	--	.923	.691	--	--	.722	.290	--	--
1860	--	.490	--	.816	--	.727	--	.892	--	.282	--	.717
1865	.830	.480	.760	--	.939	.767	.948	--	.700	.279	.567	--
1870	--	--	.776	.845	--	.811	.942	.931	--	.280	.573	.771
1875	--	.455	.783	--	--	.838	--	--	--	.271	--	--
1880	.751	.460	.735	.831	.921	.819	.915	.941	.577	.266	.554	.703
1885	--	--	.726	--	--	.784	.917	--	--	.246	.535	--
1890	.678	.414	.706	.808	.872	.774	.918	.954	.478	.232	.494	.685
1895	--	.395	--	--	--	.744	.913	--	--	.230	.448	--
1900	.596	.372	.659	.752	.877	.718	.912	.968	.394	.230	.394	.633
1905	--	--	--	--	--	--	.870	--	--	--	.356	--
1910	.443	.314	.542	.652	.822	--	.834	.900	.298	--	.303	.524

SOURCES: France: E. van de Walle, 1974; Germany: J. Knodel, 1974; The Netherlands: E. van de Walle, unpublished.

NOTES: To facilitate comparison, only administrative units of comparable population size were used; these included 9 provinces in Belgium, 86 départements in France, 55 to 71 administrative areas in Germany, and 11 provinces in The Netherlands.

Areas which recorded the highest levels were the Belgian provinces of East Flanders, West Flanders, and Limburg, the French départements of Côtes-du-Nord and Finistère, the German administrative areas of Lüneburg and Berlin, and the Dutch provinces of Noordbrabant and Limburg.

Areas which recorded the lowest levels were the Belgian province of Hainaut, the French département of Lot-et-Garonne, the German administrative areas of Schwaben, Aachen, Niederbayern, and Münster, and the Dutch provinces of Friesland, Drente, and Noord-Holland.

very different. As early as 1840, several départements had values of I_g below .400, and by 1850 it was already clear which areas would lag behind. By the turn of the century, only two départements in Brittany had values above the .700 level, while for the remainder of France the chapter on the fertility decline was closed. On the whole, France proved to be some 60 years ahead of Belgium and Germany and some 70 years ahead of the Netherlands.

Within Belgium, as shown in Table 4.3, there were large additional regional differences with respect to the pattern of the marital fertility decline. In 1846, the nine provinces had roughly the same level of I_g. In the Flemish provinces, however, the values of I_g at that time were reduced to a rather abnormally low level as a consequence of the serious economic depression. By 1856, the variation in the provincial levels was increasing, not because the fertility decline had started, but mainly because some Flemish areas were restoring their I_g values to levels that

TABLE 4.3

MARITAL FERTILITY (I_g), BY PROVINCE: 1846 TO 1970

Date	Antwerp	Brabant	East Flanders	West Flanders	Hainaut	Liège	Limburg	Luxemburg	Namur
1846	.786	.737	.793	.810	.717	.765	.773	.774	.743
1856	.799	.765	.923	.897	.722	.790	.839	.768	.745
1866	.861	.784	.930	.939	.700	.791	.863	.782	.731
1880	.837	.710	.921	.918	.577	.704	.881	.733	.618
1890	.761	.626	.849	.878	.478	.598	.872	.669	.536
1900	.661	.517	.780	.838	.394	.490	.877	.625	.469
1910	.508	.365	.594	.671	.298	.333	.822	.527	.364
1920	.403	.302	.467	.518	.277	.293	.722	.462	.350
1930	.313	.226	.344	.394	.212	.232	.592	.381	.280
1947	.308	.242	.345	.367	.270	.275	.508	.373	.325
1961	.308	.250	.303	.316	.262	.252	.416	.338	.306
1970	.242	.224	.257	.260	.259	.239	.287	.302	.271

NOTES: The values for 1920 are calculated on the average number of live births for four years only (1919, 1920, 1921, and 1922) rather than for five years centered around the census. Because of World War I, the number of live births for 1918 is unknown. The values for 1970 are based on the average number of live births for 1969 and 1970 only.
Underlined values of I_g represent initial 10% decrease below the preceding value.

were probably more typical for the period before the economic crisis of the 1840s. This increased variation in I_g levels is documented in Table 4.3. In 1846, the values varied between .717 and .810, which defines a range of only .093, whereas in 1856, after the depression, the values ranged between .722 and .923, which gives a difference of .201. After 1856, this range widens even more, but this is partly because of the start of the marital fertility decline. The first traces of it can be found in the province of Hainaut and in the Entre Sambre et Meuse region (the southern part of the province of Namur). The slight decrease in I_g recorded between 1856 and 1866 in that area of the country proved to be the start of a genuine fertility transition. In the other provinces, however, I_g either remained on the same level (Liège and Luxemburg) or continued its increase until it reached a maximum between 1866 and 1880 (provinces of Brabant, Antwerp, West Flanders, East Flanders, and Limburg). This is illustrated in Figure 4.1. In all the Flemish areas, the industrialization movement in the second half of the nineteenth century was associated with an important upward trend in marital fertility. This brought I_g into the immediate vicinity of Hutterite fertility (although combined with rather heavy restrictions on nuptiality in East and West Flanders). The reasons for this increase are not clear, but an element that may have acted in the direction of an increase is the relinquishment of lactation by the large number of mothers employed outside their homes.

Between 1880 and 1910, a marital fertility decline took place in all

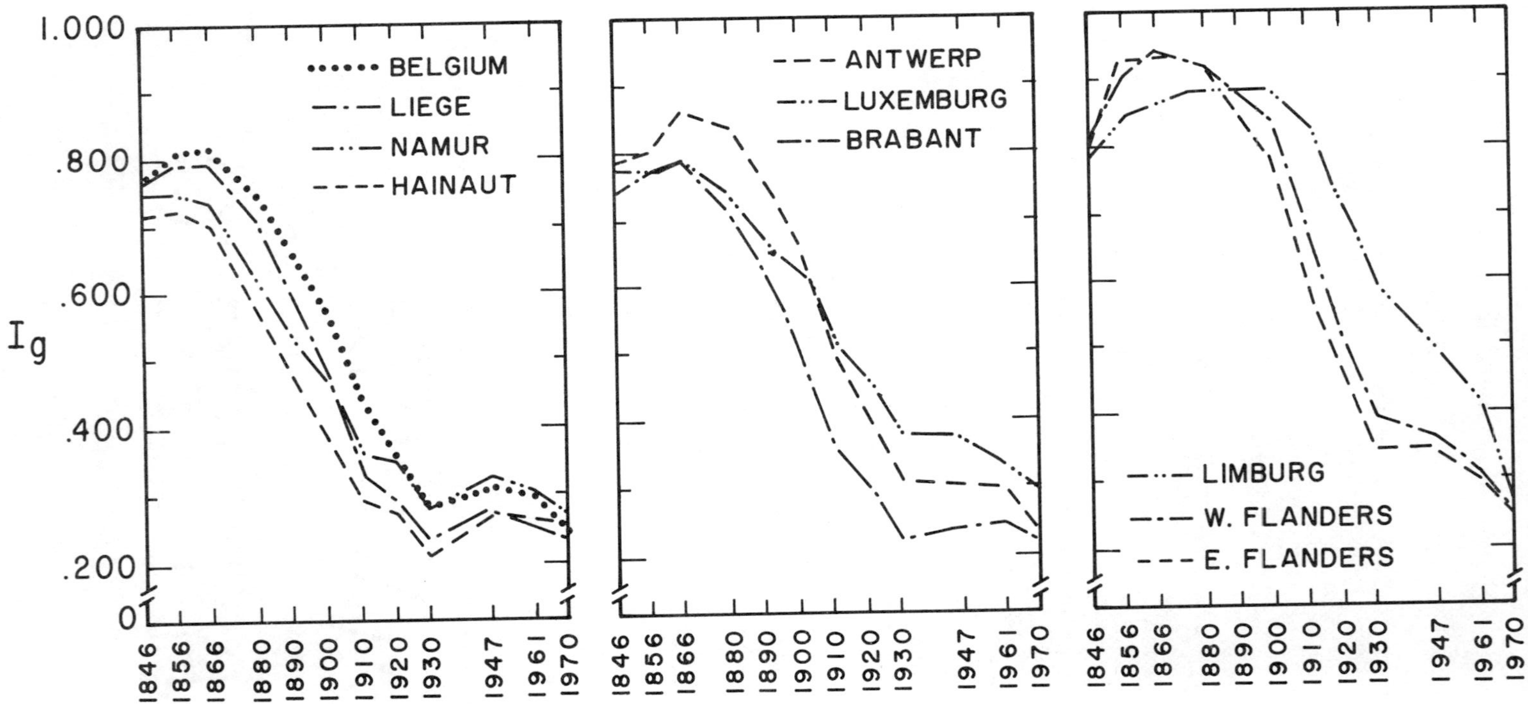

Office of Population Research, Princeton University

Figure 4.1 Marital Fertility (I_g), by Province: 1846 to 1970.

areas with the exception of Limburg. In 1910, the province of Hainaut had an I_g value of only .298 compared with .700 in 1880; its fertility transition took place 20 years before the national level came down below the .300 mark. Hainaut was followed by the province of Namur and slightly later by another Walloon province, Liège. It is worth noting that Hainaut and Liège were the most industrialized areas of Belgium; but Namur, which ranked second in the transition until 1900, was by no means an industrial leader. Apart from a small industrialized section in the upper Sambre valley, the province of Namur was predominantly rural, and it had even lost its few charcoal-operated blast furnaces during the first half of the nineteenth century.

The next three provinces to complete the fertility transition differed markedly from each other. Luxemburg was, in essence, one of the two most rural provinces of Belgium (the other being Limburg), but it had already started its fertility decline around 1866. However, halfway through the decline it was overtaken by the leading completely Flemish province of Antwerp (see Figure 4.1). The province of Brabant, which also belongs to this intermediate group, had a substantial French-speaking population in the arrondissement of Nivelles and in the capital, Brussels. (The French-speaking population accounts partly for the relatively advanced position of Brabant.)

The group of provinces that had a late decline consists exclusively of Flemish areas: East and West Flanders, and Limburg. In the former two provinces, I_g started declining slowly after 1880; but it was not until between 1900 and 1910 that the decline gained momentum. In Limburg, I_g stayed well above .800 until 1910, and its transition started only after World War I. Even after 1920, Limburg was characterized by a slow transition that contrasted strongly with the experience of the rest of Belgium. In 1961, for instance, its I_g was still higher than .400, above the level of Hainaut in 1900. Even compared with the other Flemish provinces, Limburg lagged behind considerably. In West Flanders, which ranks next to last with respect to the marital fertility decline, I_g had dropped below the .400 mark in 1930, so that Limburg was still 30 years behind even its nearest predecessor. These considerable time lags and differences occur on an extremely small geographical scale: the heart of Limburg is only 70 miles from the heart of Hainaut. Purely physical distances do not seem to have played a very significant role in Belgium's demographic history.

Beginning in 1880, it is possible to study the fertility decline by arrondissement, which gives us a clearer geographical view, as well as by province. Maps 4.1 through 4.4 show the regional pattern of the drop in I_g by arrondissement. In addition, the large urban areas of Antwerp, Brussels, Ghent, and Liège have been represented separately on each map, so as not to confuse the situation in these urban centers with the characteristics of the adjacent areas. The data on which the maps are based are presented in Table 4.4.

In Map 4.1, one can readily see that in 1880 only the arrondissement of Philippeville (Namur province) had a value of I_g below .500. Prior

TABLE 4.4

MARITAL FERTILITY (I_g), BY ARRONDISSEMENT: 1880 TO 1910

	1880	1890	1900	1910
Flanders				
Aalst	.898	.854	.834	.661
Antwerp	.810	.713	.584	.418
Bruges	.899	.870	.839	.680
Brussels	.673	.570	.470	.318
Dendermonde	1.052	.950	.903	.712
Diksmuide	.967	.886	.844	.705
Eeklo	.945	.875	.821	.629
Ghent	.845	.764	.651	.466
Hasselt	.868	.818	.865	.791
Kortrijk	.894	.853	.812	.618
Leuven	.849	.806	.791	.610
Maaseik	.930	.937	.950	.953
Mechelen	.863	.812	.743	.597
Ostend	.899	.905	.800	.651
Oudenaarde	.911	.880	.863	.658
Roeselare	.987	.949	.945	.743
St. Niklaas	1.030	.971	.902	.708
Tielt	.942	.903	.938	.797
Tongeren	.872	.850	.845	.788
Turnhout	.897	.899	.908	.823
Veurne	.921	.821	.752	.595
Ypres	.903	.852	.795	.659
Wallonia				
Arlon	.730	.650	.582	.496
Ath	.554	.480	.408	.315
Bastogne	.854	.804	.756	.651
Charleroi	.596	.478	.390	.277
Dinant	.663	.573	.511	.423
Huy	.687	.581	.491	.358
Liège	.688	.577	.470	.299
Marche	.751	.702	.643	.523
Mons	.526	.472	.382	.306
Namur	.646	.571	.485	.356
Neufchâteau	.719	.672	.623	.524
Nivelles	.707	.686	.486	.359
Philippeville	.488	.393	.365	.318
Soignies	.612	.489	.390	.310
Thuin	.539	.405	.347	.283
Tournai	.637	.556	.479	.351
Verviers	.716	.620	.500	.382
Virton	.643	.548	.541	.457
Waremme	.805	.722	.637	.464

SOURCE: Vital registration statistics and population censuses, Institut National de Statistiques - Nationaal Instituut voor de Statistiek, Brussels.

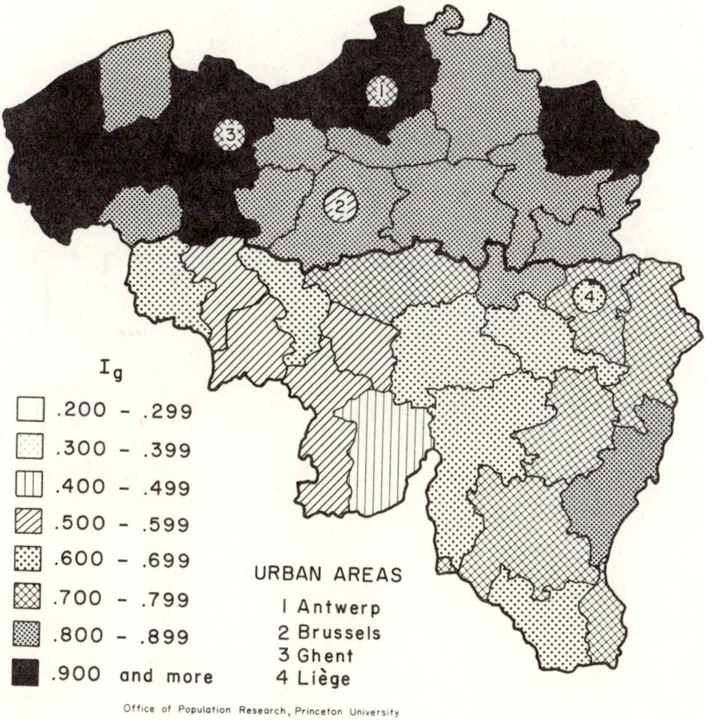

Map 4.1 Marital Fertility (I_g), by Arrondissement and Four Urban Areas: 1880.

to 1850, this arrondissement had contained some metallurgical industry, but it had become exclusively rural after 1850. Hence, the first experience of a drastic marital fertility reduction is to be found in the midst of fields and forests. By 1890 (Map 4.2), this spot of low fertility had extended and included not only the heavily industrialized arrondissements of Charleroi and Mons, but also the semi-industrialized arrondissements of Soignies and Thuin and the predominantly rural arrondissement of Ath. All these arrondissements are located in the southern part of Belgium. Outside that area, only the few communities that made up the Brussels urban district had fallen below the .500 level by 1890. By 1900, the decline had spread to Tournai, and to three other slightly industrialized Walloon arrondissements: Nivelles, Namur, and Huy. The urban area of Liège also had an I_g level below the .500 mark, but the eastern half of Wallonia, and especially the more industrialized arrondissements of Verviers and the remainder of Liège,

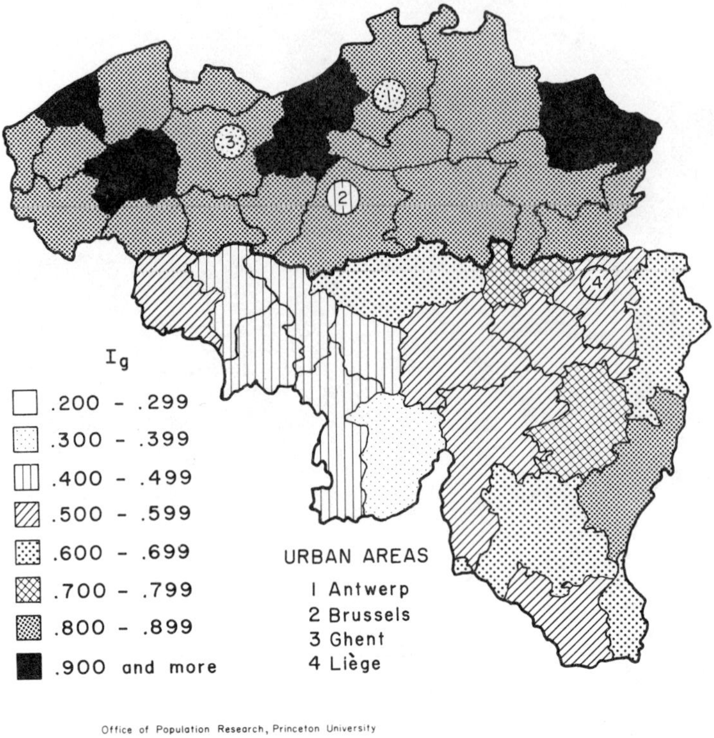

Map 4.2 Marital Fertility (I_g), by Arrondissement and Four Urban Areas: 1890.

were still above that level (Map 4.3). By 1910 (see Map 4.4), only the three Walloon arrondissements in the heart of the Ardennes (Bastogne, Marche, and Neufchâteau) were still above .500; during World War I, marital fertility finally dropped below that level.

In Flanders, the maps show predominantly dark shadings, corresponding to very high marital fertility, until 1900. Before that date, the marital fertility decline appeared only in the larger urban areas of Antwerp and Ghent. Outside these urban nuclei, the fertility transition first developed in the nonurban part of the arrondissement of Brussels, in the arrondissements of Mechelen, Louvain, and, more curiously, in two strictly rural areas of West Flanders: the arrondissements of Veurne and Ypres. Pockets of very high marital fertility were formed by the arrondissements of Tielt and Roeselare (West Flanders), Sint Niklaas and Dendermonde (East Flanders), Turnhout (Antwerp), and Maaseik, Hasselt, and Tongeren (the three arrondissements of Limburg). In the East Flanders

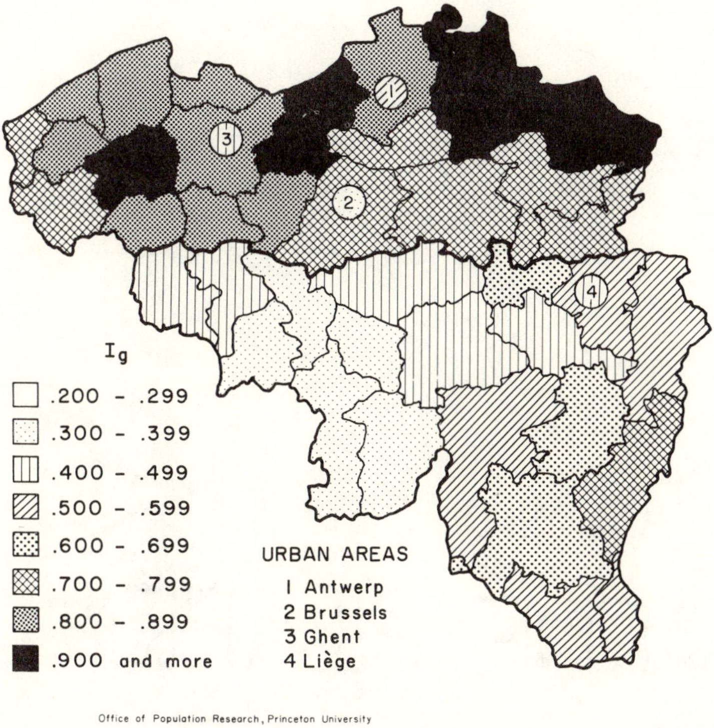

Map 4.3 Marital Fertility (I_g), by Arrondissement and Four Urban Areas: 1900.

pocket, I_g reached unity (the level of Hutterite marital fertility) in 1880. Both the East and West Flanders pockets of high fertility disappeared quickly after 1900, but, as shown in Figure 4.1, the Limburg pocket remained considerably more resistant. In fact, the steepest drop in Limburg's I_g occurred only in the period 1960–1970, as a part of a fertility decrease witnessed on the national level after 1963.

A similar picture of the decline in marital fertility can also be obtained by following the rate of change. For the period 1880–1910 we have defined this rate as follows:

$$\Delta I_g = \frac{I_g\,(1880) - I_g\,(1910)}{I_g\,(1880) - .200}$$

In this expression we have related the actual change in I_g between 1880 and 1910 to the maximum change that might have occurred. Here, the level of .200 was chosen to indicate the end of the fertility transition. The values of ΔI_g are represented in Map 4.5. Again, the map shows

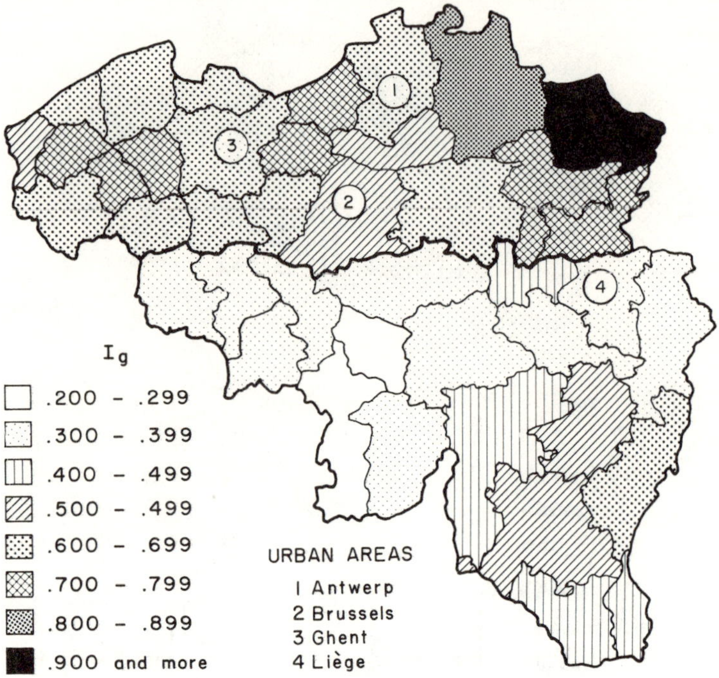

Office of Population Research, Princeton University

Map 4.4 Marital Fertility (I_g), by Arrondissement and Four Urban Areas: 1910.

how quickly marital fertility declined in the Hainaut arrondissements: more than 70 percent of the total possible fertility reduction in the arrondissements of Charleroi, Mons, and Thuin occurred in this period of 30 years. Two other arrondissements had a similar decrease: Brussels and Liège. In these, however, a substantial part of the decline is to be attributed to the presence of the urban metropolitan areas.

In Flanders, most of the arrondissements experienced less than 50 percent of their fertility transition in this period. The only exceptions are Ghent and Antwerp, and this is due to the presence of large urban areas.

On the whole, the most impressive feature on these maps is the clear distinction between the two language regions. In fact, the areas with high marital fertility and a late decline are nearly all on the Flemish side, and those with an early and faster decline are on the Walloon side. The language border separates these two demographic regimes in a

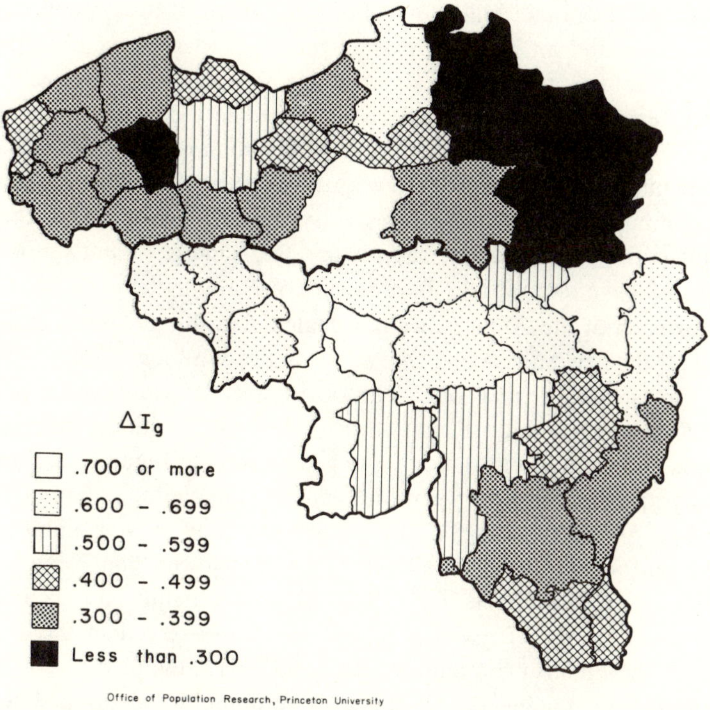

Map 4.5 Change in Marital Fertility (ΔI_g), by Arrondissement: 1880–1910.

marked way. The sharpness of this difference will be documented in the following section.

4.4 *The Fertility Decline along the Language Borders*

To show the irrelevance of physical distance in areas where two cultures meet, we have compared the fertility transitions in a geographical string of paired communities, located on either side of Belgium's main language border. This crosses the country from east to west over almost its entire length. In the random sample of 70 pairs, each pair consists of a Flemish community and its nearest Walloon counterpart. The distance between two communities in a pair never exceeds 6 miles. In some instances, the two communities within a pair are not exactly equivalent on all social and economic characteristics, but the majority of pairs in the sample are matched very well in this respect. In the aggregate, the two sets are similar: there is no significant difference between the Flemish set and the Walloon set in their average values for various social and economic indicators. For each of the 140 communities, we have calculated an index of overall fertility. Ideally, we should work with the values of I_g, but the detailed age and marital-status distribution of the female population is not available. The index used is, then, the average annual number of births per 1,000 women aged 15 to 55. (This somewhat unusual inclusion of women aged 50 to 55 is the result of the groupings used in the censuses.) Even if the measurement of fertility is not entirely satisfactory, the picture that emerges from the analysis does not leave room for doubt or misinterpretation.

For each of the 70 pairs, we have calculated the difference in fertility at each date by subtracting the value of the Walloon community from that of its Flemish neighbor. The distribution of these within-pair differences is depicted for several dates in Figure 4.2, with the distributions' means and standard deviations. As can be seen in Figure 4.2, there was hardly any difference between the Flemish and Walloon communities in 1864–1868. By 1878–1882, the distribution had moved slightly to the right, and pairs in which Walloon fertility was lower than Flemish fertility increased in number. By 1898–1902, a total shift had occurred: in only 8 out of the 70 pairs is higher fertility observed in the Walloon than in the Flemish community. By 1908–1912, the distribution moved back slightly, but nearly all Walloon communities continued to have lower fertility than their Flemish counterparts. This is not the result of a large difference along one section of the language border and a small difference along another, but represents a contrast that extended along the entire language border. In this narrow strip, 100 miles long but only 6 miles wide, we find a real demarcation line between two obviously noninteracting demographic regimes.

The more recent history of the language-border areas is also in line with the national experience. When later on fertility dropped in the Flemish regions, the within-pair differences were gradually reduced. By 1945–1949, the distribution in Figure 4.2 moved back again, and by 1959–1963 the differences had virtually disappeared.

The same experiment was also conducted along Belgium's second language border which separates Walloon villages from German-speaking ones. After World War I, a small part of German territory was annexed and added to the arrondissement of Verviers. These German-speaking areas are now generally referred to as the "East Cantons." Differences similar to those found along the Flemish-Walloon border were observed here in 1930. Here, the German villages systematically showed much higher fertility levels.

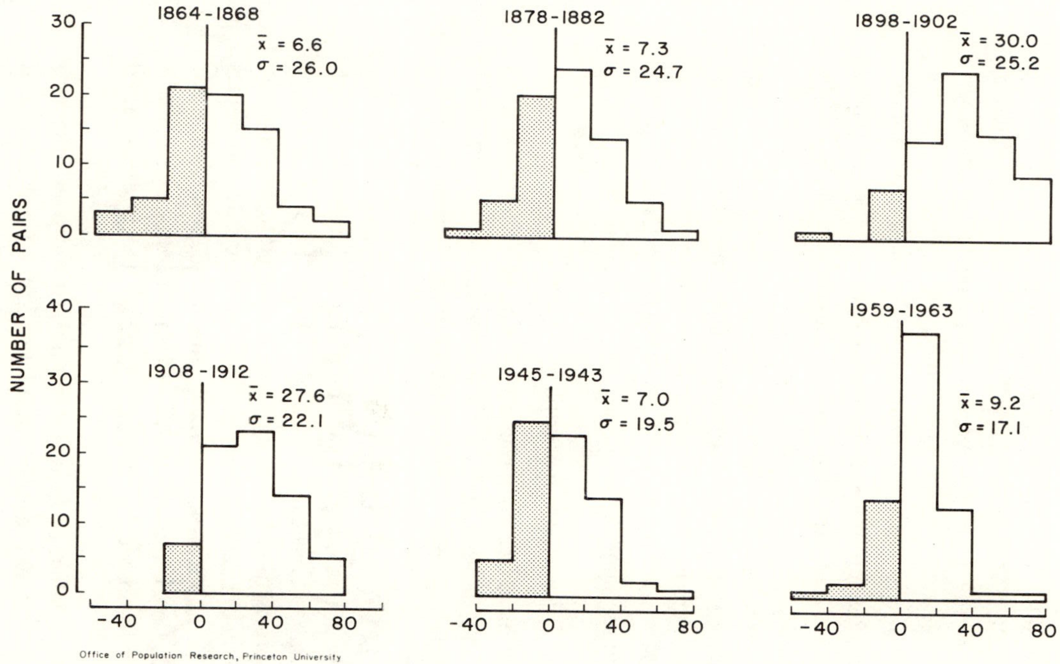

Figure 4.2 Variations in Fertility Rate, by Matched Pairs of Flemish and Walloon Communities Along the Language Border: 1864–1868 to 1959–1963.

NOTES: 70 Flemish communities were paired with 70 Walloon communities on the basis of general proximity. Negative values indicate the Walloon community had the higher fertility; positive values that the Flemish community had the higher fertility. General fertility rate defined as births per 1,000 women aged 15-55.

A third test of this nature was performed in the linguistically mixed area of Brussels. In 1910, the Brussels urban district was made up of 12 separate communities. In each of them the value of I_g could be calculated, and these values correlated with the proportion of all adults who spoke only French. (Of those enumerated as bilingual, a vast majority were originally Flemish, so the bilingual persons are excluded from the numerator of this language index.) The correlation coefficient was $-.880$, which was substantially larger than the correlation coefficient between I_g and any of a battery of social and economic indicators. Even when both language groups were living together as direct neighbors in the same streets, they had kept their cultural difference with respect to fertility in 1910.

The most important finding from this section is without doubt the fact that the largest regional difference observed in Belgium coincides completely with the language borders, whether these run from east to west (Flanders-Wallonia), from north to south (Wallonia-East Cantons) or between houses in the same city (Brussels).

4.5 *Urban-Rural Differentials in Marital Fertility*

In section 4.3 we have treated the levels of marital fertility in entire arrondissements. Only the four largest urban areas are shown separately on Maps 4.1 through 4.4. Now, we will focus more clearly on urban-rural differentials.

The rural parts of arrondissements are defined as those containing only communities with less than 10,000 inhabitants. Communities with more than 10,000 inhabitants are defined as urban. Since the censuses contain sufficient information on the age and marital status distribution of the female population, it has been possible to calculate the values of I_g for each of them. By subtraction of the numbers available for urban areas from those for the entire arrondissements, the marital status distribution can be computed for the rural sections too and converted into values of I_g.

Map 4.6 shows the values of I_g for the rural parts of arrondissements in 1910. In general, marital fertility was higher in the rural areas, and the shadings on Map 4.6 are either the same or darker than those of Map 4.4. On the Flemish side, urban-rural differentials were more pronounced. A comparison of Map 4.6 with Map 4.4 shows that 9 out of the 22 arrondissements in Flanders fall in a higher category with respect to I_g when all urban units are omitted. In Wallonia, the same holds only for 2 arrondissements (Verviers and Arlon).

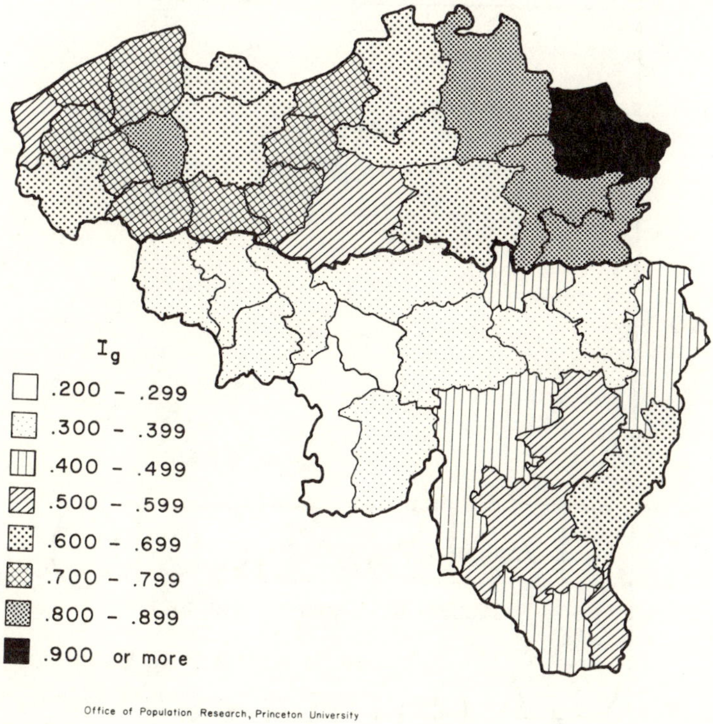

Map 4.6 Marital Fertility (I_g), by Rural Parts of Arrondissements: 1910.

A picture of the difference between urban areas can also be obtained. For this, we have grouped the urban units in six categories:

1. Provincial towns in Flanders.
2. Provincial towns in Wallonia.
3. Communities in the metropolitan areas of Antwerp and Ghent.
4. Communities in the metropolitan area of Liège.
5. Communities in the metropolitan area of Brussels.
6. Industrial towns of Hainaut province.

The evolution of I_g from 1846 until 1910 for the above is shown in Figure 4.3. The Flemish provincial towns clearly had the highest values of I_g, and their fertility decline started only after 1880. In all the other urban areas, a decline was well under way by 1866; in the Walloon provincial towns this was true as early as 1856. However, this figure shows only the trend in the average value of I_g within each category of urban communities. It may also be interesting to have a closer look

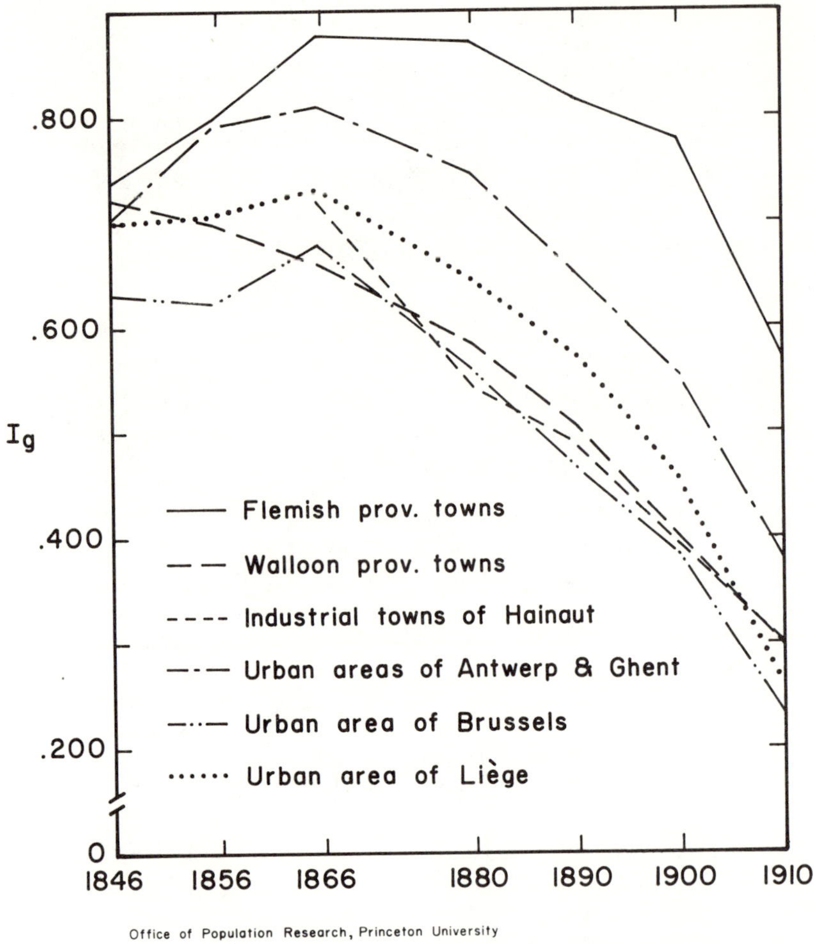

Figure 4.3 Urban Marital Fertility (I_g), by Selected Areas: 1846 to 1910.

at the variance around these averages. Figure 4.4 shows the distribution of I_g in each urban category in 1900 and 1910 for Flanders; Figure 4.5 shows the same for Wallonia. A preliminary inspection indicates that the distributions come close to the normal distribution. Hence, the normal distributions represented in these figures are only a minor simplification of the real situation, but they convey very well the large differences in dispersion around the average I_g values in each urban category.

The distribution for rural areas is included in both figures, but is represented by a dotted line, since the I_g distributions for these rural regions are based on a different unit of observation. The distributions

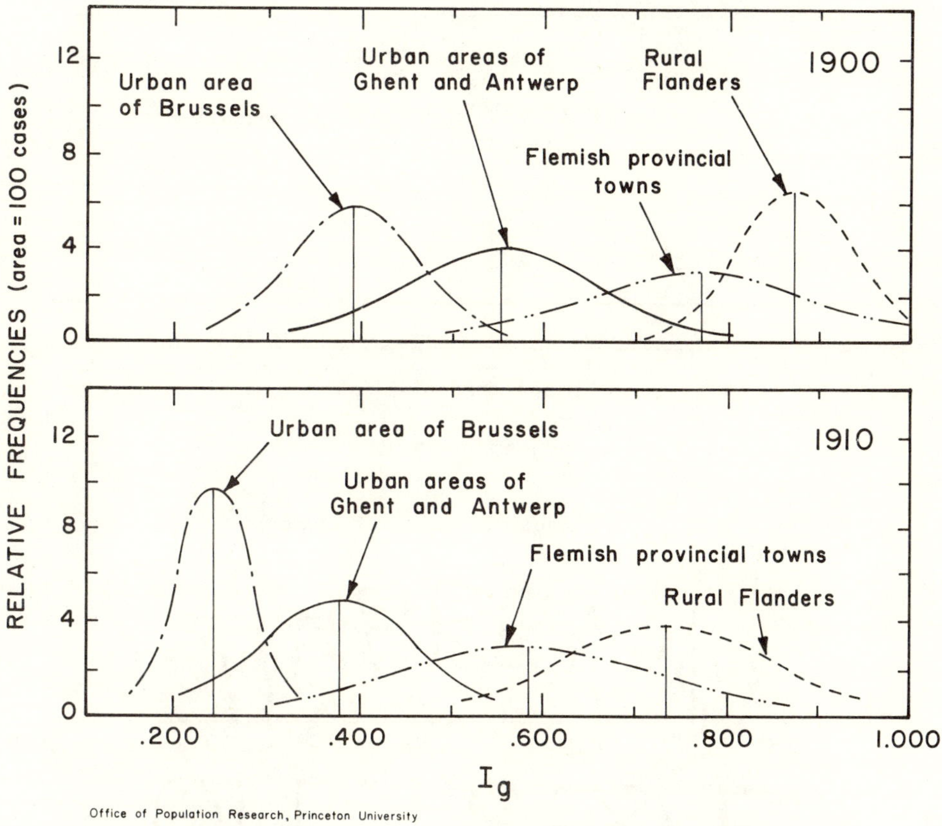

Figure 4.4 Marital Fertility (I_g), Distribution Curves by Communities within Selected Urban Areas and Rural Parts of Arrondissements, Flanders: 1900 and 1910.

for urban areas are all calculated on I_g values for administrative communities, defined as urban, whereas the distribution for rural areas is based on I_g values for the rural parts of arrondissements (pooled units of communities). This difference results only from the fact that I_g values could not be calculated for rural administrative communities separately, since the necessary information is not available. Hence, the mean of the distribution for rural areas may come very close to the true mean for the communities, but the dispersion around it may be smaller.

The information represented in Figures 4.4 and 4.5 is interesting in several respects. The most important feature is not so much the fact

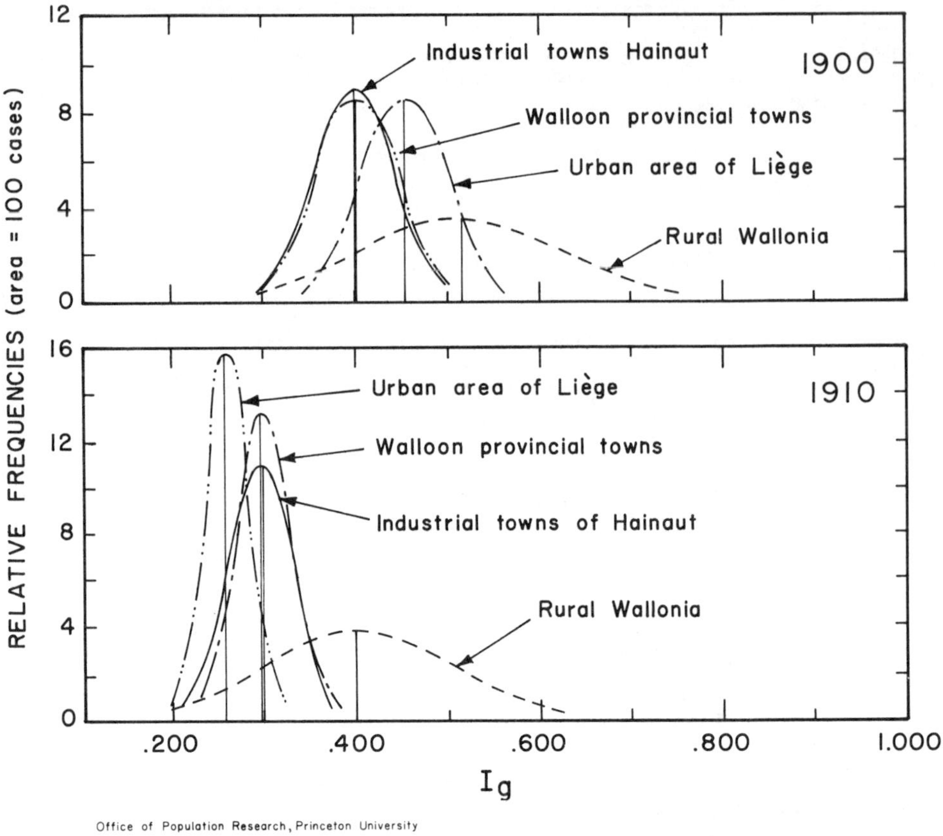

Figure 4.5 Marital Fertility (I_g), Distribution Curves by Communities within Selected Urban Areas and Rural Parts of Arrondissements, Flanders: 1900 and 1920.

that the Walloon urban areas were more advanced in the fertility transition (which we knew already), but that they formed a much more homogeneous group than the Flemish urban areas. The means of the I_g values for the different Walloon urban categories are much closer together; also the within-group dispersions are much smaller. This contrasts rather strikingly with the very large within-group and between-group dispersions in the Flemish urban areas.

To make sure that this difference between the urban areas within each language region was a reality and not merely the result of catching the two language areas in a different stage of the transition, we have also looked at the distribution for the Walloon urban areas in 1890 (at that date the Walloon urban units were approximately in the same stage as Flanders was shortly after the turn of the century). Here, the means for the Walloon groups of urban areas were close together. Moreover, the within-group dispersion was considerably smaller than in the Flemish groups in 1900 or 1910. This is documented in Table 4.5 where we compare the standard deviation of I_g in each category of urban communities at a moment when they had comparable mean values of I_g and were thus at approximately the same stage in the fertility transition.

TABLE 4.5

URBAN MARITAL FERTILITY (I_g) AT COMPARABLE LEVELS, STANDARD DEVIATIONS, SELECTED AREAS: CIRCA 1900

Type of urban community	Area	Mean value	Standard deviation	Date
Metropolitan area	Liège	.574	.069	1890
	Brussels	.587	.103	1900
	Antwerp and Ghent	.559	.092	1890
Industrial towns	Hainaut	.569	.053	1890
Provincial towns	Wallonia	.585	.090	1890
	Flanders	.574	.147	1910

There seems to be two distinct patterns of fertility transition in the Belgian urban areas. In Wallonia, the transition was fast, the urban-rural differences small, and the urban areas (industrial or not, large or small) behaved more or less as one unit. In Flanders, the urban areas followed a much more individual pattern. First, I_g dropped in the large urban area of Brussels (as might be expected from the fact that the capital contained a very high percentage of French-speaking persons). Then the transition occurred in metropolitan Antwerp and Ghent, but within these areas certain communities were significantly more advanced than others. The Flemish provincial towns followed as a third group, but with a considerable time lag and in a very heterogeneous way. By 1910, some of these provincial towns were already below the .400 level (Mechelen and Louvain), while others had not yet started (Beveren-Waas and Geel both had values of I_g of .901) and were even behind many strictly rural areas.

4.6 *The Decline of Illegitimate Fertility*

More or less parallel to the transition in marital fertility was the decline of illegitimate fertility in Belgium. This was especially steep between 1880 and 1930. The importance of this decline should not be misunderstood, however. Even before 1880, extramarital fertility was never high in Belgium, and we are speaking of a change from low to very low illegitimate fertility. Before turning to the specifics of this decline, we should cast a brief glance at extramarital fertility in Europe before 1880.

In the nineteenth century, Belgium was only a small part of a much larger area characterized by low illegitimacy. In the British Isles, the Low Countries, most of France and Spain, Switzerland, the western part of Germany, and northern Italy, the level of illegitimate fertility rarely exceeded 10 percent of marital fertility, although there were as many unmarried women in the fecund ages as there were married women. In terms of the index I_h, defined in chapter 3, all the provinces in this western European area had a value below .060. This implies that the level of illegitimate fertility was less than 10 percent of the level of marital fertility (E. Shorter, J. Knodel, and E. van de Walle, 1971, p. 387). Hence, prolonged celibacy and early widowhood did not lead to high values of extramarital fertility in most of Western Europe, even when contraception was not widespread.

In Belgium, illegitimate fertility went through essentially three stages between 1846 and 1970. In the first, between 1846 and 1890, the I_h increased in all provinces with the exception of Namur and Luxemburg (see Figure 4.6 and Table 4.6). A similar increase was also observed

TABLE 4.6

ILLEGITIMATE FERTILITY (I_h), BY PROVINCE: 1846 TO 1970

Date	Antwerp	Brabant	East Flanders	West Flanders	Hainaut	Liège	Limburg	Luxemburg	Namur
1846	.037	.068	.033	.022	.041	.035	.018	.014	.027
1856	.041	.069	.032	.027	.050	.036	.022	.015	.026
1866	.043	.068	.031	.027	.053	.041	.025	.015	.027
1880	.059	.079	.036	.032	.058	.046	.027	.014	.025
1890	.068	.070	.039	.035	.058	.046	.029	.014	.025
1900	.058	.056	.037	.034	.047	.039	.027	.012	.022
1910	.041	.039	.027	.024	.036	.031	.020	.011	.018
1920	.032	.029	.023	.020	.034	.027	.022	.010	.019
1930	.022	.023	.014	.011	.023	.022	.015	.007	.011
1947	.014	.020	.011	.008	.025	.022	.008	.007	.016
1961	.013	.021	.010	.008	.027	.023	.006	.008	.016
1970	.013	.020	.010	.008	.028	.020	.010	.011	.019

NOTE: The values of I_h are calculated on the number of illegitimate births during a five-year period centered around a census. The values for 1970 are based on the average number of births for 1969 and 1970 only.

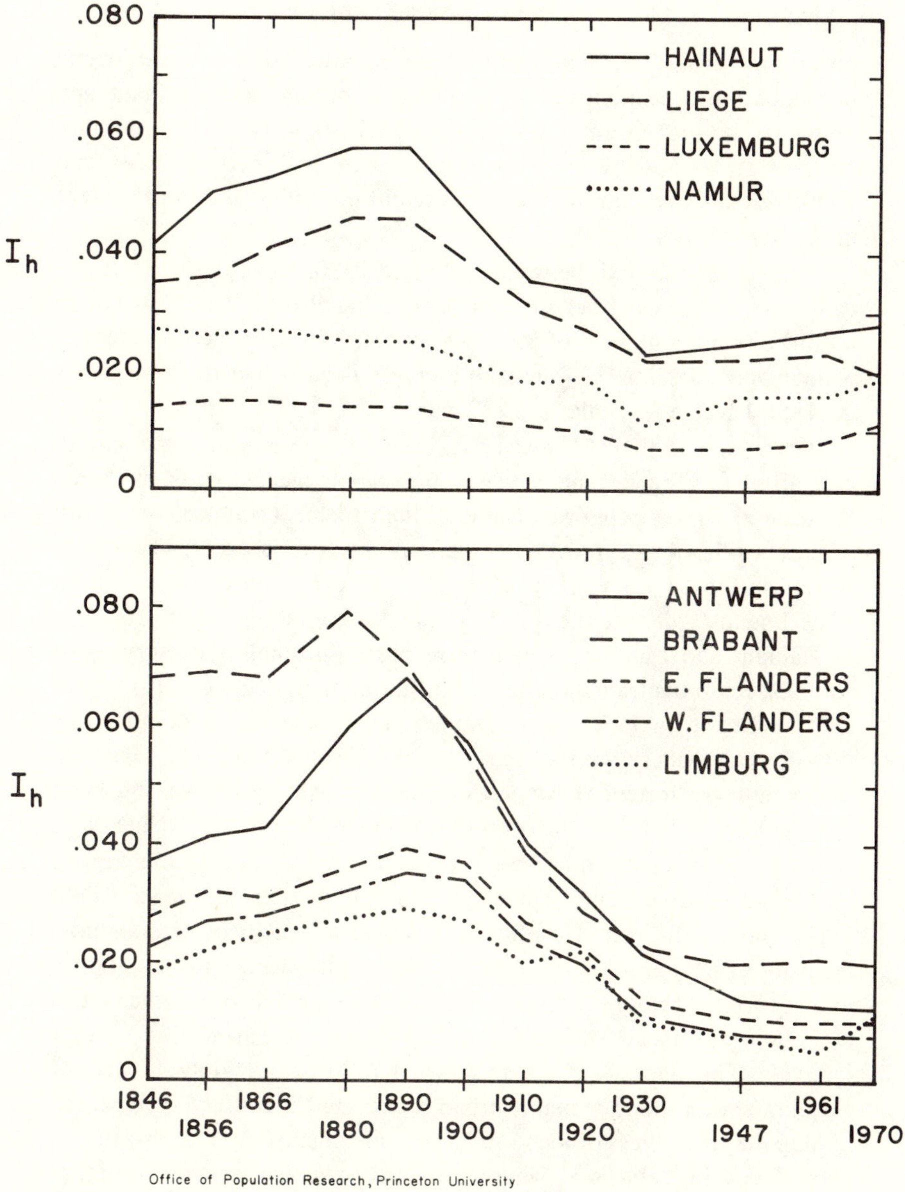

Figure 4.6 Illegitimate Fertility (I_h), by Province, Flanders and Wallonia: 1846 to 1970.

for marital fertility, especially in the Flemish area, but the upward trend in I_h was more pronounced. The Walloon provinces of Hainaut and Liège had no increase in I_g but a substantial rise in I_h. In the province of Antwerp we observe an 80 percent increase in I_h between 1846 and 1890. Marital and extramarital fertility did not follow the same pattern in this first period.

In the second period, between 1890 and 1930, I_h was reduced drastically. Aside from a brief interruption during World War I, I_h fell to a third or even a quarter of its original value. Even in the provinces of Namur and Luxemburg, where no increase occurred in the first phase, the 1930 I_h value was half the 1890 value.

One will recall that there was a definite difference in the time pattern of marital fertility decline between the two language areas, with the Walloon provinces being well ahead of their Flemish counterparts. With respect to illegitimate fertility, there is no such difference. The values plotted in Figure 4.6 show a remarkable uniformity in the time pattern of decline in I_h, despite the differences in absolute levels. The provinces of Hainaut and Limburg, which were more than half a century apart with respect to the transition in I_g both started their decline of I_h in 1890 and finished it by 1930. This implies that I_h dropped a decade later than I_g in provinces with an early marital fertility transition (Hainaut and Namur for instance), whereas in the Flemish area (East and West Flanders, and Limburg) the drop in I_h occurred before the decline of I_g.

Before we interpret this observation, we should look at the decline in I_h by arrondissement. Table 4.7 presents I_h data for 1880, 1890, 1900, and 1910. Map 4.7 illustrates this at the moment of maximum intensity (1880) and Map 4.8 shows the pattern when a substantial drop had occurred (1910). The differences between the two is rather striking: there are no areas where I_h failed to decline during this 30-year interval. The dark shadings in Map 4.7, located mainly in central Belgium and in the four major urban areas, almost entirely disappeared in Map 4.8, regardless of location. The same phenomenon is also shown very clearly in Table 4.8, where the average values and the standard deviations are reported according to the level and type of urbanization. There again, we find a uniform decline in I_h and a similar reduction in dispersion, in all types of urban communities as well as in the rural parts. In 1900, the four large urban areas had the highest values of I_h; by 1910, there was no longer a distinction between them and the other urban communities.

TABLE 4.7

ILLEGITIMATE FERTILITY (I_h), BY ARRONDISSEMENT: 1880 TO 1910

Flanders	1880	1890	1900	1910
Aalst	.025	.031	.028	.021
Antwerp	.070	.078	.063	.044
Bruges	.039	.041	.038	.028
Brussels	.093	.079	.060	.040
Dendermonde	.028	.036	.033	.027
Diksmuide	.022	.026	.024	.018
Eeklo	.031	.038	.040	.030
Ghent	.046	.045	.043	.030
Hasselt	.035	.037	.030	.025
Kortrijk	.031	.034	.034	.021
Leuven	.054	.059	.051	.040
Maaseik	.017	.019	.019	.012
Mechelen	.056	.066	.060	.042
Ostend	.052	.055	.061	.048
Oudenaarde	.034	.037	.031	.023
Roeselare	.025	.026	.025	.018
St. Niklaas	.031	.039	.040	.030
Tielt	.017	.019	.022	.013
Tongeren	.024	.026	.025	.019
Turnhout	.028	.032	.033	.027
Veurne	.026	.025	.025	.017
Ypres	.038	.041	.035	.024
Wallonia				
Arlon	.019	.017	.017	.020
Ath	.051	.048	.038	.028
Bastogne	.011	.011	.010	.018
Charleroi	.069	.066	.053	.042
Dinant	.015	.015	.014	.009
Huy	.032	.034	.031	.022
Liège	.061	.060	.051	.037
Marche	.011	.012	.009	.011
Mons	.063	.064	.048	.035
Namur	.032	.032	.028	.021
Neufchâteau	.014	.015	.015	.007
Nivelles	.045	.043	.034	.025
Philippeville	.019	.016	.013	.011
Soignies	.050	.057	.045	.037
Thuin	.060	.054	.052	.043
Tournai	.045	.043	.038	.025
Verviers	.026	.023	.016	.017
Virton	.014	.017	.011	.011
Waremme	.036	.040	.040	.034

SOURCE: Vital registration statistics and population censuses, Institut National de Statistique - Nationaal Instituut voor de Statistiek, Brussels.

In the third phase, that following 1930, the levels of I_h became even more homogeneous. Hainaut and Liège kept their slightly higher values, but the differences among the other seven provinces are almost negligible. Moreover, the evolution of I_h continued in the same direction until our last observation (for 1970). The differences between the large cities, the provincial towns, and the rural areas were further reduced.

Summarizing these findings, we observe that, at least on the national level, the Belgian population developed control of its marital fertility

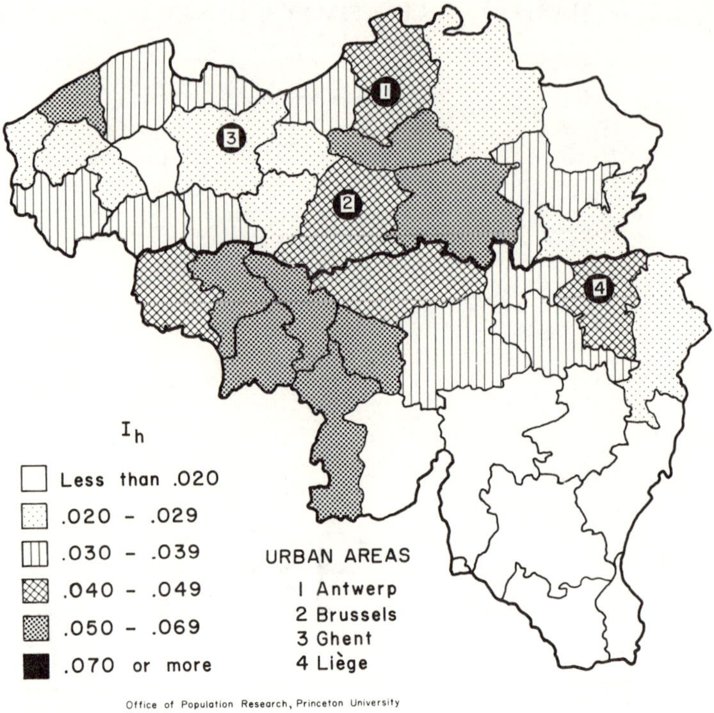

Map 4.7 Illegitimate Fertility (I_h), by Arrondissement and Four Urban Areas: 1880.

TABLE 4.8

ILLEGITIMATE FERTILITY (I_h), SELECTED AREAS VARYING IN DEGREE OF URBANIZATION: 1900 AND 1910

Degree of urbanization	Area	1900 Mean	1900 Standard deviation	1910 Mean	1910 Standard deviation
Metropolitan area	Liège	.062	.016	.033	.009
	Brussels	.061	.027	.038	.016
	Antwerp and Ghent	.066	.020	.044	.019
Industrial towns	Hainaut	.062	.019	.048	.017
Provincial towns	Wallonia	.033	.014	.027	.011
	Flanders	.046	.015	.033	.013
Rural area	Wallonia	.028	.014	.021	.009
	Flanders	.031	.009	.024	.008

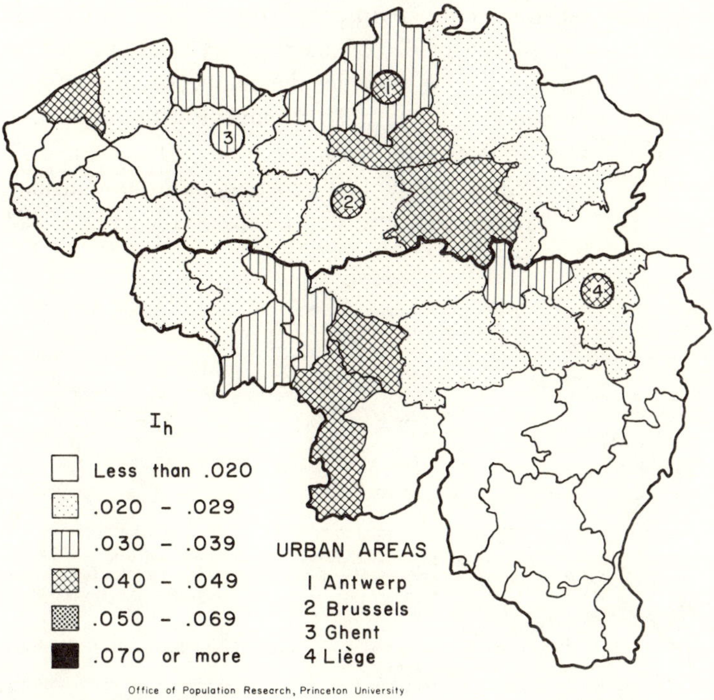

Map 4.8 Illegitimate Fertility (I_h), by Arrondissement and Four Urban Areas: 1910.

and illegitimate fertility at approximately the same time and to the same degree. A similar observation can also be made for other western European countries; the parallelism between the time series of I_g and I_h is particularly striking for the Netherlands, Germany, Switzerland, and Denmark (E. Shorter, K. Knodel, and E. van de Walle, 1971, p. 378). This shows undeniably that both phenomena shared a common element: the increased practice and effectiveness of contraception. We still have to account, however, for the lack of parallelism between the two time series when the national aggregate is broken down into separate subregions. Mechanisms that could account for the divergence between I_g and I_h must be linked to the different nature of marital and illegitimate fertility. A closer look at the statistical meaning of an illegitimate birth may, therefore, be helpful.

In the index I_h we relate a certain number of illegitimate births to a weighted number of unmarried women. This view of illegitimacy is distorted by the fact that not all conceptions outside wedlock lead to an illegitimate birth, since a certain proportion of them will result in a legitimate birth as a consequence of marriage. The extent of this phenomenon will therefore greatly influence the number of illegitimate births and consequently also the index I_h. To document this more specifically, let us suppose that we deal with two populations, called A and B, and that in both populations exactly 100 conceptions occur outside wedlock (see Table 4.9). Suppose also that all these conceptions lead to a

TABLE 4.9

ILLEGITIMACY, PERCENTAGE BIRTHS CLASSED ILLEGITIMATE, BASED ON TWO THEORETICAL DISTRIBUTIONS OF CONCEPTIONS OUTSIDE OF MARRIAGE

	Population A			Population B		
	A_1	A_2	A_3	B_1	B_2	B_3
Number of births	30	10	60	30	60	10
Percentage illegitimate	75.0	25.0	--	33.3	66.7	--

NOTES: Each population consists of 100 conceptions outside wedlock.
A_1 and B_1 refer to adulterous or incestuous conceptions leading to illegitimate births which cannot be recognized (except in very rare instances) or legitimized.
A_2 and B_2 refer to nonadulterous and nonincestuous conceptions leading to illegitimate births which can be recognized and legitimized (legitimation implies recognition).
A_3 and B_3 refer to conceptions which result in legitimate births because marriage occurs between the time of conception and delivery.

live birth. Some of these conceptions (in our example, 30 in both A and B) are adulterous or incestuous. According to Belgian law, these births cannot be recognized by the mother (since the adulterous or incestuous nature may not show) and can certainly not be legitimized, since marriage between the parents is excluded. The 30 births in cells A_1 and B_1 of Table 4.8 are illegitimate children who can, in principle, never appear in the statistics of recognition and legitimations. The second group of births occurs to single women (or widows) who can, theoretically, marry the father of their child since the relationship was neither defined as adulterous (even if the father was a married man) nor incestuous. If mariage occurs before the birth of the child, the birth will be registered as legitimate. Only if no marriage occurs before the birth will the child be included among the illegitimate. But, unlike those in cells A_1 and B_1, these illegitimate births may be recognized by either parent and may be legitimized if the parents marry. If such a child is recognized, it will have a family (either one or both parents) and will also inherit certain rights. If it is legitimized, it has the same rights as any other legitimate children subsequently born to the same parents. In practice, the mother will very often recognize a nonadulterous illegitimate child. Hence, if we take the sum of recognitions (either immediate or later) and of legitimations (of children who had not already been recognized), we shall have a good idea of the number of illegitimate children that belong to categories A_2 and B_2 in Table 4.9. Late recognitions and legitimations do not necessarily occur just to infants, however, but to older children as well. Therefore, we have to take the mean age of these groups into account in relating them to the total number of illegitimate births.

The total number of illegitimate children can be broken down approximately, then, into two categories (A_1 and A_2), and a percentage can be established for each cell. Now we can compare population A and B again. Suppose that in A a very small fraction of nonadulterous (and nonincestuous) conceptions result in illegitimate births, while the majority of them result in legitimate births because of shotgun marriages. Of the total number of illegitimate children, only 25 percent in our example belong to category A_2. Suppose that in population B, to the contrary, very few legitimate births result, since shotgun marriages do not occur, and the majority of the 70 nonadulterous conceptions appears in the illegitimate category. Then, cell B_2 contains 66.7 percent of all illegitimate births compared with 25 percent in A_2. The distribution between the first two categories is thus seen to be largely dependent on the relative frequency of illegitimate conceptions that result in legitimate births (cells A_3 and B_3); and of these we have no idea, for there are no statistics showing the number of births in the first eight or nine months of the mother's marriage before the year 1962.

Let us now look at the statistics of recognition and legitimations that give the approximate breakdown into categories A_1 and A_2 for the nine provinces for 1851–1860 and for 1901–1910. The percentage of nonrecognized (A_1) and recognized or legitimized (A_2) illegitimate births are given in Table 4.10. The figures in this table show very clearly an important decrease in the nonrecognized group. At first sight, this might suggest that there had been a decrease in adulterous (or incestuous) relationships. Moreover, a drop in A_1, from 63.3 percent to 29.5 percent for Belgium as a whole, would imply that the middle of the nineteenth century was an epoch of considerable immorality, and that the start of the twentieth century was an era of great virtue. This interpretation of Table 4.10 is, of course, hard to maintain. In addition,

TABLE 4.10

ILLEGITIMATE BIRTHS, PERCENTAGE NONRECOGNIZED (A_1) AND RECOGNIZED OR LEGITIMIZED (A_2), BY PROVINCE: 1851 TO 1860 AND 1901 TO 1910

Area	1851-1860		1901-1910	
	A_1	A_2	A_1	A_2
Province				
Antwerp	56.8	43.2	30.7	69.3
Brabant	61.0	39.0	30.7	69.3
East Flanders	71.5	28.5	36.6	63.4
West Flanders	79.9	20.9	42.1	57.9
Hainaut	54.5	45.5	9.3	90.7
Liège	57.3	42.7	19.9	80.1
Limburg	71.7	28.3	42.7	57.3
Luxemburg	73.2	26.8	43.6	56.4
Namur	72.2	27.8	24.3	75.7
Belgium	63.3	36.7	29.5	70.5

NOTE: For definitions of A_1 and A_2 see Table 4.9.

the provinces where the authority of the church was least accepted (Hainaut and Liège), and where a morality was developing that paid much less attention to Catholic principles regarding marriage and procreation, would have had by far the lowest levels of illegitimacy due to adultery. This makes the assumption about the decrease in adulterous offspring even more untenable.

It is much more likely that the mechanism described in Table 4.9 is at work: the number of prenuptial conceptions that were not legitimized through precipitated marriages must have increased considerably. This would account for (1) the sharp increase in the proportion of illegitimate births that were recognized later on (cell A_2 of Table 4.9 and 4.10); and, to some extent also, (2) the substantial increase in I_h during the period 1846–1890.

The increase in I_h before 1890 may also be partly attributed to the fact that the index I_h is not entirely independent of the mean age at marriage. Let us document this by a simple example. Suppose that population A has a mean age at marriage of 27 years and that some prenuptial relations start during a period of, say, two years before marriage. These relations result in a number of illegitimate births. In population B, the mean age at marriage is 24 years and in this population some prenuptial relations also start two years before marriage, resulting in the same number of illegitimate births as in population A. In calculating the index I_h, one relates now an identical number of illegitimate births for both populations to a larger number of unmarried women in population A and to a smaller number of unmarried women in population B. With an identical behavior (the same incidence of prenuptial relations occurring during the same period before marriage), population A would have a smaller value of I_h than population B. Hence, when the mean age at marriage is lowered or I_m increased, one would automatically expect an increase in I_h. This increase is then a result of the definition of I_h and does not correspond to a change in prenuptial behavior at all. The extent to which this mechanism is responsible for the actually observed increase in I_h is unknown.

To summarize, the increase of I_h between 1846 and 1890 was probably due to three factors:

1. A large proportion of conceptions occurring outside wedlock may have resulted in illegitimate births because of a reduction in the incidence of shotgun marriages (mechanism documented in Tables 4.9 and 4.10). This phenomenon seems to be more typical for those areas with a less-traditional orientation such as Hainaut and Liège and applies to a considerably smaller degree in more strongly Catholic provinces such as Limburg, East Flanders, West Flanders, and Luxemburg.
2. Prenuptial sexual relations may have increased, leading to higher values of I_h in these areas that were breaking away from the traditional Malthusian marriage pattern, and that developed higher levels of secularization (especially Hainaut and Liège).
3. A lowering of the mean age at marriage would have reduced the quantity (number of unmarried women) in the denominator of I_h and inflated automatically the value of this index of illegitimate fertility. Again, the decrease in the mean age at marriage (or the increase in I_m) was particularly strong in the provinces of Hainaut, Liège, Antwerp, and Brabant, which also had the highest values of I_h in 1880–1890.

Since we have no means to study the impact of the first two factors in any statistical detail, we have no idea to what extent the statistical mechanism mentioned in point three can be held responsible for the upswing in I_h prior to 1890. Stated in other terms, the increase in I_h in certain areas is definitely linked to the three factors mentioned above, but we have no additional information that would enable us to calculate specific weights for each of the factors separately.

After 1890, the values of I_h are subject to a continuous reduction.

As stated earlier, this drop was most probably caused by increased use and effectiveness of contraception. However, this explanation does not account for the fact that I_h dropped in nearly all areas at the same time, whereas I_g, which is equally affected by increased contraception, dropped much earlier in certain areas than in others. The discrepancy between the timing of the reduction in I_g and the timing of the reduction in I_h is very difficult to explain, since we have no quantitative idea about the impact of the three factors associated with the evolution of I_h. As a result, we have no basis to favor one explanation over another. The early drop in I_h combined with the late reduction in I_g in Limburg or the reverse situation in Hainaut remains a puzzling issue.

4.7 *The Decline of Overall Fertility*

One will recall from Section 3.2 that the index of overall fertility (I_f) is expressed in terms of its components in the following way:

$$I_f = I_g \cdot I_m + I_h \, (1 - I_m)$$

and that in the case of negligible illegitimate fertility this expression reduces to

$$I_f = I_g \cdot I_m$$

Values of I_f for the Belgian provinces are represented in Figure 4.7 and Table 4.11. As a consequence of their early reduction in marital

TABLE 4.11

OVERALL FERTILITY (I_f), BY PROVINCE: 1846 TO 1970

Date	Antwerp	Brabant	East Flanders	West Flanders	Hainaut	Liège	Limburg	Luxemburg	Namur
1846	.311	.325	.296	.295	.319	.330	.290	.334	.325
1856	.318	.329	.302	.311	.335	.330	.306	.316	.318
1866	.366	.361	.356	.372	.354	.342	.335	.320	.331
1880	.415	.356	.375	.387	.312	.311	.374	.318	.296
1890	.385	.310	.359	.373	.269	.285	.350	.284	.252
1900	.349	.273	.363	.386	.246	.250	.376	.277	.244
1910	.289	.205	.295	.324	.198	.184	.380	.256	.216
1920	.222	.168	.221	.235	.179	.161	.321	.213	.189
1930	.198	.145	.199	.222	.155	.149	.320	.203	.178
1947	.197	.158	.210	.216	.195	.177	.287	.207	.209
1961	.222	.182	.208	.215	.207	.188	.281	.233	.224
1970	.178	.161	.182	.187	.193	.171	.204	.201	.190

NOTES: The values for 1920 are calculated on the average number of live births for four years only (1919, 1920, 1921, and 1922) rather than for five years centered around the census. Because of World War I, the number of live births for 1918 is unknown. The values for 1970 are based on the average number of births for 1969 and 1970 only.
Underlined values of I_f represent initial 10% decrease below the preceding value.

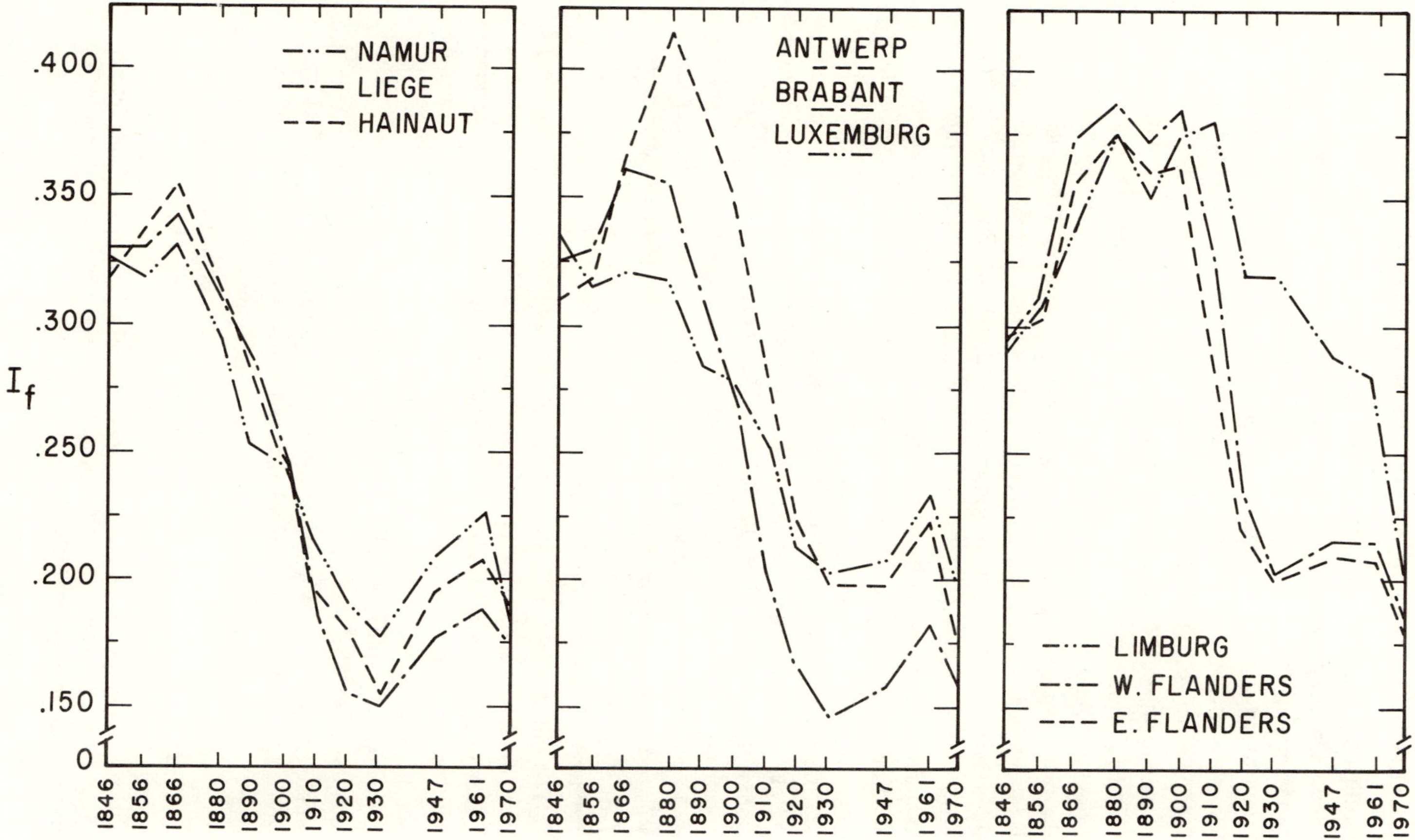

Office of Population Research, Princeton University

Figure 4.7 Overall Fertility (I_f), by Province: 1846 to 1970.

fertility (I_g), all Walloon provinces had a swift reduction of I_f after 1866. On the Flemish side, however, I_f increased substantially, and more than I_g (see Figure 4.1). This additional increase was caused primarily by the rise of I_m in the second half and especially in the last decade of the nineteenth century. Put another way, to estimate I_f in Wallonia between 1866 and 1910, one would multiply the rapidly decreasing values of I_g by slowly increasing values of I_m. To obtain I_f for Flanders up to 1890, one multiplies steadily increasing values of both I_g and I_m. As a result, a large gap between the overall fertility levels of the two language regions becomes visible, the original difference in I_g being magnified through the effect of I_m. With comparable mortality, this difference in I_f would have been translated directly into much higher growth rates in Flanders. In fact, adult mortality was slightly higher in Flanders, and infant mortality was nearly twice as high in Flanders as in Wallonia. Yet, despite its mortality disadvantage, the Flemish population's share of the total population grew steadily from 1860. In 1866, leaving the arrondissement of Brussels out of the picture,[4] there were 52 persons in Flanders for every 48 in Wallonia. Despite some migration from Flanders to Wallonia, these numbers were 55 and 45 respectively by 1910; in 1947 the discrepancy had grown to 61 and 39, and by 1970, the proportions had stabilized around 64 and 36. Fertility was not the only factor in this differential growth; the early decline of I_g in Wallonia also resulted in an older population, which in its turn had a negative impact on the growth rate.

The differences that came into existence during the fertility transition contributed in some degree to a shift in the political and economic balance. After World War I, when the demographic differences became fully apparent in the age compositions, Walloon public opinion became sensitized by a flood of pessimistic reports and newspaper articles. The term "demographic suicide" appeared regularly in the 1930s. The qualification "old" was applied to the Walloon population and industry alike, and the lack of a larger segment of younger people was held responsible for the stagnation of the traditional Walloon sectors of economic activity. The coal pits closed gradually, primarily because of the irregularity of the coal layers and because of competition from imported coal or, later on, other sources of energy; the string of industrial towns

[4] The arrondissement of Brussels contains the urban area that became increasingly French-speaking as a large number of originally Flemish-speaking inhabitants or immigrants adopted French as their own language.

in Hainaut suffered from severe decay as the new chemical industry established itself elsewhere. At each step, part of the blame was laid on the demographic situation, even when only slightly economic factors were at work. The culminating point of this movement was the report of the French economist and demographer A. Sauvy in 1962 on the Walloon demographic situation. The pronatalist policy formulated in this report was to be implemented primarily through differential child allowances for the two language regions (A. Sauvy, 1962, pp. 39-46). This was obviously unacceptable to the Flemish politicians. Demographic trends soon eliminated, however, the imbalance that the Sauvy report had intended to correct. The report was shelved as it became increasingly apparent that Flemish fertility was moving quickly to the same order of magnitude as Walloon fertility. By 1970 this trend was completed and the difference in I_f became negligible. The evolution of fertility had created a major political issue in its course, but the solution came as quickly in the 1960s as the problem had emerged in the early 1900s.

4.8 *Contraceptive Practice and Fertility Decline*

We may infer from the data on marital fertility that contraceptive practice became more and more widespread from the 1860s on in the province of Hainaut and in the southern part of Namur. Gradually thereafter, contraceptive practices must have been adopted extensively in the rest of Wallonia, in the Flemish urban areas, and finally in the Flemish countryside. At any rate, Caudelier was seriously wrong when he claimed as late as 1900 that contraception was not spreading and that nuptiality was the only significant factor (Caudelier, 1900, p. 190).

In this context two important questions were raised:

1. What sorts of methods were used to achieve this unprecedented degree of fertility control?
2. Why did couples decide to limit their offspring quite suddenly in the last decades of the nineteenth century, when their parents and ancestors had either not raised the question or had been obliged to accept a steady growth of their families?

In this section we will primarily discuss the first problem and will present a more detailed analysis of the second question in chapter 5.

In the rich and superbly documented classic work on the medical history of contraception, N. E. Himes puts forward the thesis that the decline in fertility was a direct result of the modernization and the democratization of contraceptive use. On the basis of clinical and demographic evidence, mainly for the United States, he claims that the fertility transition was the consequence of an extensive diffusion of scientific knowledge of birth control (N. E. Himes, 1936, pp. 333-394). To him, the desire to control conception is "a well-nigh universal culture-trait, universal, that is, in time and space" (N. E. Himes, 1936, p. 421).

A different view is defended by P. Ariès (1960, pp. 311-327). To him, the desire to control fertility was by no means universal, but fluctuated from society to society and over time, depending on the permissiveness or restrictiveness of the dominant moral code. It has only been since the seventeenth century that the moral codes of Western civilization began to change. The ancient culture of Nature and Fertility survived within Christianity, which in its turn stressed the immorality of any act that would disturb the succession of events as embodied in the Natural Order. Births and deaths were givens. Not only according to the prevailing value system, but also according to general and popular belief, nobody could or should ever alter his fate. The widespread adoption of birth control in France at the start of the nineteenth century is, in Ariès' opinion, the consequence of a drastic change in mentality. The fatalistic outlook that prevailed in Europe for centuries yielded to a rational view that was not only able to distinguish between sexuality and procreation, but also able to draw conclusions from this distinction. There was, furthermore, no need for contraceptive innovation: coitus interruptus had only to be extended from extramarital relations to behavior within wedlock.

From Himes one obtains the impression that couples were always aware of the fact that children had to be made (and that they were always trying to prevent this), whereas Ariès defends the position that parents were simply getting children, until they found out quite recently that they could chose not to. To Himes, the goals were clearly defined, only the means were lacking or ineffective. To Ariès, the means were available, only the ends were not defined strongly enough.

We can see room for both points of view. We should not forget that Himes was concerned mainly with the Anglo-Saxon situation in his chapter on the democratization of contraception, whereas Ariès focused primarily on the French situation in which a fertility decline took place at a time when no substantial improvements in contraceptive techniques had been made. It may well be that France and England (or the U.S.)

belonged sociologically to two different types. In France, the new reproductive goals were defined earlier and more clearly (a favorable mentality developed even in the villages), and the motivation was more pronounced. The help of a modern contraceptive technology was not needed, since coitus interruptus was probably known. As a result, fertility declined gradually and the process was completed silently before the moral authorities became fully aware of its consequences. In England, to the contrary, the goals were not defined as clearly, nor were they achieved through Malthusian restrictions on nuptiality. Fertility control within wedlock remained more or less absent until the second half of the nineteenth century, and the change in mentality did not grow as easily as in France. Motivations being less pronounced, the new fertility attitudes had to be propagated more actively through certain pressure groups. The pattern of dispersion was less silent and gradual over time, but moved with shocks. The Bradlaugh-Besant trial (1877), throwing the issue of birth control into the open, is perhaps the best example of such a shock.

Belgium took characteristics of both the French and English examples and developed some of its own as well. As in England, the evolution of fertility was sudden, and I_g fell from very high levels. Unlike England, the neo-Malthusian pressure groups, seeping into Flanders from across the Dutch border or emerging in a few circles in Wallonia, hardly had a chance to grow into fully developed organizations. Stengers' history of these groups is very clear on this point: the neo-Malthusians remained a small set of inspired and motivated individuals, but they were boycotted by Catholics, Liberals, and Socialists alike (J. Stengers, 1971, pp. 1119-1138). In this way, the sudden fertility decline was by no means a response to an event like the Bradlaugh-Besant trial, nor the result of propagation by organized pressure groups. Rather, just as in France, it was a silent process.

The Belgian story is also curious in other respects. On the side of technological innovation, the Belgian contribution was extremely meager. The only prominent figures in this respect were a clergyman and a medical doctor, who both lived, strikingly enough, in the province of Hainaut. The first, the Reverend Alphonse Lecomte, apparently had a substantial knowledge of human biology, and in 1873 was ready to publish an important text on the problems of periodic infecundity associated with the normal menstrual cycle. His work on the matter was swiftly taken out of circulation after a negative report from his bishop and from Rome. The potential of the rhythm method was not resurrected by Rome until the 1930s. The second prominent individual, Dr. Mascaux, was, according to Stengers, the most outspoken person in a small group of Walloon neo-Malthusians. He was the inventor of a condomlike device, lubricated with a contraceptive paste. This device—the "cone of Dr. Mascaux"—was manufactured across the border in France, but its marketing was by no means a success. Advertisements for other forms of condoms were also printed but stayed mostly tucked away in corners of newspapers. On the whole, the general public associated them with venereal diseases and prostitution. Belgian law was instrumental in giving condoms this particular image: contraceptive devices could not be sold openly and not at a profit, so condoms had to be marketed as prophylactics devised for protection against venereal diseases. Consequently, no respectable husband would ever think or dare to use a condom in his marital relations. The vulcanization of rubber may have been a great technological step forward in condom manufacturing, but vulcanized or not, condoms retained their dubious associations in Belgium.

What else is then left in the prerhythm era? Abortion, withdrawal, and abstinence. Abortion leads us directly into the vast field of speculation. There is no doubt that it was practiced (in fact, the Flemish referred to abortionists as *Engeltjesmaaksters* or "Angel makers"), but nobody has any idea about its incidence. Abstinence and coitus interruptus were filling the rest of a large vacuum. Abstinence can hardly be considered as psychologically advisable, and coitus interruptus also belongs to the category of sexually unsatisfying methods. This makes one point very clear: when the population of Wallonia and Flanders started to control their fertility, they did so at great sexual expense. Hence, the motivation for birth control must have been larger in the second half of the nineteenth century than in the first half. It seems that, contrary to Himes' opinion, the motivations were not constant over time or space.

If coitus interruptus was the most important method, was it then introduced from France, or was the method reinvented and diffused within the country itself? If we are to believe literature and newspapers, the French were responsible. A Flemish author, Stijn Streuvels, renowned for his rather realistic descriptions of Flemish rural life shortly after the turn of the century, quotes the "French method" and refers to the "tricks" one could learn in France (S. Streuvels, 1927, p. 832).

However, evidence of this sort is seldom conclusive. It hints at a possibility, without disproving any alternative. In fact, it is possible that coitus interruptus was revived logically and that the label "French method" was applied to it later on. One could expect that the "French method" was not adopted to the same degree in all strata of the Flemish population. It may well be that the French-speaking Flemish bourgeoisie adopted the method first, and that it spread to the other layers later—the more rural, Catholic, and Flemish-nationalistic individuals being the last affected. Then the origin was not located in France, but among the Francophone bourgeoisie.

At any rate, whether we have to look across the border or within the country to find the source, it is clear that coitus interruptus was among the principal methods responsible for the fertility decline. As late as 1966, a national fertility survey found that 40.7 percent of all couples were still practicing coitus interruptus. In Flanders, this percentage was 43.7, in Wallonia 32.3, and in Brussels 34.1 (R. Cliquet, 1969, statistical appendix, p. 15). These percentages can easily be taken as approaching a western European maximum for the time. In fact, one has to go back as far as the 1920s and 1930s to find comparable figures in the English and American surveys. In 1971, coitus interruptus was still cited by 36.1 percent of all married Belgian women aged 30 to 34 as the method currently used and by 53.0 percent as a method used at some time.

What factors are responsible for this relative conservatism with respect to contraceptive use? First, the Catholic authorities voiced strong opposition, initially against the notion of family limitation in general, and after the 1930s, against all contraceptive techniques other than the rhythm method. Let us follow this story chronologically, drawing on J. Stengers' historical analysis (J. Stengers, 1971, pp. 1164-1174).

In 1907, the demographer Camille Jacquart discussed the demographic situation in great detail with a key figure in the Belgian Catholic church, Father Vermeersch. A month later, elaborate statistical tables on Belgian birth rates appeared on the desk of the Primate of Belgium, Cardinal Mercier. In 1908, Vermeersch drafted a paper entitled "Against the Progress of Immorality," and on the basis of this document the Belgian bishops decided to proclaim guidelines for the parish clergy to counteract the "plague of Onanism." Before the guidelines were made public, Mercier in 1909 acted on his own behalf: a pastoral letter was read in the churches of his Archdiocese of Mechelen. The gist of his letter can be paraphrased as follows: Belgium is joining France on the decadent path of onanism, a healthy population is succumbing to the spread of the neo-Malthusian disease; in short, the nation faces a catastrophe. Mercier offered the following alternative: the world is large enough to feed generations of increasing size; only, the earth's wealth has to be conquered by work, courage, and ingenuity; this conquest requires a large amount of "moral energy," and the seedbed for this energy is to be found in the spirit of solidarity and sacrifice typical of large families. Mercier's letter received nationwide circulation, and shortly thereafter very explicit instructions were given to the parish clergy: they must interrogate in the confessional and advise women not to cooperate in marital relations involving the use of any form of contraception.

The trend was apparently firmly set. In 1914, a similar letter from the German bishops was read in all the churches of Germany. In 1919, the French Bishops followed. In 1918, Father Vermeersch left Mechelen to take the chair of moral theology at the Gregorian University in Rome, and according to Stengers, there are indications that Vermeersch was largely responsible not only for the basic ideas, but also for the actual text of the Papal Encyclical "Casti Cannubii" of 1930.

Clearly, the Belgian church had taken the lead in the western European Catholic drive against contraception. Stengers offers the following hypothesis to explain this phenomenon: the fertility transition in Belgium occurred in a country where the Catholic church had maintained a strong moral authority. Unlike France, Belgium took only a few decades to reduce marital fertility to unprecedented low levels in nearly all regions of the country, and church reactions had no opportunity to take the path of "laxist" theology. The church was facing a rapid spread of both onanism and secularization at the same time.

At the time of Mercier's reaction, the control of fertility was already in a very advanced stage, and the tide could not be turned. The most that could be achieved was a slowdown in the diffusion of contraceptive practice among the more faithful Catholics. The situation could have been different if the church had been alerted earlier in the process. Contemporary demographers did not grasp the significance of the fertility trends very quickly, however. As we have seen, Caudelier was still pointing at the nuptiality factor in 1900, when levels of I_g had dropped considerably in Wallonia and had started their downward trend in Flanders a decade earlier. Later on, they were willing to recognize that marital fertility was the responsible factor, but then the marital fertility transition was nearing its end. Ironically, if Belgian demographers had devised an appropriate measure of marital fertility, rather than following the trends in overall fertility, they would have come to a correct diagnosis by 1880; the moral authorities could then have taken action at a time when I_g values were around the .600 level. Of course, nobody knows what the outcome would have been in these circumstances, but it is nevertheless interesting to note that a demographer like Jacquart, with direct ties to the top church authorities, could have provoked a much earlier reaction simply by pressing his analysis of overall fertility further to the level of marital fertility.

The position of the Belgian Socialist party vis-à-vis contraception and fertility regulation was also not favorable. Within that party, the classic Marxist view tended to dominate: a strong party depends on a strong proletariat, and a declining fertility will adversely affect the growth of the Socialist-voting lower classes. In addition, Socialist leaders were well aware of the regional differences in the fertility decline, and the fact that population growth was considerably higher in predominantly Catholic Flanders than in predominantly Socialist Wallonia was not viewed with enthusiasm. Occasional neo-Malthusian arguments were voiced and tolerated within the party; but the defenders of contraception remained very few and did not belong to the party elite. As a result, the Socialist leader Emile Vandervelde, who had so carefully analyzed the social and economic situation before World War I, remained conspicuously silent on matters regarding population in the 1920s.

With the church openly hostile to fertility control and with Walloon socialists fearing a demographic diminution of their region, one could hardly expect that the legal provisions in Belgium would become more liberal or more permissive with respect to the spread of contraception. In fact, the distribution of contraceptive devices or information were criminal offenses falling under title VII of the Penal Code. This title contained, in addition to the spread of contraceptives, the following offenses: abortion, infanticide, kidnapping, bigamy, adultery, pornography, prostitution, and rape. Sales of and propaganda for contraceptives remained regulated by that title until as late as 1973. Before that date, the only way around the highly restrictive legal provision was to strip devices of their contraceptive connotations. The condom became a prophylactic against venereal infections, the pill a medicine, and the IUD a prosthetic device.

The spread of contraception in Belgium can be typified in the following way: it was a silent process, and the matter was hardly discussed publicly in a positive way. Moreover, as there were no important neo-Malthusian pressure groups within or outside the political party structures, legislation on contraceptive sales and information remained oppressive until 1973. In this setting, a general climate of shame developed; the only free outlet (and presumably the prime source of information) was a particular type of joke. Yet, despite the lack of modernization of contraceptive usage, a swift decline in marital fertility occurred in most of the country. This means that motivations must have been sufficiently strong to push nearly the entire population of fecund couples to the sexually less satisfying forms of contraception. The factors that could have conditioned this motivation are studied in the next chapter.

References—Chapter 4

Ariès, P. 1960. Interprétation pour une histoire des mentalités. In *La prévention des naissances dans la famille; ses origines dans les temps modernes,* by H. Bergues et al., pp. 311-327. Paris: INED, Presses Universitaires de France.

Bourgeois-Pichat, J. 1965. Les facteurs de la fécondité non dirigée. *Population* 20:383-424.

Caudelier, R. 1900. *Les lois de la population et leur application à la Belgique,* p. 190.

Cliquet, R. 1969 Kennis, gebruik en effectiviteit van anticonceptie in België. *Bevolking en Gezin* 19:1-62.

Duchène, J., and Lesthaeghe, R. 1975. Essai de reconstitution de la population belge sous le régime francais: quelques charactéristiques démographiques de la population féminine. *Population et Famille* (Brussels).

Jain, A., Hsu, T. C., Freedman, R., and Chang, M. C. 1970. Demographic aspects of lactation and postpartum amenorrhea. *Demography* 7:255-270.

Henry, L. 1961. Some data on natural fertility. *Eugenics Quarterly* 8:81.

Himes, N. 1963. *The medical history of contraception.* 2nd ed. New York: Gamut.

Knodel, J. 1974. *The decline of fertility in Germany, 1871–1939.* Princeton: Princeton University Press.

Léridon, H. 1973. *Aspects biométriques de la fécondité humaine.* Paris: Presses Universitaires de France.

Lesthaeghe, R. 1974. Een demografisch model voor de oostvlaamse landelijke populatie in de 18e eeuw. *Tijdschrift voor Nieuwste Geschiedenis* 1:61-100.

Retel-Laurentin, A. 1967. Influences de certaines maladies sur la fécondité. *Population* 4:841-860.

Romaniuk, A. 1967. La fécondité des populations congolaises. *Éditions Mouton.* Paris.

Sauvy, A. 1962. Le problème de l'économie et de la population en Wallonie; conditions du développment économique et mesures à prendre en vue d'un renouveau général. *Revue de Conseil Économique Wallon* (Liège) 54-55:39-46.

Shorter, E., Knodel, J., and van de Walle, E. 1971. The decline of non-marital fertility in Europe, 1880–1940. *Population Studies* 25:375-393.

Stengers, J. 1971. Les pratiques anticonceptionelles dans le mariage au XIXe siècles; problèmes humains et attitudes religieuses. *Revue Belge de Philosophie et d'Histoire* 49:403-481, and 1119-1174.

Streuvels, S. 1972. De teleurgang van de waterhoek (1927). In *Volledig werk*, vol. 3. Brugge: Desclée de Brouwer.

Tack, G. 1973. *Een demografische studie van Walem, 1674–1755*. Unpublished dissertation. Ghent: Rijksuniversiteit Gent.

van de Walle, E. 1974. *The female population of France in the nineteenth century*. Princeton: Princeton University Press.

van de Walle, E., and Knodel, J. 1967. Breast-feeding, fertility and infant mortality: an analysis of some early German data. *Population Studies* 21:109-131.

CHAPTER 5: Factors Associated with the Fertility Decline—A First Approach

In 1934, the French demographer A. Landry started his volume on the "demographic revolution" with the following question: "If, generally speaking, reproduction remained uncontrolled for centuries, why did it change? . . . Why did fertility change in France after a certain point in time and why did this change occur at different moments in other countries?" (A. Landry, 1934, p. 37). For the first time the question was clearly defined; it has been a central problem of modern demography ever since.

In this chapter we shall take up Landry's question literally and apply it to the history of fertility in Belgium. We shall first set up a theoretical framework linking a series of social and economic variables to our dependent variable, marital fertility. Then, on the basis of this framework, several of the variables will be operationalized. Unfortunately, some background variables require measurements that cannot be obtained from the Belgian statistical material; therefore, we will have to restrict ourselves to those variables that can be operationalized either directly or through a reasonable proxy. The empirical verification in this chapter will be of a simple nature: we want to explore the network of relationships involving just two or, at most, three variables simultaneously. Later on, when these simple relationships are verified, rejected, or altered, we shall continue with the construction of a more complete regression model.

5.1 *The Definition of the Theoretical Framework*

The level of marital fertility can fluctuate considerably despite the total absence of any conscious practice aimed at its regulation. One can thus speak of fluctuations within the limits of "natural" fertility. In the period that we are covering here, however, the change in marital fertility was by far too pronounced to consider it a change from one level of "natural" fertility to another. Clearly some form of conscious and voluntary fertility regulation must have appeared. Such unprecedented alteration in behavior calls for a closer inspection of a series of variables that are thought to condition the adoption of fertility control.

The use of contraception presupposes the following elements:

1. Knowledge of method. Individual couples must have knowledge

about procedures that will prevent births in an effective way, and there must be sufficient communication between spouses to employ a procedure successfully.

2. Acceptability of concept. Either the notion of contraception or at least some particular contraceptive method must be culturally and ethically acceptable. This is not universally so: the Hutterites, for example, regard contraception as a religious offense, and more important in the Belgian context, so does the Catholic church (except for the rhythm method).
3. Acceptability of cost. Contraceptives that imply the purchase of devices must be within a couple's economic reach. Cost does not apply in the same sense to nonappliance techniques, but these, together with some appliance methods, may have a psychological or a physiological "price" when their use involves some sexual or physical inconvenience.
4. Willingness and ability to make conscious calculations. Conscious contraceptive behavior generally appears when couples want to postpone a pregnancy or to terminate further childbearing. In other terms, contraception is applied when couples are willing and able to make an assessment of their desired family size and can evaluate to some extent the feasibility of a next pregnancy in the perspective of their present family size, their prospective fertility potential, and their current and future socioeconomic or psychological situation. Conscious calculations of this sort must be, at least to some degree, culturally acceptable, and a certain minimum of rationality must be present in assessing the impact of various constraints.
5. Recognition of advantage. Fertility regulation must be advantageous in an economic, social, or psychological sense. The costs of childbearing and rearing may be considered too large with respect to family income; or, expressed in other terms, parents may consider a large number of offspring as hampering a current or future standard of living. Not only their own economic or social well being, but also that of the children they already have may be taken into account. An example of such a consideration is embodied in A. Dumont's theory of social capillarity: even when parents cannot raise their own social status, they may want to give their children the maximum opportunity for upward social mobility by restricting their efforts to a reduced number of off-

spring. The variables involved in "calculation" of this nature have been studied by several authors. R. Easterlin (1972, p. 6), for example, defined the demand for children as a function of income and cost constraints relative to the current and prospective utility of children. By the latter variable, Easterlin understands "a preference map which expresses the household's estimation of the degree of satisfaction attached to various possible combinations of children and other economic goods." As a result, such factors as the prospective supplement of income from children's labor, or the old-age security parents may later receive, enter into the calculation.

6. Absence of contra-indicating demographic factors. Given that fertility falls to some extent within the calculus of conscious choice, several demographic factors may play a role in the decision process. In a setting characterized by a late marriage, the reproductive span is considerably shortened and situations leading to an excessive family size will not arise as frequently as in a setting characterized by early marriage. Since couples generally desire a number of *surviving* children, the levels and trends in infant and childhood mortality may also affect decisions regarding fertility.

The various elements outlined so far cluster around two central issues. The first deals with rational thought, or the cultural and ethical acceptability of bringing fertility within the framework of conscious choice. The second involves the terms of the calculation itself and centers around the balance of advantages and disadvantages of high versus reduced fertility.

5.2 *Rationality and Fertility*

Behavior will be considered as rational insofar as it pursues possible ends within existing conditions by means best adapted to realize the ends. The ends are generally the maximization of certain returns. These returns may be of an economic nature (income, profit), or of a social nature (status, authority, power); in addition they will generally involve a psychological dimension (satisfaction, gratification).

Fertility behavior will be labeled rational if the following conditions are met:

1. Couples are aware of the fact that they are responsible for their

own children and believe that they have the right to intervene in the fertility process.

2. Couples are capable of formulating expectations regarding their future fertility in the context of their social and economic position.
3. Couples are willing to translate these expectations into means for the successful attainment of their own chosen ends. In other words, they must be aware that they have the potential power to intervene in the fertility process.

According to P. Ariès, the first condition has not always been met. In ancient cultures as well as in medieval Christianity, all phenomena were believed to be regulated by a Natural Order or by Divine Providence. The elements that made up these concepts were interdependent, and the idea that man had the right or ability to intervene and act consciously with regard to these elements was not known (P. Ariès, 1960, pp. 326-327). The same laws regulated the human life cycle, temperament, and character traits, the seasons of the year, and the course of the stars. In ancient cultures, fertility of land, animals, and people was linked to omens of various sorts. Important decisions were made only after consultation with augurs. Many of these characteristics were apparently taken over by Christianity in different forms. The omens based on chance were generally eliminated; instead, the individual's fate was placed in the hands of Divine Providence. Certain magical beliefs and practices were suppressed; others, however, acquired the status of pious devotions, giving rise to magico-religious beliefs. In this way an entire hagiographic collection of saints developed in order to cure an equally lengthy series of diseases and ills, including sterility.

The belief that couples have the right to intervene in their fertility can be associated with (1) the dissociation of procreation from sexual gratification; (2) the disappearance of magico-religious beliefs, rituals, and superstitions; (3) the emergence of a value system centered around individual rights; and (4) the rise of the conviction that individual's have the right, and eventually the obligation, to take their own fate and that of their families into their own hands.

Given that individuals may decide what is best for themselves and the persons for whom they assume responsibility, they must also be able to specify certain goals and decide which of the alternatives would yield the highest economic, social, or psychological returns. In other words, they must indulge in calculations.

Apparently, these conditions were gradually being met in certain areas and in certain social groups in Western Europe by the eighteenth century. The French gave three names to the degree of rationality applied to the fertility process: *politique* (decision-making), *calculs* (evaluation), and *économie conjugale* (maximization of returns through fertility limitation). In 1751, Prémontval, a French populationist, complained that "it is only *la politique* which decides whether one is going to have more or less children." In 1763, Turmeau de la Morandière referred to "the infamous *économie*," whereas Mesance felt in 1788 that "the *calculs* were responsible for celibacy and for not wanting more than two children" (P. Ariès, 1960, pp. 317-318). There is also clear statistical evidence of fertility control at the time of these authors. The bourgeoisie of Geneva definitely practiced conscious fertility limitation (L. Henry, 1956, p. 178) and, in the decades following the French Revolution, so did several French villages. The French may not have been among the industrial leaders, but they were among the first to apply rational forms of decision-making to fertility behavior on a national basis.

What happened in Belgium? In the last decades of the eighteenth century, it was quite obvious that the Belgian bourgeoisie were well acquainted with the new French philosophies and ideas. Within the Austrian Low Countries and the Principality of Liège, this acquaintance manifested itself in the form of political demands and in the breakdown of adherence to religious authority. This elite formed a seedbed from which a strong anticlerical movement grew and eventually matured as the Liberal party after independence in 1830. Whether the bourgeoisie applied the same rationalistic principles to more intimate matters, however, is not clear: there are no studies so far that systematically explore their ideas on family formation or that follow their demographic characteristics. In fact, we have to wait until a second and far more fundamental wave of rationalism spread and reached larger segments of the population. This occurred after 1860 and was carried largely by the entirely new political and ethical ideology of socialism.

In contrast with this ideology, however, all sorts of superstitious devotions and pilgrimages still persisted, mainly in the countryside, throughout the nineteenth century. These expressions of popular devotions were a thorn in the flesh of the socialists. Non-Catholics saw them as a way to keep large segments of the population locked up in passive ignorance and as a means for keeping the rural proletariat separate from the urban proletariat.

Economic rationality, social awareness, and political emancipation of the less educated emerged only in the second half of the nineteenth century, whereas traditional forms of belief were quite resistant. Without doubt, the breakthrough occurred first in Wallonia, probably shortly after 1850. In Flanders, the evolution came later and developed more slowly, probably as a result of several centuries of economic backwardness and a different pattern of industrialization. But, there too, this new rationality seems to be linked to the increase of secularization.

To summarize, the degree of rationality applied to fertility probably overlaps substantially in Belgium with the spread of secularization. Moreover, the dimension of Catholic versus non-Catholic may not only have caused some differentiation with respect to the acceptability of the notion of fertility-centered calculations in general, but it is clear that this dimension was of great importance with respect to the use of specific contraceptive techniques as well. In fact, not only calculations had to be made, but also appropriate means to control fertility had to be chosen. This task certainly did not become easier for the Catholic segments of the population after 1910, when all forms of onanism were strongly attacked by the Church officials.

The overlap between *économie conjugale* and secularization could not have been complete, however. Fertility among the Catholic population declined too, and it is obvious that other variables affected Catholic fertility in just the same way as they affected the fertility of the more secularized.

5.3 *Elements of the Calculation*

We will now focus on the various elements that may interfere in the assessment of the degree to which fertility control may be advantageous. In doing so, we will not be able to place the discussion on the level of individual couples, but we will try to indicate the general direction of the elements of the calculation during the second half of the nineteenth century.

The first element concerns the utility of children. Here we will indicate whether or not the terms of the calculation were changed by alterations in prospective income earned by children and in future old-age security.

Were parents expecting a supplement of income from their children's labor? This question has often been positively answered in agricultural societies. In a situation where marriage was late, it may well be that the children who were still at home contributed substantially to the family income and also to the care of younger siblings. With increasing urbanization, industrialization, and geographical mobility, however, and with a reduction of the age at marriage, this expectation may have become weaker. If we are comparing the Flemish group of rural semi-agricultural or semi-artisanal workers of the late nineteenth century with the Walloon industrial proletariat, we find indications of a higher value placed on children for their utility in the Flemish group: employment rates among children, regardless of sex, were much higher in Flanders. It was customary for children to give their full pay to their mother (something that husbands did not always do). In the Walloon group, wages were generally much higher. Wives of the Borinage workers, for example, did not often engage in any activity other than housekeeping, and small-scale gardening; consequently, they tended to look after their children themselves rather than leaving this task to a relative, neighbor, or another child. Moreover, when children started working, a portion of their income could be saved to allow them to form a household of their own, and, in the Walloon group, this was done at much younger ages than in the contrasting Flemish group.

Did parents expect some form of old-age security from their children? As far as security in the form of shelter and care, we have already indicated in Section 3.9 that the households of the late eighteenth and early nineteenth century had a remarkably modern structure: apparently some older people could join the household of a child or other relative, but many did not or could not. The notion, often encountered in the literature, that parents could count on their surviving offspring for care and shelter, tends to be overstated, at least in the Belgian context. This does not exclude the possibility of help in the form of money or kind, however. On this we lack documentation, and it would be difficult to estimate to what degree this element contributed to the subjective evaluation of the utility of children. However, in the more Catholic areas, where the lack of help from children to parents was more negatively viewed than elsewhere, it may well be that this element of old-age security played a more important role. On the other hand, we would expect that Belgium's early development of a social-security and pension system would have increased the independence of the elderly and consequently reduced their expectation of help from children. On the whole, we are left with the impression that the prospective utility of children as perceived by parents was decreasing rapidly in the nineteenth century.

Let us now look at the constraints: income and costs. On the income side, there is no doubt that average real income was increasing almost without interruption during the second half of the nineteenth century. Between 1846 and 1886, real income nearly doubled in Belgium. This increase was most pronounced in the coal and metallurgical industries, where real income tripled. In these sectors, the rise was coupled with a considerable shortening of labor time. In the mechanized textile industries, too, there were important improvements with respect to income and labor time between 1850 and 1870; an acceleration of this trend occurred after 1880. Indications of a general rise in real income after 1854 are a reduction of the proportions of the workers' budgets that were devoted to food expenditures and an increase in the consumption of meat, butter, and wheat (H. van der Wee, 1972, pp. 203-204). Regionally, the increase of real income was definitely more pronounced in Wallonia than in Flanders, and was clearer in the urban areas than in the rural ones. In fact, we have to wait until after the agricultural crisis of the 1880s before tangible income improvements appeared in those areas that had resisted the increasing trend of industrialization. By the twentieth century, however, the trend was firmly set in all areas and, although substantial differences had developed, nearly everyone benefited from the improvements.

It is also clear that the costs of child rearing were steadily rising, particularly those linked to the growing desire for what economists usually call "high quality children." This desire was probably not entirely new in the nineteenth century, but it could materialize only in that century as a result of the unprecedented increase in real incomes. As early as the seventeenth century we find definite traces in Western Europe of a gradual shift toward a more child-oriented society. This was especially pronounced in the growing concern about all matters related to education and, in medicine, in the development of pediatrics. Fundamental alterations in the social stratification system in the second half of the nineteenth century—the gradual shift away from an ascribed to an achieved status system; the opening up of new businesses, trades, and occupations; and the spread of education—were increasingly responsible for soaring costs of child rearing and for a reduction in the demand for children. Through the mechanism of social capillarity, parents who could not yet realize their own status aspirations would do whatever was in their power to help their children climb higher on the social stratification scale. A. Sauvy (1960, p. 388) argued that low fertility was more indicative of a child-oriented society than high fertility, and that fertility limitation was primarily the expression of "altruistic malthusianism."

To summarize, we would basically agree with the elements and mechanisms described by the model of H. Leibenstein (1957, p. 163) where the utility of children is declining and the expense increasing, and where the effect of rising income supports the desire for "high quality children." In nineteenth-century Belgium this would definitely result in a decrease in the demand for children, first in those areas where real incomes rose early and where opportunities for social mobility increased as a result of rapidly changing occupational structures. In short, we would expect a decrease in the number of children desired, especially where industrialization and urbanization progressed more quickly.

Let us now see how the evolution of infant mortality and of nuptiality in the second half of the nineteenth century and the first decade of the twentieth century may have affected the terms of the calculation.

A fall in infant and childhood mortality should intensify the effect of a drop in the number of children wanted. More specifically, if the object is to have a set number of surviving children, parents would have to produce fewer births to realize the desired number. Given that couples would not immediately have a tangible indication that infant mortality was declining, a time lag should develop between the start of an infant-mortality decline and the start of a fertility decrease. Such a time lag has been expected by several authors (H. Habakkuk, 1972, pp. 63-65; G. Ohlin, 1973, p. 6; T. P. Schultz, 1973, pp. 12-13). Other authors see it slightly differently: according to H. Leibenstein (1957, p. 164), the decline in infant mortality would first increase the number of "child-utility years," and, with it, the desired and actual number of children. Fertility would consequently increase during the first phase. This increase is labeled the "infant mortality hump" by Leibenstein. During a second phase, the costs of caring for this extra load would be realized and fertility would decline.

Whatever the mechanism postulated, these authors expect a cause-effect relationship and a time lag between the two phenomena. This time lag follows a well-defined sequence: the infant mortality drop precedes the fertility decline. We shall see later on whether this conjecture holds in the Belgian example.

The next variable to be considered is the marriage pattern. Three hypotheses can be adopted to link nuptiality to fertility.

In hypothesis A, one would argue that nuptiality changes first and breaks away from the Malthusian pattern of late and nonuniversal marriage. This happens under the pressure of several exogenous variables of an economic, social, or legal nature. In this context we have already pointed out Hofstee's theory concerning the effects of proletarization and Habakkuk's hypothesis regarding the decline of inheritance systems based on primogeniture (see Section 3.6). With a decline in overall celibacy, the reproductive potential rises for the total population, and with a decrease in age at marriage the reproductive span is widened for individual couples. With a longer exposure to fertility, couples may reach their desired number of children sooner, i.e., at a time well before the woman's menopause. Other things being equal, earlier marriage opens up a greater need for spacing births and for truncating reproduction. This hypothesis has been invoked by Hofstee and Peterson (1960, pp. 334-347) to explain the course of the fertility transition in the Netherlands.

In the second hypothesis, B, the sequence of events is reversed. The change in nuptiality does not occur before the alteration of marital fertility. Instead, the increase in the control of fertility within wedlock permits the decrease in the mean age at marriage and the drop in celibacy. In this hypothesis, when the fertility of couples is brought under greater control, the Malthusian marriage pattern gradually loses its fertility regulatory function, and a natural tendency to marry earlier and more universally can be released. This form of explanation has been applied to the French situation by J. J. Spengler (1938, p. 73) and to the data of Austro-Hungarian Empire by P. Demeny (1968, p. 516).

In the third hypothesis, C, nuptiality and marital fertility are not causally linked to each other; rather, their relationship is spurious as they are both responding to the same exogenous conditions. In Habakkuk's example, the shift from an inheritance system based on primogeniture toward a system of equal sharing may increase nuptiality intensity among younger and previously disadvantaged siblings; it may also lead to a drop in marital fertility, since parents wish to prevent excessive subdivision of property. A single exogenous factor, here the inheritance system and its changes, is separately responsible for the change in marriage pattern and the change in reproductive behavior. Hence, the dependent variables bear no direct relation to each other. Other factors, such as industrialization and urbanization, can similarly be taken as a common set of causes of the shifts in nuptiality and in marital fertility, again deleting any causal interpretation of the correlation between the two dependent demographic variables.

From this it is obvious that the nuptiality factor can be taken as a causal antecedent, vis-à-vis marital fertility change, only if hypothesis A applies. An increase in fertility potential caused by earlier marriage should then result in "excess fertility" and this would lead to an increasing use of contraception. In this instance one would expect the nuptiality change to occur before the fertility decline. Conversely, if the drop in I_g comes before the increase in I_m, we can be sure that the change in nuptiality did not trigger the transition of I_g. The most one could then say in defense of hypothesis A is that nuptiality may have subsequently reinforced the marital fertility trend, but that it does not rank among the original causes initiating the marital fertility transition.

5.4 *Empirical Analysis: The Measurement Problems*

With the theoretical framework and the discussion of the previous sections in mind, we shall now consider the empirical problems more closely. In doing so, we will be severely limited in the sense that several variables which we have conceptually identified so far cannot be readily operationalized. As a result, the problem of operationalization will turn up in several subsequent sections. Second, we shall refrain from using any but simple models in this chapter. Rather than taking up several exogenous factors simultaneously, we shall limit ourselves to a preliminary examination of the relationship between no more than two independent variables and a single dependent variable. In this way, the elementary relationships can be studied in depth. A more complex network of relationships will eventually be built using the insights gained at this preliminary stage.

In the work to come we are going to deal with what is statistically known as causal inference. This term is rather misleading since, using non-experimental data, no statistical procedure is capable of proving or disproving that a relationship is solely asymmetric or causal. In many instances, however, one is willing to accept that a relationship is asymmetric on the basis of theoretical (and not on the basis of purely statistical) considerations. Phrased slightly differently, results from regression analysis can be given a causal interpretation only when one is willing to accept the existence of a theoretical causal model on a priori grounds. In the following sections, we felt that such grounds existed and that we would somewhat underinterpret our results if we were to continue to treat them solely as mere indicators of associations rather than asymmetric effects.

At first, empirical tests will concern the relationship between rationality and the decline in marital fertility. In Section 5.2 we argued that the increasing application of a more rational rather than traditional outlook to certain elements in life, and more particularly to fertility behavior, coincided substantially with the process of secularization in Belgium. We shall first take several different ways of operationalizing this variable and associate these ways with the decline in I_g.

We have also argued that the other elements involved in the assessment of desired fertility, namely the increase of potential income, the desire for "high quality children," and the decreasing utility of children, are associated with industrialization, urbanization, increasing social capillarity, and modernization of the occupational structure. The association between these latter variables and marital fertility will constitute the second topic for empirical testing.

From here, we shall move on to the infant-mortality thesis as expressed by Leibenstein, Easterlin, Ohlin, and Schultz. More specifically, we shall try to find out whether the time lag between the declines in infant mortality and in marital fertility emerged in the expected direction, and whether traces can be found of the "infant mortality hump." Then, a test will be made of hypotheses A through C, which state the possible theoretical relationships between nuptiality and marital fertility. Our aim will be to find out whether the relationship between I_g and I_m or *EM* is spurious, and, if this proves to be untrue, whether nuptiality changes can be taken as causally antecedent to changes in marital fertility. Finally, two more independent variables will be related to marital fertility: language homogeneity and the degree of literacy. These two sociological variables do not appear in our general theoretical framework, but we assume that these variables have a particular impact on marital fertility when dealing with the Belgian situation.

In all this analysis, we should not forget that we lose information and simplify considerably. The first important loss occurs when we drop the direct measurement of certain variables and proceed on the basis of "proxies," or operationalized variables that measure the true variable in an indirect fashion. In this way, not only will we have to substitute the level of secularization for the rationality variable, but we will also have to decide which particular statistical operationalization of secularization will best measure this phenomenon. Hence, we have a double source of measurement error: (1) the use of "proxies" (secularization instead of rationality); and (2) the operationalization itself (should we measure secularization through frequencies of Sunday mass attendance, Easter duty fulfillment, or voting behavior?)

The list of measurement problems is not yet complete. Our preliminary piecemeal approach, taking each pair of variables separately, is useful, but can be very misleading. Hence, we must eventually look at the whole picture together, using multivariate forms of analysis rather than ordinary correlation coefficients. But then, several other statistical problems will emerge. Among these, the collinearity problem will be very important: when we are dealing with several exogenous variables at the same time, it will be difficult to isolate their separate effects on the endogenous variables, especially when the exogenous variables are highly correlated among themselves.

Finally the scope of this book is restricted to the use of ecological data. For the most part our analyses are based on data for arrondissements, that is, on units that range from 50,000 to around 500,000 inhabitants. They cannot, therefore, be taken as evidence of the processes operating on the level of individuals, but only as evidence of relationships at the aggregate level. With these restrictions in mind, we shall now tackle the empirical relationships.

5.5 *Secularization and Fertility*

If we mean by secularization the gradual breaking away from organized religion and the decrease of participation and involvement in the religious community, the best available operationalization would lie in statistics concerning such events as Sunday mass attendance or Easter practice (Easter confession and communion). If we mean by secularization the shift away from the principles embodied in Catholic ideology, we should do better by looking at another form of operationalization. In this instance, voting behavior may qualify as a proxy, since, in Belgian social history, votes for the Liberal and Socialist parties had the clear connotation of being the expression of nonreligious or antireligious sentiments.

Both forms of operationalization have their own statistical shortcomings. Measurement through voting behavior is a rather roundabout procedure. In individual cases, a person with a definite adherence to the Catholic religion may vote for a Socialist or the Liberal party on strictly political grounds and not on ethical issues. This could have occurred if he attached great importance to universal suffrage or to the rights of workers to organize themselves in labor unions (which would shift the vote to socialists) or to the safeguarding of private enterprise (which would provoke a Liberal vote). Obviously, measurement error of this nature affects our operationalization.

On the other hand, the relative frequency of Sunday mass attendance or fulfillment of Easter duties may be "lagged" measurements. Many agnostics would continue their Sunday and Easter duties simply because of social pressure of various forms. As the Belgian stereotype goes, one may go to church "to show a new hat," or "in order not to offend Catholic patrons of one's business," or simply to do one's spouse a favor and to maintain an image of conjugal solidarity vis-à-vis religion. Operationalization through criteria based on public religious performances may thus lead to a substantial underestimation of secularization, especially in the nineteenth and early twentieth centuries, when social pressures were far from negligible.

The hypothesis that measurement through church attendance or Easter duty fulfillment may not accurately describe the level of secularization seems to hold when empirical data are examined. For various years around the turn of the century we possess data on the proportion *nonpascantes* for parishes in the provinces of West Flanders (W. Rombauts, 1971, pp. 180-187), Luxemburg, and Namur (C. Pourbaix, 1973, Appendix). In addition, we have the results of the first elections held according to the system of universal male suffrage in 1919. These data on the proportion Communist, Socialist, and Liberal (i.e., non-Catholic) votes are not available by parish or community, but solely by election canton. But, after recalculating the proportions of *nonpascantes* by election canton, the two sets can be compared. This is done on Figure 5.1 in the form of a scattergram. In the cantons where the non-Catholic vote is anywhere below 50 percent of the total vote, we observe less than 7 percent of *nonpascantes*. Only in the cantons where the threshold of 50 percent non-Catholic votes is exceeded do we find percentages of *nonpascantes* beyond the 7 percent level. In short, the percentage of non-Catholic votes ranges from 6 percent to about 70 percent, whereas the percentage of *nonpascantes* ranges only from less than 1 percent to 26 percent. This marked difference between the distributions of both variables results in a high degree of curvilinearity of the relationship shown on Figure 5.1. Hence, the operationalization of the level of secularization before World War I through Easter duty fulfillment would cause serious problems in the sense that it would fail to distinguish between areas with lower overall levels of secularization and areas with much higher levels. Consequently, the operationalization through voting behavior is preferred in the subsequent analysis when we are dealing with pre-World War I data.

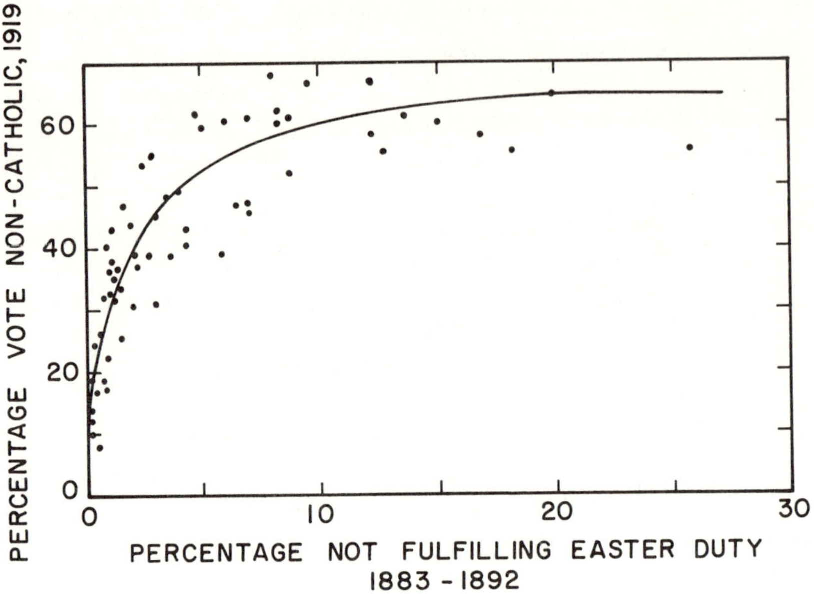

Office of Population Research, Princeton University

Figure 5.1 Secularization, Relation Between Non-Catholic Vote, 1919, and Easter Duty Fulfillment, 1883–1892, Cantons of West Flanders, Namur, and Luxemburg.

If, however, more recent data were to be analyzed, both forms of operationalization would qualify. R. De Smet and R. Evalenko (1956, p. 100) have shown for the 1950 elections that the relationship between voting behavior and Sunday mass attendance has become much stronger. The correlation coefficient between the Catholic vote and Sunday mass attendance is +.93 in the Walloon cantons and +.73 in the Flemish cantons. Clearly, the original curvilinear relationship gradually becomes linear over time, and the degree of secularization already expressed in the voting behavior of 1919 (see Table 5.1) shows up increasingly in the form of lower frequencies of adherence to Catholic practices during the following decades.

Having made a choice on how to operationalize secularization, we are now in a position to explore the relationship between secularization and fertility. This can be done through a correlation analysis between the non-Catholic vote in 1919 and I_g or I_h in 1910. In doing so, we are prepared to accept that the election results of 1919 reflected fairly well the political situation 9 years earlier. But, we would probably be on weaker ground if we were to take the 1919 election results as repre-

TABLE 5.1

PERCENTAGE VOTE NON-CATHOLIC, BY ARRONDISSEMENT: 1919

Flanders		Wallonia	
Aalst	38.2	Arlon	60.2
Antwerp	52.2	Ath	64.4
Bruges	29.7	Bastogne	40.6
Brussels	53.4	Charleroi	79.0
Dendermonde	40.3	Dinant	48.2
Diksmuide	27.4	Huy	72.9
Eeklo	33.9	Liège	77.5
Ghent	51.2	Marche	49.8
Hasselt	24.2	Mons	78.5
Kortrijk	45.2	Namur	63.2
Leuven	42.9	Neufchâteau	46.8
Maaseik	19.6	Nivelles	71.8
Mechelen	42.1	Philippeville	58.5
Ostend	48.4	Soignies	75.4
Oudenaarde	48.6	Thuin	71.3
Roeselare	24.3	Tournai	67.0
St. Niklaas	30.4	Verviers	64.0
Tielt	16.0	Virton	61.2
Tongeren	33.5	Waremme	65.9
Turnhout	22.6		
Veurne	44.2		
Ypres	29.0		

SOURCE: R. Desmet, R. Evalenko, and W. Fraeys, 1958, appendix.

NOTES: Level of secularization is defined as the percentage of votes non-Catholic in the 1919 election.
Non-Catholic vote refers to Socialist, Liberal, and Communist votes.

sentative of the level of secularization for any period prior to 1910. The fact that secularization is measured 9 years later than the level of fertility poses a small methodological problem, but there is no way to proceed otherwise.

The results of the comparison between secularization and fertility are shown in Table 5.2 in the form of correlation coefficients computed on the basis of data for arrondissements. These coefficients show undeniably that the secularization variable cannot be overlooked: it is responsible for a substantial proportion of the variance of I_g and I_h in both language regions. The relative change in marital fertility (ΔI_g) over the period 1880–1910 is also highly correlated with secularization. Only the relative change in illegitimate fertility (ΔI_h) seems to have followed a more independent path. Clearly, the degree of secularization

TABLE 5.2

SECULARIZATION, CORRELATION WITH SELECTED FERTILITY MEASURES, FLANDERS AND WALLONIA: CIRCA 1910

Area	Correlation coefficients between level of secularization and			
	I_g 1910	I_h 1910	ΔI_g 1880-1910	ΔI_h 1880-1910
Flanders (N = 22)	-.830	+.637	+.787	+.343
Wallonia (N = 19)	-.836	+.803	+.890	+.501

NOTES: Level of secularization is defined as the percentage of vote non-Catholic in the 1919 election.

ΔI_g is defined as $\frac{I_{g1880} - I_{g1910}}{I_{g1880} - .200}$. ΔI_h is defined as $\frac{I_{h1880} - I_{h1910}}{I_{h1880}}$.

must be maintained in our set of predictors; only, as we shall see later on, it will be very difficult to separate its effect from that of other independent variables with which secularization shows a high degree of collinearity.

5.6 *Industrialization, Urbanization, and Fertility*

In Section 5.3 we argued that the increasing desire for "high quality children," the increased costs of child rearing, and the mechanism of social capillarity are among the prime causes of the fertility decline. Since none of these variables can be operationalized directly at the aggregate level, we have to make the crucial step from main theory to auxiliary theory again. This operation is done on the basis of the argument that these variables are positively associated with the degree of industrialization and urbanization. We would expect that the desire for "high quality children" and their upward mobility would be most clearly perceived in areas with increasing industrialization and urbanization.

Statistically, the degree of industrialization and urbanization has been measured by arrondissement through three variables:

1. The percentage of the male active population engaged in agriculture.
2. The index of occupational structure, or the logarithm of the ratio between occupational categories typical for modern industry and those occupations characteristic of the occupational structure of the nineteenth century (see Section 2.5).

3. The percentage of the population living in communities with more than 10,000 inhabitants.

These three variables are very highly correlated with each other. Essentially, they each measure a common phenomenon. Taking advantage of these correlations, we have extracted the common dimension statistically through principal component analysis. When the correlations between separate indicators of a single phenomenon are high, the principal component will explain a high proportion of their common variance, and it can then be substituted for the three original indicators. This seems to hold well in our case since the principal component explains more than 84 percent of their common variance (see Table 5.3). By

TABLE 5.3

INDEX OF INDUSTRIALIZATION AND URBANIZATION, CONSTRUCTED BY PRINCIPAL COMPONENT ANALYSIS, TESTS OF ADEQUACY, FLANDERS AND WALLONIA: 1890 TO 1910

Area	Date	Correlation between principal component and: Percentage males in agriculture	Log. occupational structure	Percentage inhabitants in urban communities	Percentage of sum of variances of three indices, explained by principal component
Flanders (N = 22)	1890	--	--	--	84.2
	1900	--	--	--	89.9
	1910	-.927	+.981	+.921	91.8
Wallonia (N = 19)	1890	--	--	--	97.2
	1900	--	--	--	95.7
	1910	-.951	+.998	+.847	95.7

NOTE: These operations were performed on the basis of the principal component computer program designed and kindly made available by L. Polissar.

taking the principal component as a new variable, the index of industrialization and urbanization (see Table 5.4), we lose hardly any information embodied in the three original variables. In addition, we reduce measurement error and save several degrees of freedom when it comes to introducing other variables in further multivariate analysis. It should be stressed, however, that the logarithm of the index of occupational structure was defined in a different way for the two language areas (see Section 2.5). As a consequence, the new variable is statistically not comparable between Flanders and Wallonia. When a comparison across the language border has to be made, we shall rely on the percentage of males engaged in agriculture (see Table 5.5), which is

TABLE 5.4

INDEX OF INDUSTRIALIZATION AND URBANIZATION, BY ARRONDISSEMENT: 1890 TO 1910

Flanders	1890	1900	1910
Aalst	-.229	-.168	-.112
Antwerp	.747	.819	.910
Bruges	.103	.154	.137
Brussels	.633	.639	.690
Dendermonde	-.062	-.102	-.012
Diksmuide	-.273	-.461	-.538
Eeklo	-.227	-.217	-.277
Ghent	.320	.318	.293
Hasselt	-.162	-.257	-.229
Kortrijk	.207	.149	.047
Leuven	-.076	-.079	-.035
Maaseik	-.449	-.317	-.284
Mechelen	.186	.260	.450
Ostend	.200	.364	.374
Oudenaarde	-.259	-.354	-.384
Roeselare	-.071	.037	.029
St. Niklaas	.264	.201	.202
Tielt	-.444	-.390	-.514
Tongeren	-.094	-.240	-.233
Turnhout	-.148	-.100	-.071
Veurne	-.130	-.154	-.246
Ypres	-.038	-.103	-.198
Wallonia			
Arlon	-.562	-.167	-.071
Ath	-.435	-.427	-.463
Bastogne	-.929	-.871	-.923
Charleroi	1.121	1.105	.997
Dinant	-.353	-.378	-.413
Huy	.327	.309	.328
Liège	.988	.873	.861
Marche	-.755	-.699	-.812
Mons	.812	.743	.703
Namur	.245	.200	.194
Neufchâteau	-.564	-.637	-.660
Nivelles	-.184	-.318	-.306
Philippeville	.042	.014	-.021
Soignies	.467	.466	.594
Thuin	.335	.293	.389
Tournai	-.272	-.111	-.048
Verviers	.432	.191	.192
Virton	-.274	-.224	-.311
Waremme	-.439	-.300	-.232

SOURCE: Population censuses of 1890, 1900, and 1910, Institut National de Statistique - Nationaal Instituut voor de Statistiek, Brussels.

NOTE: The composite index of industrialization and urbanization, being the principal component of three other indices, cannot be used for comparisons of time or comparisons between the language regions. It states only the relative position of an arrondissement with respect to other arrondissements of the same language region and at a particular point in time. If comparisons across time and across language regions have to be made, one should use the percentage of males in agriculture. This variable is the strongest correlate of the composite index.

TABLE 5.5

PERCENTAGE MALES IN AGRICULTURE, BY ARRONDISSEMENT: 1890 TO 1910

Flanders	1890	1900	1910
Aalst	65.3	44.6	38.7
Antwerp	13.4	9.3	6.4
Bruges	46.9	30.9	28.7
Brussels	23.5	14.0	3.2
Dendermonde	33.2	37.7	29.2
Diksmuide	59.6	49.0	51.9
Eeklo	63.3	43.7	42.9
Ghent	31.1	25.4	20.1
Hasselt	49.1	46.5	45.2
Kortrijk	27.3	19.1	14.9
Leuven	54.0	40.9	35.9
Maaseik	69.8	46.7	43.4
Mechelen	49.8	31.3	21.6
Ostend	35.1	21.7	20.0
Oudenaarde	64.7	44.1	40.6
Roeselare	42.0	31.3	26.5
St. Niklaas	38.4	30.0	23.2
Tielt	57.8	40.4	48.0
Tongeren	40.9	39.5	40.3
Turnhout	69.6	44.6	44.8
Veurne	49.3	35.6	41.1
Ypres	44.8	39.8	39.0
Wallonia			
Arlon	31.3	29.4	21.8
Ath	43.7	43.2	40.6
Bastogne	43.0	50.4	51.9
Charleroi	4.0	3.2	3.1
Dinant	30.9	30.6	31.0
Huy	17.5	16.5	17.2
Liège	5.5	5.6	4.1
Marche	39.6	41.4	33.0
Mons	11.7	10.9	8.7
Namur	15.8	17.1	15.0
Neufchâteau	38.4	41.5	40.9
Nivelles	23.2	23.5	21.1
Philippeville	23.3	23.8	20.3
Soignies	20.4	16.8	13.1
Thuin	15.0	15.1	13.3
Tournai	26.8	24.7	20.3
Verviers	15.5	17.8	13.8
Virton	27.6	31.4	30.7
Waremme	31.1	31.4	30.7

SOURCE: Population censuses of 1890, 1900, and 1910, Institut National de Statistique - Nationaal Instituut voor de Statistiek, Brussels.

the best remaining correlate of the composite index of industrialization and urbanization.

The strength of the relationship between these indicators of urbanization and industrialization and marital fertility levels or changes is presented in Table 5.6. This table gives the proportion of the variance of I_g or ΔI_g explained by the independent variables. The original zero-order or multiple correlation coefficients are given in parentheses (zero-order correlation coefficients are shown with + or − signs). The table is composed of two segments, one for each of the language areas. Each

TABLE 5.6

MARITAL FERTILITY MEASURES (I_g AND ΔI_g), PROPORTION OF VARIANCE EXPLAINED BY INDICATORS OF INDUSTRIALIZATION AND URBANIZATION, FLANDERS AND WALLONIA: 1890 TO 1910

Area	Indicator	Date	I_g 1890	I_g 1900	I_g 1910	I_g 1880-1900	I_g 1890-1900	I_g 1880-1910	I_g 1890-1910	I_g 1900-1910
Flanders (N = 22)	Percentage males in agriculture + log. occupational structure	1890	.362 (.601)	--	--	.605 (.778)	.699 (.836)	.535 (.731)	.571 (.755)	--
		1900	--	.516 (.718)	--	--	--	--	--	.521 (.722)
		1910	--	--	.532 (.730)	--	--	--	--	--
	Index of industrialization and urbanization	1890	.406 (-.637)	--	--	.629 (+.793)	.712 (+.844)	.586 (+.766)	.630 (+.794)	--
		1900	--	.541 (-.736)	--	--	--	--	--	.486 (+.697)
		1910	--	--	.488 (-.698)	--	--	--	--	--
	Index of industrialization and urbanization + level of secularization	1910	--	--	.744 (.863)	--	--	--	--	--
	ΔPercentage males in agriculture + Δlog. occupational structure	1890-1900	--	--	--	.150 (.387)	.282 (.531)	--	--	--
		1890-1910	--	--	--	--	--	.342 (.585)	.428 (.654)	--
		1900-1910	--	--	--	--	--	--	--	.477 (.691)
Wallonia (N = 19)	Percentage males in agriculture + log. occupational structure	1890	.450 (.671)	--	--	.662 (.814)	.452 (.672)	.701 (.837)	.600 (.775)	--
		1900	--	.517 (.726)	--	--	--	--	--	.600 (.775)
		1910	--	--	.663 (.814)	--	--	--	--	--
	Index of industrialization and urbanization	1890	.364 (-.603)	--	--	.640 (+.800)	.453 (+.673)	.699 (+.836)	.609 (+.780)	--
		1900	--	.505 (-.711)	--	--	--	--	--	.597 (+.773)
		1910	--	--	.631 (-.795)	--	--	--	--	--
	Index of industrialization and urbanization + level of secularization	1910	--	--	.716 (.846)	--	--	--	--	--
	ΔPercentage males in agriculture + Δlog. occupational structure	1890-1900	--	--	--	.319 (.565)	.307 (.554)	--	--	--
		1890-1910	--	--	--	--	--	.484 (.696)	.413 (.643)	--
		1900-1910	--	--	--	--	--	--	--	.422 (.650)

NOTES: The values in parentheses are the zero-order or multiple correlation coefficients, i.e. the square root of the values mentioned first.

ΔI_g is defined as $\frac{I_{g1880} - I_{g1910}}{I_{g1880} - .200}$

segment is made up of four quadrants, depending on the nature of the variables. Since all tables in the subsequent sections are similarly designed, these quadrants can be labeled systematically in the following way:

Quadrant A	*Quadrant B*
Levels of independent variables against *levels* of dependent variables	*Levels* of independent variables against *relative changes* of dependent variables
Quadrant C	*Quadrant D*
Relative changes of independent variables against *levels* of dependent variables	*Relative changes* of independent variables against *relative changes* of dependent variables

The results in Quadrant A of Table 5.6 indicate that the level of industrialization and urbanization has the expected negative relationship with I_g. In Flanders, 36 to 53 percent of the variance in I_g is explained, and when the impact of secularization is added, nearly three-quarters of the regional variance of I_g in 1910 is determined. In Wallonia, the relationship tends to be even stronger.

Also, the correlation coefficients show an increase over time. This should not be surprising: the more the transition progresses, the more the levels of I_g become independent of their pretransitional levels, and the more they correspond with the differentiation along the industrialization and urbanization dimension. This is especially obvious in Wallonia, where, as we indicated before, marital fertility started to decline earlier than in Flanders.

In Quadrant B, we have correlated the values of ΔI_g for various periods with the levels of industrialization and urbanization at the outset of each period. As the values of ΔI_g are less affected by the pretransitional levels of marital fertility than the values of I_g, the coefficients of determination (R^2) are generally higher in Quadrant B than in Quadrant A. In Flanders, 48 to 71 percent of the variance between arrondissements in ΔI_g is explained, and the same order of magnitude also prevails in Wallonia. The ultimate test is performed in Quadrant D. There, the coefficients of determination are substantially lower, especially when relative change rates of I_g for the period 1880–1900 are predicted. When ΔI_g is predicted for the decade after the turn of the century, 48 percent of the variance is determined in Flanders and 42 percent in Wallonia on the basis of the relative changes in the indices of occupational structure alone.

On the whole, the relationship between industrialization-urbanization and the marital fertility decline cannot be denied. Clearly, the values of I_g were decreasing first in areas with the highest degree of modernization of the occupational structure. Even where we are incapable of refining the specific nature of the relationship, it seems that the economic variables have had a marked effect on the transition of marital fertility in Belgium. How large this influence has been is difficult to say at this stage. To answer this question more explicitly, we will need the results from a multivariate approach presented in the next chapter.

After identifying two obviously crucial independent variables (secularization and industrialization-urbanization), we should be able to answer another question at this point: was there a regional pattern of deviation from the predicted values of I_g or ΔI_g, or were the regression residuals scattered more or less randomly over the territory of the two language areas? Or, stated in other terms, were there adjacent arrondissements that were either more advanced or more backward with respect to the marital fertility decline, once we have eliminated the general effect of industrialization-urbanization and of secularization? An answer to this problem is given on Maps 5.1 through 5.4. On the maps we have indicated the standardized residuals emerging in four regressions. These standardized residuals are defined as follows:

$$\frac{\begin{pmatrix}\text{Observed value of} \\ I_g \text{ or } \Delta I_g\end{pmatrix} - \begin{pmatrix}\text{Predicted value of} \\ I_g \text{ or } \Delta I_g\end{pmatrix}}{\text{Standard deviation of (observed-predicted values)}}$$

The value of this standardized residual for the arrondissement of Brussels, for example, in the regression linking I_g 1910 with the index of industrialization and urbanization is -1.61. This means that the predicted value of I_g 1910 was considerably higher for Brussels than the observed value; the level of marital fertility in the arrondissement was already reduced below the level that one might expect given the degree of industrialization and urbanization. The arrondissements that were more advanced with respect to the marital fertility transition are indicated on our map by no shading or by a light shading; the arrondissements that were still lagging behind in the marital fertility transition, after eliminating the effect of the independent variables, are indicated by darker shadings.

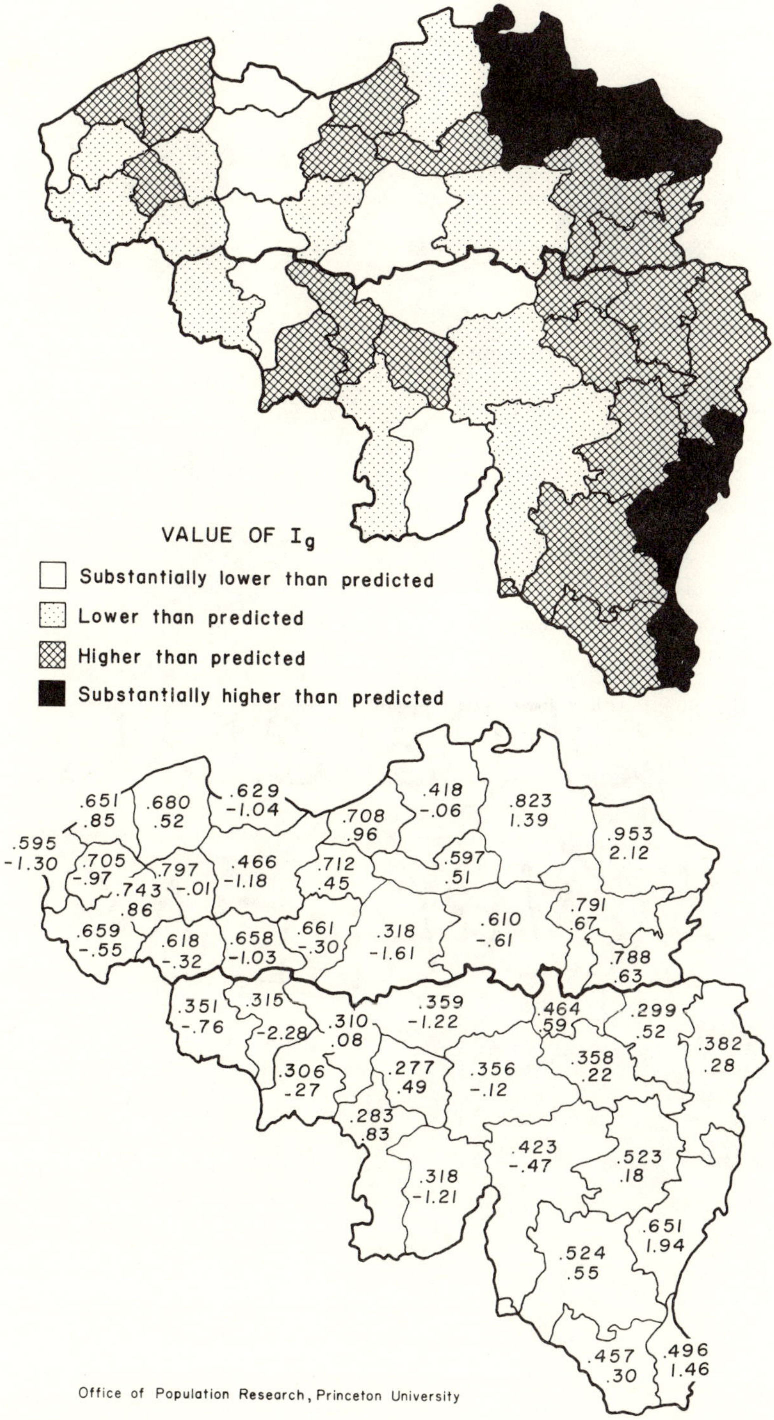

Map 5.1 Marital Fertility (I_g), Deviations from Predicted Value (prediction based on index of industrialization and urbanization in 1910), by Arrondissement: 1910.

NOTE: Separate regressions for each language area.

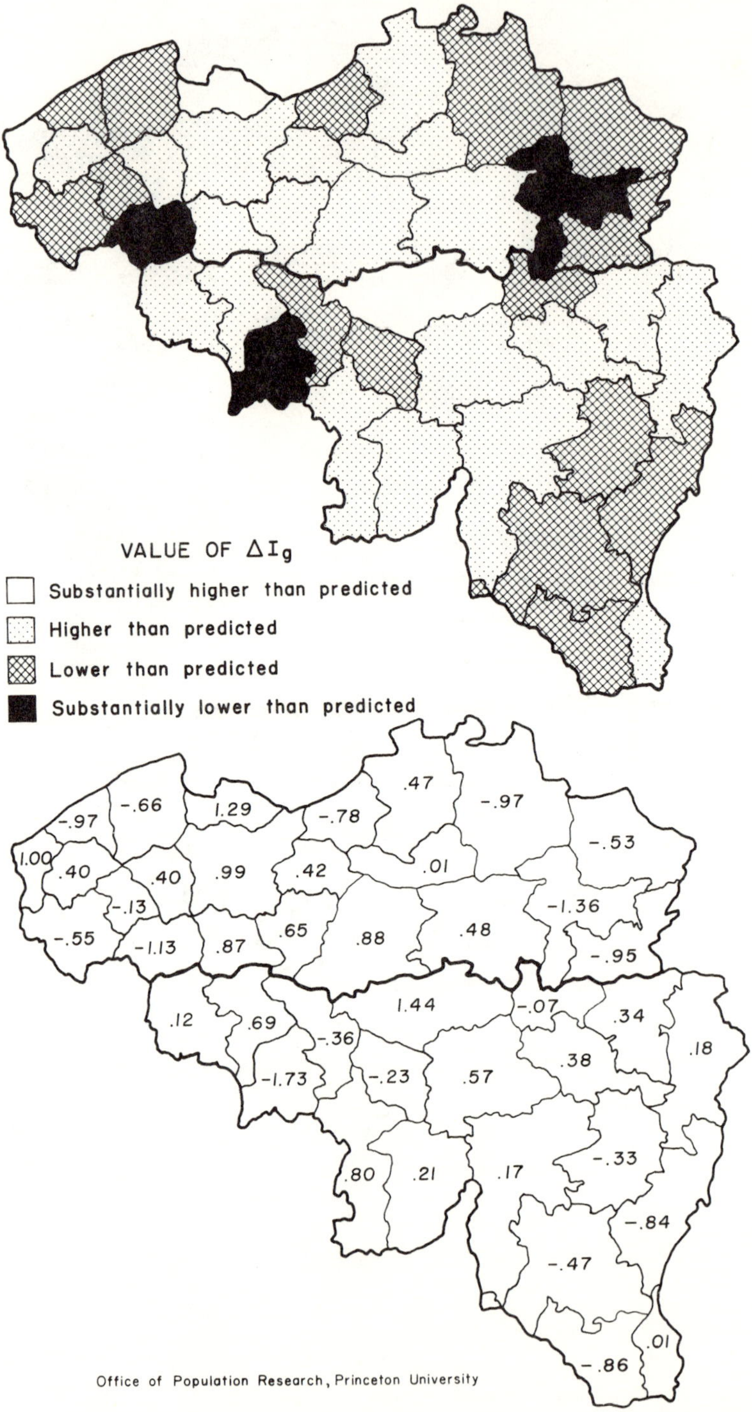

Map 5.2 Change in Marital Fertility (ΔI_g), Deviations from Predicted Value (prediction based on index of industrialization and urbanization in 1890), by Arrondissement: 1880–1910.

NOTE: Separate regressions for each language area.

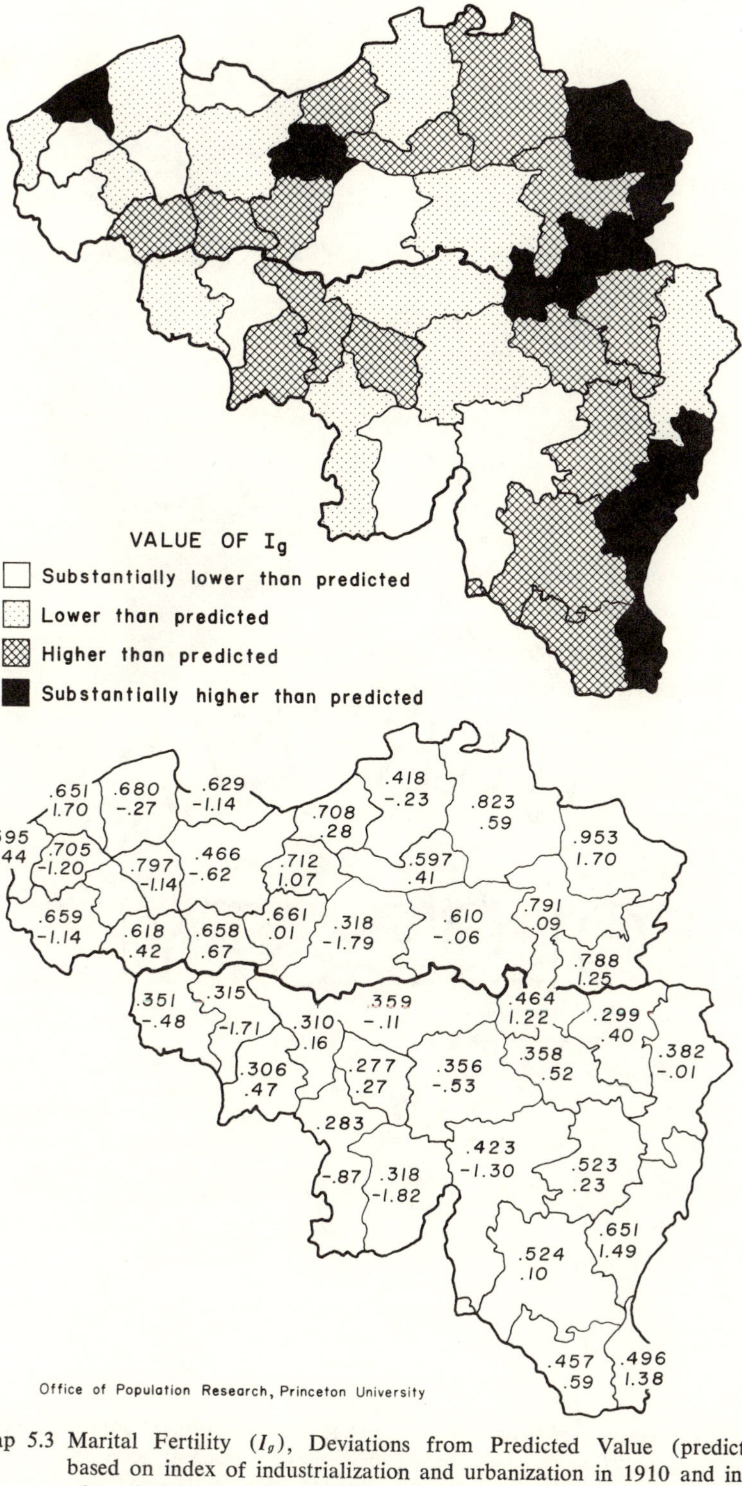

Map 5.3 Marital Fertility (I_g), Deviations from Predicted Value (prediction based on index of industrialization and urbanization in 1910 and index of secularization in 1919), by Arrondissement: 1910.

NOTE: Separate regressions for each language area.

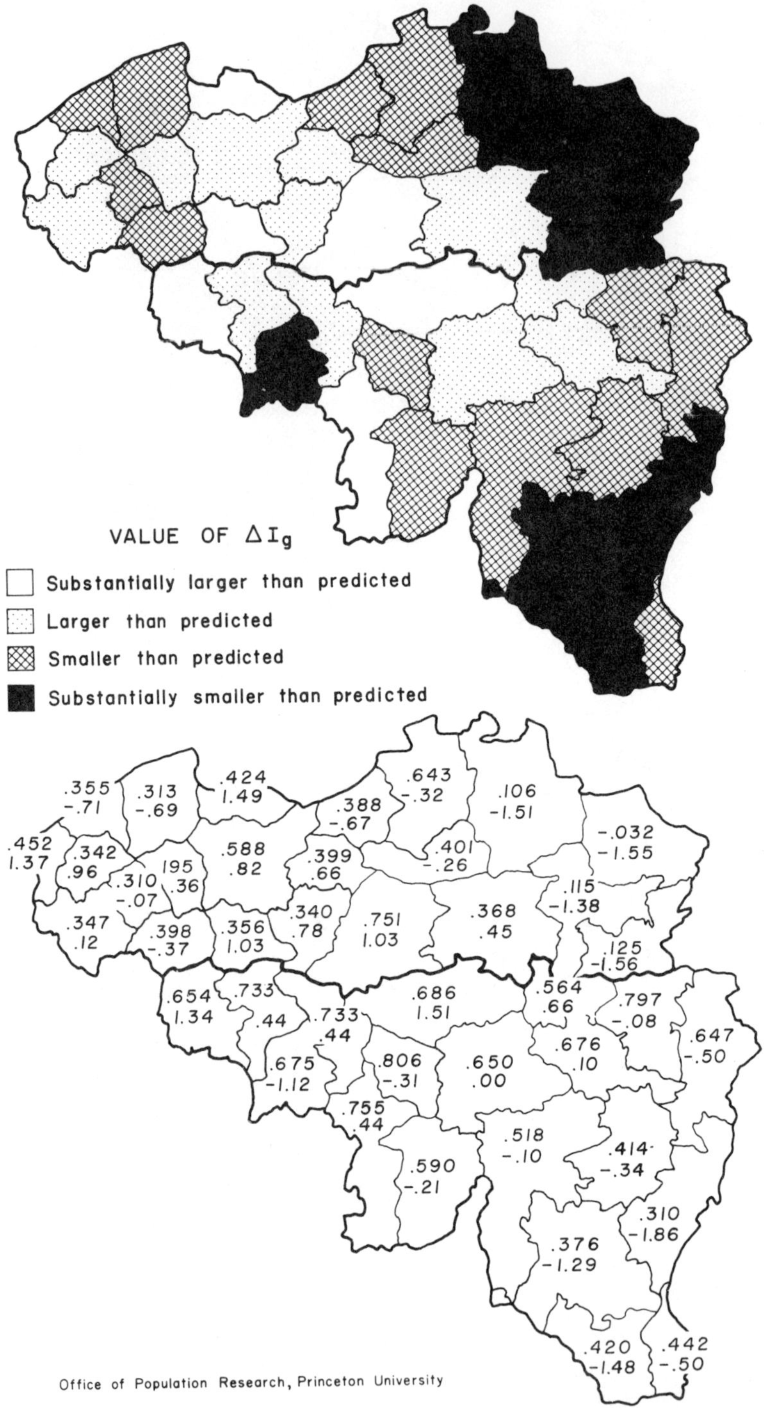

Map 5.4 Change in Marital Fertility (ΔI_g), Deviations from Predicted Value (prediction based on change in male proportion in agriculture, 1890–1910, and change in logarithm of the index of occupational structure, 1890–1910), by Arrondissement: 1880–1910.

NOTE: Separate regressions for each language area.

The general pictures emerging from these maps where the values of I_g or ΔI_g are predicted on the basis of the level of industrialization and urbanization (and also on the basis of the level of secularization in Map 5.3) are consistent on one major point: all the arrondissements in the eastern part of Belgium, from Limburg to southern Luxemburg, have residuals that indicate a definitly slower marital fertility decline than could be expected on the basis of the degree of industrialization-urbanization (and secularization). In Wallonia, we also find darker shadings in a few arrondissements of the province of Hainaut. The relationship between I_g (or ΔI_g) and the independent variables becomes slightly curvilinear at very low levels of I_g (or at very high levels of ΔI_g), however. This slight curvilinearity is the result of the fact that these arrondissements (e.g., Mons and Charleroi), with the highest levels of industrialization in the nation, can hardly be expected to have extremely low levels of marital fertility, even though they had the lowest level in the whole of Belgium. In fact, if these two arrondissements had had a slightly higher score on the industrialization-urbanization variable, one would have obtained nearly zero fertility according to the linear regression line for Wallonia, which is of course impossible. The other arrondissements of Hainaut, those of Walloon Brabant and those of the province of Namur, show a faster marital fertility decline than could be expected on the basis of the regression with industrialization-urbanization (and secularization). It seems, then, after controlling for the two major independent variables, that a certain geographical dispersion pattern could have had an effect in Wallonia: the control of marital fertility started in the Hainaut and Entre Sambre et Meuse area; it spread gradually to Walloon Brabant and in the direction of the other arrondissements of Namur. After that, it seems that the Liège and Verviers areas were affected, and finally the arrondissements in the province of Luxemburg started to decline. This interpretation of the geographical pattern of the residuals holds only insofar as they are not correlated with other variables. Hence, in the subsequent sections we shall see whether we can find another explanation for this apparently geographical dispersion phenomenon.

In Flanders, the arrondissements containing a large urban center (Brussels, Antwerp, and Ghent) show a tendency to be more advanced with respect to marital fertility control than could be expected from the regression line. This was not so for Wallonia, where the arrondissement of Liège, containing the fourth major urban area of Belgium, was lagging behind. The Limburg arrondissements (Hasselt, Maaseik, and Tongeren) and the adjacent arrondissement of Turnhout show a very strong resistance to marital fertility control. To a smaller degree, this was also true for the West Flanders arrondissements of Ostend and Bruges. On the whole, however, the arrondissements of Brabant, East Flanders, and the remainder of West Flanders, i.e., the western part of Dutch-speaking Belgium, either conform with the general trend or are slightly more advanced than could be expected on the basis of their level of industrialization and urbanization. Especially the arrondissements of Veurne, Diksmuide, and Ypres, three predominantly rural arrondissements located along the West Flanders border with France, have residuals indicative of a more advanced marital fertility transition. This seems to be in line with the thesis that fertility regulation practices might have been imported from France. But, the finding that the East Flanders arrondissement of Eeklo, located along the Dutch border, has residuals equally indicative of a more advanced position, does not correspond to the "import thesis." To summarize, it seems that the three large urban areas were the centers of the geographical dispersion of fertility control in Flanders, whereas Limburg remained the major resisting area. The "import thesis" cannot be rejected on the basis of the geographical distribution of the residuals in Flanders, but the evidence in support of this thesis does not seem to be as strong as it was in Wallonia.

Let us now see if we can expect a similar relationship between illegitimate fertility and the index of industrialization and urbanization. From Section 4.6 we know that the values of I_h declined after 1890, and we also know that several mechanisms were at work. In simplifying the matter somewhat, it appears that the degree of industrialization and urbanization has two opposing influences on illegitmate fertility:

1. The old Malthusian rule about illegitimate fertility breaks down in the more urban and more industrialized areas. A larger number of illegitimate conceptions are not legitimized through a marriage preceding the birth, I_h values are higher, and the correlations in Quadrant A of Table 5.7 are positive.
2. Practices of fertility regulation appear first in the urban and industrial regions; these practices are applied to sexual relations outside as well as within wedlock. In this case, the level of I_h goes down first in these areas after the peak around 1880–1890, and

a positive correlation emerges with ΔI_h in Quadrant B of Table 5.7.

As the correlation coefficients in Quadrant A are substantially larger in the two language areas than in Quadrant B, it seems that the first effect

TABLE 5.7

ILLEGITIMATE FERTILITY MEASURES (I_h AND ΔI_h), CORRELATION WITH INDEX OF INDUSTRIALIZATION AND URBANIZATION, FLANDERS AND WALLONIA: 1880 TO 1910

		Correlation coefficient between index of industrialization and urbanization and			
		I_h			ΔI_h
Area	Date	1890	1900	1910	1880-1910
Flanders (N = 22)	1890	+.827	--	--	+.372
	1900	--	+.833	--	--
	1910	--	--	+.794	--
Wallonia (N = 19)	1890	+.750	--	--	+.512
	1900	--	+.728	--	--
	1910	--	--	+.723	--

NOTES: The index of industrialization and urbanization is defined as the principal component of three variables: 1) the percentage of the active male population engaged in agriculture; 2) the index of occupational structure, or the logarithm of the ratio between occupational categories typical for modern industry and those typical of the nineteenth century; and 3) the percentage of the population living in communities with more than 10,000 inhabitants.

was dominating the second effect. This ties in with the finding in Figure 4.5 showing a substantial increase in I_h before 1880 in Hainaut and Liège, the most industrialized provinces in Belgium, and in Antwerp and Brabant, the most urbanized ones. Subsequently, as fertility control appeared and as I_h fell back from its peak levels just before the turn of the century, a positive correlation emerged between ΔI_h 1880–1890 and the index of urbanization and industrialization.

5.7 *Infant Mortality and Marital Fertility*

The history of infant mortality in Belgium is a research topic on its own. In this section, we have to limit ourselves to a brief description of the orders of magnitude involved and to the relationship that infant mortality might possibly bear to the decline of marital fertility.

First, regional differences with respect to infant mortality were extremely large throughout the nineteenth century, especially during the last decades. In the four years centered around 1890, the infant mortality rate, defined as the number of deaths before age 1 per 1,000 live births in the same period, varied from 260 in several West Flanders arrondissements to about 100 in the Walloon arrondissements of Thuin and Philippeville. Most of this very large variation is attributable to the heterogeneity of Flemish infant mortality rates. This is clearly shown in Map 5.5 and in Table 5.8, where these rates are presented by arrondisse-

TABLE 5.8

INFANT MORTALITY RATE, BY ARRONDISSEMENT: 1890 TO 1910

Flanders	1890	1900	1910
Aalst	151	146	143
Antwerp	197	186	153
Bruges	182	194	158
Brussels	184	168	157
Dendermonde	203	201	170
Diksmuide	264	242	214
Eeklo	161	175	144
Ghent	232	228	191
Hasselt	150	141	107
Kortrijk	191	218	178
Leuven	136	128	113
Maaseik	156	160	154
Mechelen	193	150	143
Ostend	267	286	240
Oudenaarde	139	138	105
Roeselare	211	247	227
St. Niklaas	246	243	204
Tielt	167	171	161
Tongeren	157	142	132
Turnhout	150	140	125
Veurne	269	248	203
Ypres	214	225	178
Wallonia			
Arlon	154	150	130
Ath	118	100	86
Bastogne	119	137	92
Charleroi	140	149	117
Dinant	117	110	91
Huy	123	106	85
Liège	154	136	120
Marche	128	115	82
Mons	125	115	88
Namur	137	124	101
Neufchâteau	123	112	87
Nivelles	131	123	99
Philippeville	108	100	73
Soignies	129	120	95
Thuin	107	124	98
Tournai	140	139	103
Verviers	163	145	112
Virton	137	112	92
Waremme	119	113	96

SOURCE: Vital registration statistics, Institut National de Statistique - Nationaal Instituut voor de Statistiek, Brussels.

NOTE: Infant mortality rate is defined as the number of deaths before age 1 per 1,000 live births.

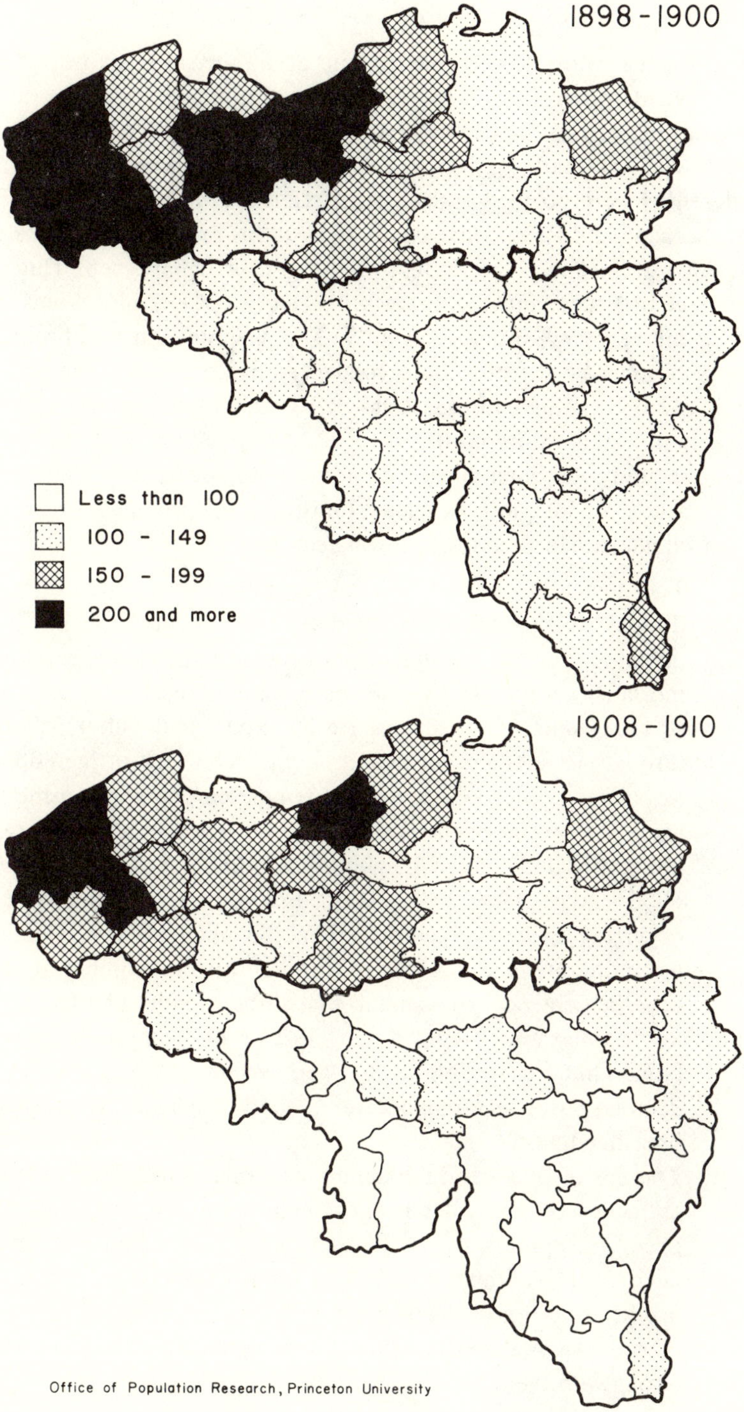

Map 5.5 Infant Mortality Rate, by Arrondissement: 1898–1900 and 1908–1910.

ment for the whole of the country. It can be seen that six out of eight West Flanders arrondissements had infant mortality rates above the 200 level at the turn of the century and that three out of the six arrondissements of East Flanders fall in this category. Most of these regional differences were not new, but can be found also in the Napoleonic era (J. Duchène and R. Lesthaeghe, 1975). In his report to the minister of the interior in Paris, the prefect of the Escaut département (later the province of East Flanders) expressed as early as 1807 his astonishment about the very high infant mortality. The phenomenon was brought to the government's attention by several persons after him. The situation probably deteriorated further after 1870, and there was no sign of a drop in infant mortality until about 1903. In 1907, the first attempt was made to study the phenomenon in a more systematic way. The author of the study, C. Jacquart, restricted himself to the provinces of East and West Flanders. He cited the following causes:

1. The decrease, or total lack, of lactation. In a series of reports drafted by the provincial medical commissions, the decline of lactation is nearly always mentioned as the prime cause of infant mortality. Very shortly after birth, infants received a concoction of milk, water (not always fresh), flour, and butter, often fed through an infected bottle and nipple. This lack of lactation was associated with the high rates of female participation in the labor force. As soon as the mother started work in the factory, the infant was left with a neighbor, grandmother, or another child (C. Jacquart, 1907, pp. 19-32). In a sample of 6,312 live births occurring to women employed in the linen industry, an infant mortality rate of 403 was found, and of the total number of deaths, 46.3 percent occurred in the first three months of life. Slightly lower rates were found among infants of mothers employed at home, but, according to P. Verhaegen (1902, 2, p. 9), the *dentellières* or lace-makers were equally negligent with respect to breastfeeding.
2. The use of opiates. In Flanders widespread use was made of an extraction of poppy heads or of opiate syrup, locally called "slaapgoed" (sleeping syrup). This extraction was commonly given to keep crying infants and children quiet. The use of opiates may not have been a cause of death in itself, but it cut off the normal alarm system through which infants indicate that something is wrong with them.

3. The pollution of drinking water. In many parts of Flanders a serious problem of drinking water existed until after World War I, when water supplies collected in the Ardennes were distributed over the entire territory. Before that period, the countryside remained exclusively dependent on local artificial wells. In the alluvial plains of Polders, for instance, the impermeable clay layers polluted the water very severely. In addition, the drinking water of the urban centers was often taken from canals that were becoming increasingly polluted by industrial or organic wastes (e.g., retting of flax).

Obviously, several social and environmental factors may have been responsible for the very high infant mortality rates in the western part of the country. Very specifically, the use of opiates may show that the local mentality was not highly child-oriented.

As previously indicated, infant mortality rates did not decline in Belgium before the turn of the century. This means that, with the exception of Limburg, the decline in marital fertility preceded the change in infant mortality. There was a time lag between the start of the change in the two phenomena, but this time lag goes in the opposite direction from what would be expected on the basis of the hypotheses of Leibenstein, Ohlin, et al. As a result, it is difficult to argue that the drop in infant mortality was among the factors that contributed to the start of the marital fertility transition in Belgium. Not only is the time lag reversed, but also there is not even a strong correlation between infant mortality levels and marital fertility in cross sections. The various correlation coefficients are presented in Table 5.9. The values of these coefficients are low in both language regions and in all four quadrants of the table. Moreover, when there is some association, the sign of the coefficient is often in the opposite direction to what could be expected on the basis of the theses of Leibenstein, Ohlin, or Schultz. Particularly in Flanders, there is a negative relation after 1900 between infant mortality rates and levels of I_g (Quadrant A) instead of the expected increasing value. Even when the relative changes in both variables are compared, hardly any association can be found (Quadrant D). In Wallonia, the highest correlation coefficients are found in Quadrant D, but the sign indicates that arrondissements with the greatest reduction in infant mortality are the ones that tended to have the smallest decrease in marital fertility.

TABLE 5.9

MARITAL FERTILITY MEASURES (I_g AND ΔI_g), CORRELATION WITH INFANT MORTALITY MEASURES, FLANDERS AND WALLONIA: 1880 TO 1910

			Correlation coefficients							
			I_g				ΔI_g			
Area	Measure	Date	1880	1890	1900	1910	1880-1900	1890-1900	1900-1910	1890-1910
Flanders (N = 22)	Infant Mortality ($_1q_0$)	1890	+.250	+.085	-.156	-.252	+.419	+.432	+.363	+.260
		1900	+.351	+.235	-.005	-.152	+.275	+.318	+.304	+.227
		1910	+.343	+.246	+.025	-.100	+.240	+.291	+.262	+.188
	Relative change in infant mortality ($\Delta _1q_0$)	1890-1900	-.282	-.362	-.337	-.267	+.243	+.168	+.125	+.100
		1900-1910	+.050	-.010	-.032	-.123	+.041	-.007	+.086	+.110
Wallonia (N = 19)	Infant mortality ($_1q_0$)	1890	+.273	+.218	+.094	-.031	+.009	+.167	+.266	+.230
		1900	+.314	+.235	+.135	+.064	+.086	+.202	+.219	+.208
		1910	+.228	+.127	+.001	-.112	+.198	+.280	+.369	+.341
	Relative change in infant mortality ($\Delta _1q_0$)	1890-1900	-.086	.026	.102	.154	-.331	-.296	-.325	-.325
		1900-1910	-.064	.024	.141	.280	-.244	-.283	-.443	-.401

NOTE: $\Delta _1q_0(t,\ t+x)$ is defined as $\dfrac{_1q_0(t) - {_1q_0}(t+x)}{_1q_0(t) - 0.050}$. ΔI_g is defined as $\dfrac{I_{g1880} - I_{g1910}}{I_{g1880} - .200}$.

Hence, on the basis of the reversed time sequence and on the basis of the lack of correlation in the cross sections, we suspect that the decline in infant mortality played a rather insignificant role in the history of the marital fertility transition in Belgium. Most probably, other factors were already conditioning marital fertility in the direction of a decline before the weight of an infant mortality reduction could be felt.

5.8 *Nuptiality and Fertility*

In Section 5.3 we presented three hypotheses linking marriage patterns to marital fertility. In hypothesis A, a decrease in the mean age at marriage occurs first and the resulting increase in the length of the reproductive span would then be a factor contributing to the gradual adoption of fertility control. In hypothesis B, marital fertility declines before nuptiality changes, and later on, the classic Malthusian function of late and nonuniversal marriage gradually weakens. Finally, according to hypothesis C, the two phenomena are independent, and any statistical relationship between them is spurious and caused by the fact that both nuptiality and martial fertility are responding to a common set of other social, economic, or cultural determinants.

The first element that may help in making a choice among these alternatives is the time sequence of the start of the nuptiality changes and the marital fertility transition. After setting the 1856 levels of I_g and I_m at 100 and expressing the values for later years in terms of this index, we see that heterogeneity develops among the provinces with respect to this time sequence. This is shown on Figure 5.2. In the province of Luxemburg, the indices of I_m and I_g evolve in a more or less parallel way: the upward movement of I_m and the downward trend in I_g both take off at approximately 1866. In the provinces of Liège and Brabant (and also in Hainaut and Antwerp, which are not shown on Figure 5.2), the upward trend in I_m seems to precede the decline in I_g by just a few years. In the remaining Flemish areas, and most clearly in Limburg, the nuptiality change is definitely well under way before the decline in I_g occurs. Hence, there is only a very weak indication of a time lag in Wallonia, whereas there are stronger indications that the nuptiality change occurred before the marital fertility change in the Flemish areas. At any rate, on the basis of what is shown on Figure 5.2, hypothesis B receives no support in either language area.

A second method for determining which of the three hypotheses corresponds best to the data consists of introducing a third variable that is known to have a considerable influence on both nuptiality and marital fertility . We can then test in what direction the statistical control of this variable influences the original correlations between nuptiality and marital fertility. These original correlation coefficients are presented in Table 5.10. There, nuptiality is measured as the proportion of ever-married females aged 20 to 24 (*EM*) and marital fertility is expressed as I_g. If we compare the order of magnitude of the coefficients by language area, it becomes obvious that the relationships are stronger in Wallonia than in Flanders. This is especially so in Quadrants C and D where the relative change rate in the proportion ever-married (ΔEM) is highly correlated with I_g and with ΔI_g in Wallonia. Also, the signs of the coefficients in Quadrants C and D are always in the expected direction in Wallonia, but not in Flanders. This hints that the nuptiality and marital fertility changes in Flanders are more likely to be spuriously related (strategy C): when the original correlations between *EM* (ΔEM) and I_g (ΔI_g) are low, the partial correlation between them will be more likely to approach the zero level once we have controlled for the presumed common causal factor influencing both *EM* (ΔEM) and I_g (ΔI_g).

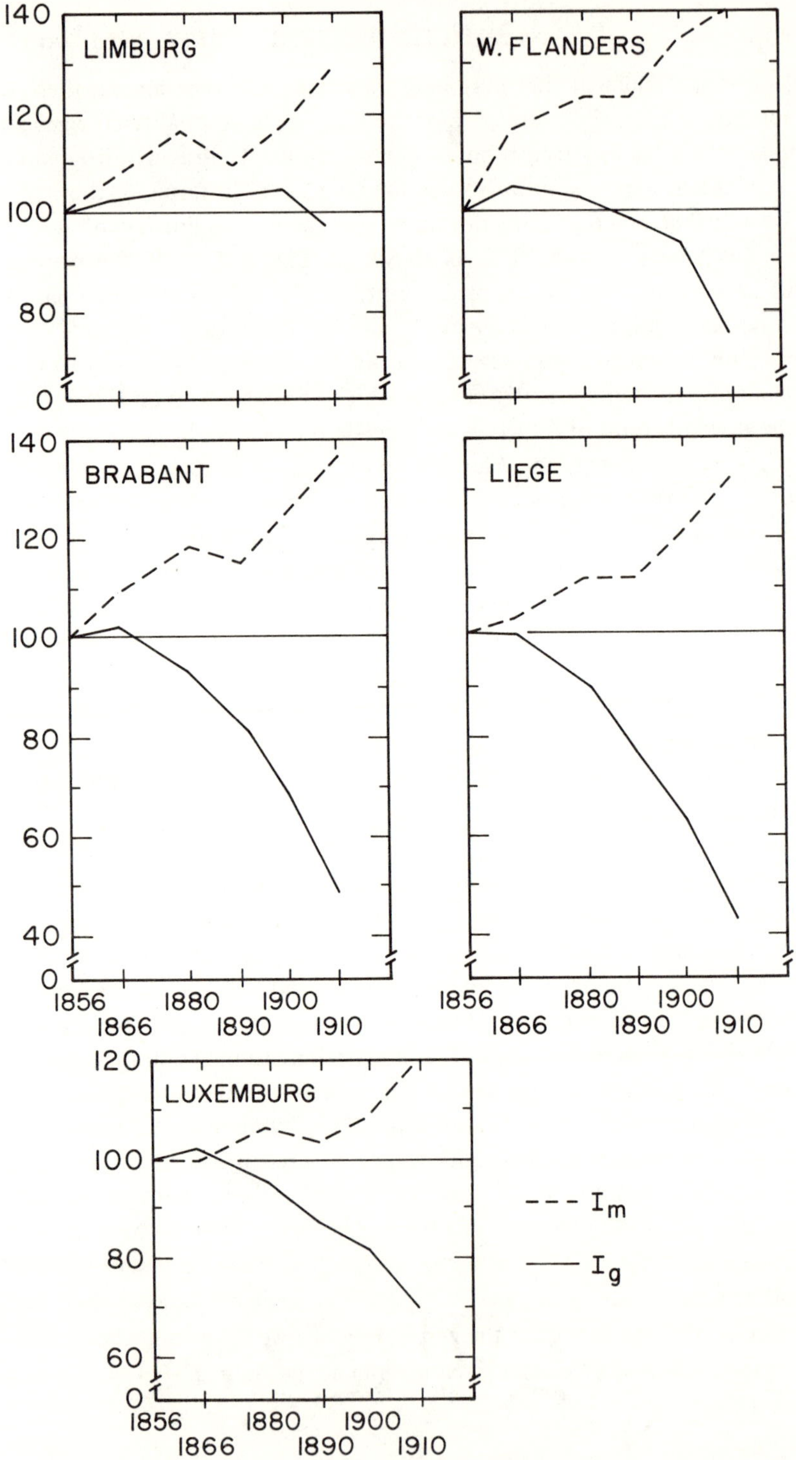

Office of Population Research, Princeton University

Figure 5.2 Marital Fertility (I_g) and Proportion Married (I_m), Levels Relative to 1856, Selected Provinces: 1856 to 1910.

TABLE 5.10

MARITAL FERTILITY MEASURES (I_g AND ΔI_g), CORRELATIONS WITH MEASURES OF PROPORTION EVER-MARRIED AGED 20-24 (EM AND ΔEM), FLANDERS AND WALLONIA: 1880 TO 1910

			Correlation coefficients							
			I_g				ΔI_g			
Area	Measure	Date	1880	1890	1900	1910	1880-1900	1890-1900	1900-1910	1890-1910
Flanders (N = 22)	EM	1880	-.558	-.587	-.698	-.591	+.635	+.701	+.434	+.536
		1890	-.305	-.385	-.587	-.650	+.640	+.715	+.569	+.668
		1900	-.327	-.383	-.596	-.631	+.640	+.742	+.549	+.656
		1910	-.316	-.376	-.574	-.583	+.617	+.709	+.495	+.604
	ΔEM	1880-1900	+.452	+.415	+.248	+.010	-.067	-.005	+.113	+.123
		1890-1900	-.193	-.158	-.271	-.228	+.267	+.374	+.193	+.256
		1900-1910	+.025	+.001	+.059	+.136	-.061	-.107	-.153	-.154
		1890-1910	-.191	-.136	-.200	-.109	+.196	+.262	+.065	+.122
Wallonia (N = 19)	EM	1880	-.714	-.692	-.773	-.706	+.762	+.639	+.466	+.562
		1890	-.688	-.728	-.764	-.695	+.788	+.585	+.483	+.550
		1900	-.764	-.787	-.822	-.752	+.812	+.580	+.503	+.562
		1910	-.781	-.794	-.836	-.755	+.803	+.579	+.465	+.539
	ΔEM	1880-1900	-.716	-.781	-.765	-.696	+.765	+.459	+.473	+.491
		1890-1900	-.789	-.798	-.819	-.748	+.778	+.518	+.482	+.522
		1900-1910	-.635	-.608	-.662	-.555	+.575	+.443	+.201	+.317
		1890-1910	-.792	-.787	-.823	-.733	+.758	+.526	+.409	+.481

NOTE: $\Delta EM_{t,\, t+1}$ is defined as $\frac{EM_{t+1} - EM_t}{.800 - EM_t}$. ΔI_g is defined as $\frac{I_{g1880} - I_{g1910}}{I_{g1880} - .200}$.

Let us now see what happens with the correlations of Table 5.10 once a third variable is introduced. As a common determinant of nuptiality and marital fertility we have chosen the logarithmic index of occupational structure, the principle indicator of industrialization and the most powerful correlate of *EM* and I_g. The results are given in Table 5.11. There, hypotheses A, B, and C, linking nuptiality and marital fertility, are rewritten to allow for the influence of occupational structure. On the right-hand side, *EM* (ΔEM) and I_g (ΔI_g) are supposed to be related in a spurious way (hypothesis C), and the correlation between them (r_{23}) is the product of the correlations between each of them and the occupational structure. Hence, we expect that $r_{23}=r_{12}\, r_{13}$, or, in terms of partial correlations, that $r_{23.1}=0$ (i.e., the correlation between *EM* and I_g reduces to zero once the effect of occupational structure is controlled for).

For each of the models, we have indicated in the first column the size of the correlation coefficient (r) corresponding to the spurious relation

TABLE 5.11

MARITAL FERTILITY (I_g), PROPORTION EVER-MARRIED AGED 20-24 (EM), AND OCCUPATIONAL STRUCTURE RELATIONSHIP TESTED IN THREE CAUSAL MODELS, FLANDERS AND WALLONIA: 1880 TO 1910

					$x_1 \to x_3 \to x_2$			$x_1 \to x_2 \to x_3$			$x_1 \to x_2$, $x_1 \to x_3$		
					Hypothesis A			Hypothesis B			Hypothesis C		
Area	x_1	x_2	x_3	Date	r_{12}	r'_{12}	diff.	r_{13}	r'_{13}	diff.	r_{23}	r'_{23}	diff.
Flanders	Log. Occup. Structure	I_g	EM	1880	-.519	-.354	.165	.634	.290	.344	-.558	-.329	.299
				1890	-.447	-.257	.190	.653	.169	.484	-.369	-.225	.144
				1900	-.714	-.466	.248	.784	.425	.359	-.595	-.560	.035
				1910	-.644	-.465	.179	.794	.377	.417	-.586	-.511	.075
	Log. Occup. Structure	ΔI_g	ΔEM	1880-1900	-.052	.035	.087	-.023	.770	.793	-.067	.027	.094
				1890-1910	.081	.206	.125	.025	.749	.724	.122	.154	.032
				1890-1900	.312	.312	.000	.117	.835	.718	.374	.261	.113
				1900-1910	-.083	-.076	.007	.116	.611	.495	-.153	-.046	.107
	Log. Occup. Structure	ΔI_g	ΔEM	1880-1900	-.026	.186	.212	-.013	.387	.400	-.067	.072	.139
				1890-1910	.060	.480	.420	.059	.491	.432	.122	.336	.214
				1890-1900	.195	.579	.384	.217	.521	.304	.374	.302	.072
				1900-1910	-.069	-.064	.005	.009	.448	.439	-.153	-.029	.124
Wallonia	Log. Occup. Structure	I_g	EM	1880	-.537	-.471	.066	.660	.383	.277	-.714	-.354	.460
				1890	-.619	-.534	.085	.734	.451	.283	-.728	-.454	.274
				1900	-.704	-.663	.046	.804	.583	.224	-.822	-.617	.205
				1910	-.768	-.577	.191	.764	.580	.184	-.755	-.587	.168
	Log. Occup. Structure	ΔI_g	ΔEM	1880-1900	.619	.670	.051	.513	.809	.296	.765	.542	.223
				1890-1910	.372	.565	.193	.272	.774	.502	.481	.437	.044
				1890-1900	.347	.614	.267	.318	.670	.352	.518	.411	.107
				1900-1910	.154	.447	.292	.090	.766	.676	.201	.342	.141
	Log. Occup. Structure	ΔI_g	ΔEM	1880-1900	.266	.671	.405	.513	.348	.165	.765	.234	.531
				1890-1910	.264	.608	.344	.292	.548	.256	.481	.333	.148
				1890-1900	.078	.524	.446	.271	.151	.120	.518	.079	.439
				1900-1910	.129	.434	.305	.087	.641	.554	.201	.278	.077

NOTES: Best fits are underlined.

$\Delta EM_{t,\ t+1}$ is defined as $\frac{EM_{t+1} - EM_t}{.800 - EM_t}$. ΔI_g is defined as $\frac{I_{g1880} - I_{g1910}}{I_{g1880} - .200}$.

(dotted lines in the figures of Table 5.11). In the second column one will find the predicted value (r') of that correlation coefficient, calculated as the product of the correlation coefficients represented by full arrows. Finally, the third column contains the absolute difference between r and r'. The analysis is performed on the levels corresponding to Quadrants A, B, and D (levels against levels, levels against changes, changes against changes).

Now, we shall see where the differences between r and r' are minimal. For hypothesis B, they are by far too large; hence, hypothesis B should be rejected. This is similar to our earlier conclusion based on the time sequences in Figure 5.2. The results in Table 5.11 do not directly indicate, however, that hypothesis C should be preferred over hypothesis A.

In Wallonia, both hypotheses seem to qualify equally well, and since we found no clear indication of a time lag between the start of the changes in nuptiality and marital fertility, we cannot make a choice between A and C. The results for Flanders are not very powerful in discriminating between the two alternatives, either. The only additional fact is that the differences between r and r' linked with hypothesis C are generally smaller in Flanders than in Wallonia.

To summarize our findings so far, it is obvious that we are justified in claiming that the nuptiality changes were not a response to the marital fertility transition. For Wallonia we cannot decide between the remaining alternatives, whereas for Flanders we prefer hypothesis C, which states the independence of nuptiality from marital fertility. In the next chapter, we introduce exogenous variables, other than the index of occupational structure, to examine this problem more closely.

There remains the relationship between nuptiality and illegitimate fertility. As a starting point, we should recall Dupâquier's three Malthusian rules in Section 3.6:

1. No conceptions outside wedlock.
2. No sharing of one dwelling by more than one couple.
3. No marriage without "establishment" (i.e., the availability of an independent means of living).

In Sections 3.9, 3.10, and 3.11 we argue that various factors were instrumental in reducing the impact of rule 3, leading to a gradual decrease in the mean age at marriage. We should then expect that the areas that broke away earlier from the Malthusian marriage pattern (rules 2 and 3), should also be the areas where the impact of rule 1 is felt to a smaller degree. In other words, one would expect a positive association between any measure of nuptiality intensity and illegitimate fertility. At first sight, this expectation comes out very well if the proportion of ever-married women aged 20-24 is correlated with I_h (see Table 5.12, Quadrant A). Also a marked positive correlation emerges in both language areas. However, when we bear in mind that the index of illegitimate fertility I_h is to some extent statistically dependent on the nuptiality intensity, we should be very careful in explaining the full strength of the correlation coefficients by referring to behavioral components. As indicated in section 4.6, we have no means of assessing more precisely to what degree a lower mean age at marriage (or a higher value of EM) provokes automatically a higher value of I_h.

TABLE 5.12

ILLEGITIMATE FERTILITY MEASURES (I_h AND ΔI_h), CORRELATION WITH PROPORTION EVER-MARRIED AGED 20-24 (EM), FLANDERS AND WALLONIA: 1880 TO 1910

		Correlation coefficients between EM and				
		I_h				ΔI_h
Area	Date	1880	1890	1900	1910	1880-1910
Flanders (N = 22)	1880	+.763	--	--	--	+.257
	1890	--	+.679	--	--	--
	1900	--	--	+.818	--	--
	1910	--	--	--	+.745	--
Wallonia (N = 19)	1880	+.675	--	--	--	+.406
	1890	--	+.726	--	--	--
	1900	--	--	+.709	--	--
	1910	--	--	--	+.657	--

NOTE: ΔI_h 1880-1900 is defined as $\frac{I_{h1880} - I_{h1910}}{I_{h1880}}$; all values of ΔI_h 1880-1910 are positive.

Consequently, the correlation coefficients in Table 5.12 are at the same time reflecting the effects of a breakdown of Dupâquier's Malthusian rules and the strictly statistical dependence of I_h on nuptiality. This confusion may be very unfortunate, but we have no means to eliminate it on the basis of the available information.

The results in Table 5.12 bear striking similarities to the correlations between industrialization-urbanization and I_h of ΔI_h (see Table 5.7, Section 5.6). There, too, it was found that the correlation coefficient kept its positive sign when ΔI_h became the dependent variable, but that the magnitude of the coefficient went down considerably in Quadrant B compared to Quadrant A. Hence, nuptiality changes and changes in the occupational structure or degree of urbanization seem to have remarkably similar effects on I_h and ΔI_h. This finding becomes less remarkable, however, if we know that the industrialization-urbanization factor largely determines the pace of the nuptiality change and that, consequently, these two variables are closely correlated themselves. Once more, the presumed causal link between independent variables conditions the outcome of the correlation analysis with respect to the dependent variable, I_h or ΔI_h. In this perspective, a part of the effect of industrialization-urbanization on I_h or ΔI_h may have gone through the intermediate variable nuptiality. A fuller exploration of this subject will be taken up again in chapter 6, since a multivariate approach is clearly necessary.

5.9 *Language Homogeneity and Marital Fertility*

We have already detected a fundamental difference in the marital fertility transition between the Walloon and the Flemish areas (see Section 4.4). This difference emerged not only along the language border, but also in the various communities that make up the Brussels urban area. As a result, we may also expect that certain linguistic minorities either in Flanders or in Wallonia could have a different pattern of marital fertility decrease and could exercise an influence on the level of I_g in the arrondissements.

In Flanders, such linguistic minorities were found in the middle-sized and large urban areas. They consisted mainly of well-educated bourgeoisie and of industrial entrepreneurs who had gradually adopted the French language during the eighteenth and nineteenth centuries. As these groups formed a leading social class, they were often imitated by others in their immediate environment; the use of the French language was a major instrument through which upward social mobility was manifested. Also, the Flemish dialects, characterized by substantial differences in vocabulary and pronounciation, did not qualify as a teaching language. In the Netherlands a standard form of Dutch was adopted, but in Flanders it was the French language that was chosen as the basis for all teaching in secondary schools and universities. In fact, no courses were offered in Dutch in the two universities located in Flanders until after World War I, and even then the argument was voiced that Dutch was totally unfit for scientific use. For these two related reasons, a fairly large segment of the Flemish population became Francophone, and this trend continued until about World War I. After that date, the trend was reversed, but the phenomenon continued to have very serious political implications in the 1930s and 1940s.

What is, however, more important for the study of the marital fertility decline is that between 1880 and 1910 an influential social group had developed that kept itself culturally distinct on the basis of education, upward social mobility, and earning capacity. As this group was breaking away from almost all forms of the traditional Flemish ways of life, including the use of the language, it may very well be that this Francophone, bilingual group was also breaking away from traditional attitudes and behavior with respect to fertility.

With the above in mind, we shall try to operationalize the concept of language censuses held jointly with the population censuses. For Flanders, the index of language homogeneity will be defined as the proportion of persons above age 15 who have a speaking and writing knowledge of only Dutch (or Flemish). This definition serves us doubly well. Apart from the upper classes, certain groups of laborers acquired some command of French. They, too, are excluded from the numerator of the index of language homogeneity. These groups were made up primarily of seasonal laborers who worked in France for substantial periods of time. Obviously, during their stay in France, some achieved an elementary command of the language, and, as this was valued positively in the Belgian context at the turn of the century, it is most unlikely that they would fail to report that knowledge when the census agents came around. According to the import thesis, this group of laborers may have introduced certain forms of contraception at home.

Another element that influences the index of language homogeneity is the presence of a few predominantly Walloon villages in Flemish arrondissements and vice versa. As the language border did not completely coincide with the borders of the arrondissements, we find, for example, small Walloon communities in the southern parts of the arrondissements of Kortrijk, Oudenaarde, and Tienen, and Flemish communities in the arrondissements of Waremme and Liège. From the study of fertility in the sample of villages along the language border (Section 4.4), it is clear that this element should be taken into account as well.

Flemish communities were not the only non-Francophone groups in Wallonia: there were some German dialects spoken along the German and Luxemburg borders. This was especially the case in a large part of the arrondissement of Arlon and to a lesser degree in Bastogne and Verviers. The use of these dialects decreased considerably between 1880 and 1910 in favor of French. Though a substantial German-speaking area was annexed after World War I and added to the arrondissement of Verviers, this does not affect our indices of language homogeneity, since we do not go beyond 1920. Wallonia also contained a non-negligible population of migrants from Flanders or from other European nations. In general, these persons achieved a certain command of French quickly, as there was very little opportunity to use their own language outside their family circle. By far the greatest proportion of bilingual individuals were not original Walloons who had learned Dutch, but immigrants who had learned French. Consequently, our index of language homogeneity for Walloon areas has been defined as the proportion of persons above age 15 with a knowledge of French (or of a Walloon dialect) only. Data for these indices are presented in Table 5.13 and are illustrated in Maps 5.6 and 5.7. They show that knowledge and use of French increased considerably in Belgium as Flanders became less homogeneous and as Wallonia became more homogeneous with respect to language.

There remains the problem of the communities that make up Brussels.

TABLE 5.13

LANGUAGE HOMOGENEITY, BY ARRONDISSEMENT: 1880 TO 1910

	1880	1890	1900	1910
Flanders				
Aalst	91.6	89.6	86.8	89.0
Antwerp	84.5	80.4	72.2	73.6
Bruges	89.7	87.2	81.4	79.5
Brussels	57.0	45.1	37.0	35.0
Dendermonde	92.2	92.6	90.0	91.1
Diksmuide	93.3	90.7	88.9	88.5
Eeklo	94.4	93.2	91.1	92.2
Ghent	86.9	82.2	78.9	78.0
Hasselt	80.2	84.5	79.9	81.4
Kortrijk	73.7	71.8	65.8	66.1
Leuven	84.4	80.1	75.1	76.6
Maaseik	89.0	90.7	87.5	87.9
Mechelen	90.5	88.4	84.2	84.4
Ostend	87.0	88.2	77.3	76.5
Oudenaarde	83.6	82.0	75.3	79.9
Roeselare	92.6	91.8	87.1	88.7
St. Niklaas	93.5	93.7	90.6	89.9
Tielt	92.8	93.4	88.9	90.3
Tongeren	80.2	77.1	70.6	72.4
Turnhout	95.1	94.1	90.1	90.5
Veurne	90.0	86.5	79.3	80.2
Ypres	74.3	69.2	63.3	67.5
Wallonia				
Arlon	46.3	55.6	61.6	67.5
Ath	94.2	92.8	93.3	92.8
Bastogne	89.6	88.6	88.6	90.0
Charleroi	95.3	94.7	93.1	92.6
Dinant	99.3	98.9	98.6	98.4
Huy	99.0	98.6	97.8	98.0
Liège	89.1	86.1	85.0	86.7
Marche	99.4	99.0	98.7	98.8
Mons	98.2	98.4	97.7	96.6
Namur	99.4	97.4	96.9	96.9
Neufchâteau	98.7	98.3	97.7	97.7
Nivelles	97.7	95.9	94.6	94.2
Philippeville	99.5	99.0	99.1	98.2
Soignies	88.3	87.7	86.5	87.1
Thuin	98.9	98.8	98.0	97.0
Tournai	97.4	95.8	94.9	94.1
Verviers	82.2	80.4	66.5	80.4
Virton	97.4	97.0	96.8	96.7
Waremme	83.5	82.6	81.0	80.9

SOURCE: Population censuses of 1880, 1890 1900, and 1910, Institut National de Statistique - Nationaal Instituut voor de Statistiek, Brussels.

NOTE: The index of language homogeneity is defined as the ratio of the population aged 15 and older which speaks only the language of the area (Dutch in Flanders, French in Wallonia) to the total population aged 15 and older.

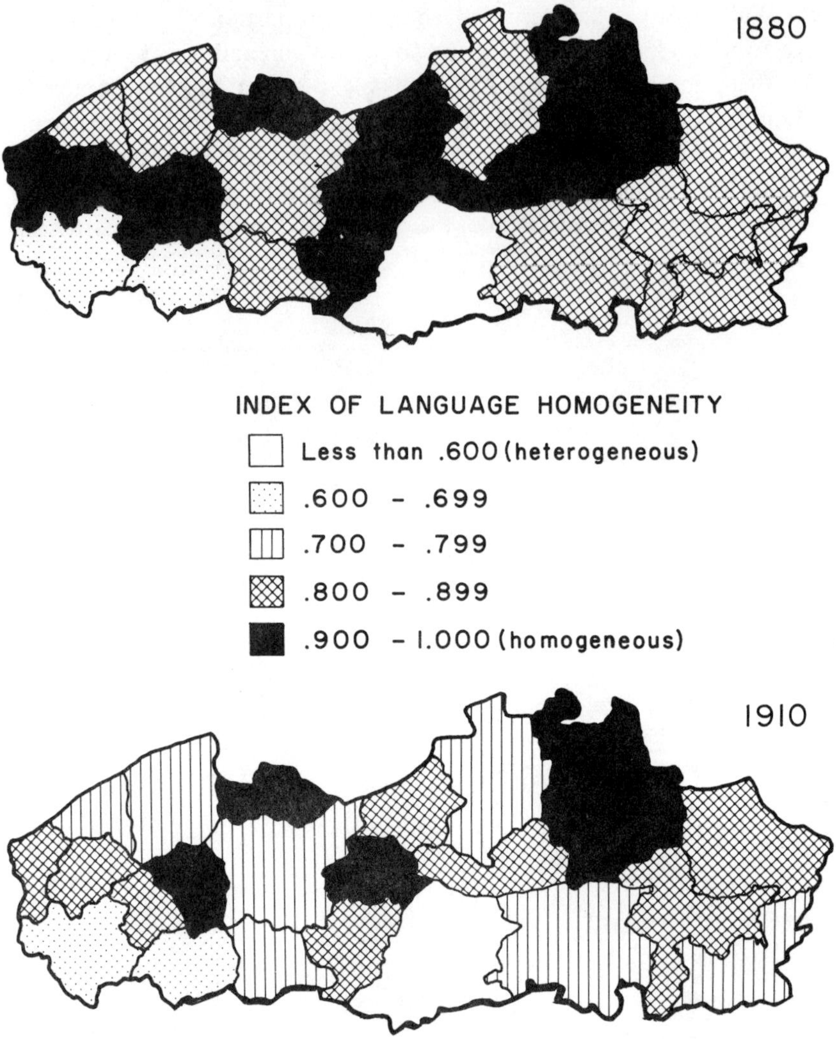

Office of Population Research, Princeton University

Map 5.6 Language Homogeneity, Percentage Speaking Dutch, by Arrondissement, Flanders: 1880 and 1910.

Around 1900 these communities contained more persons who spoke only French than persons who were either bilingual (predominantly of Flemish origin) or Flemish-speaking. In the rest of the Brussels arrondissement, however, the situation was reversed. If the index of language homogeneity is calculated on the basis of the total arrondisse-

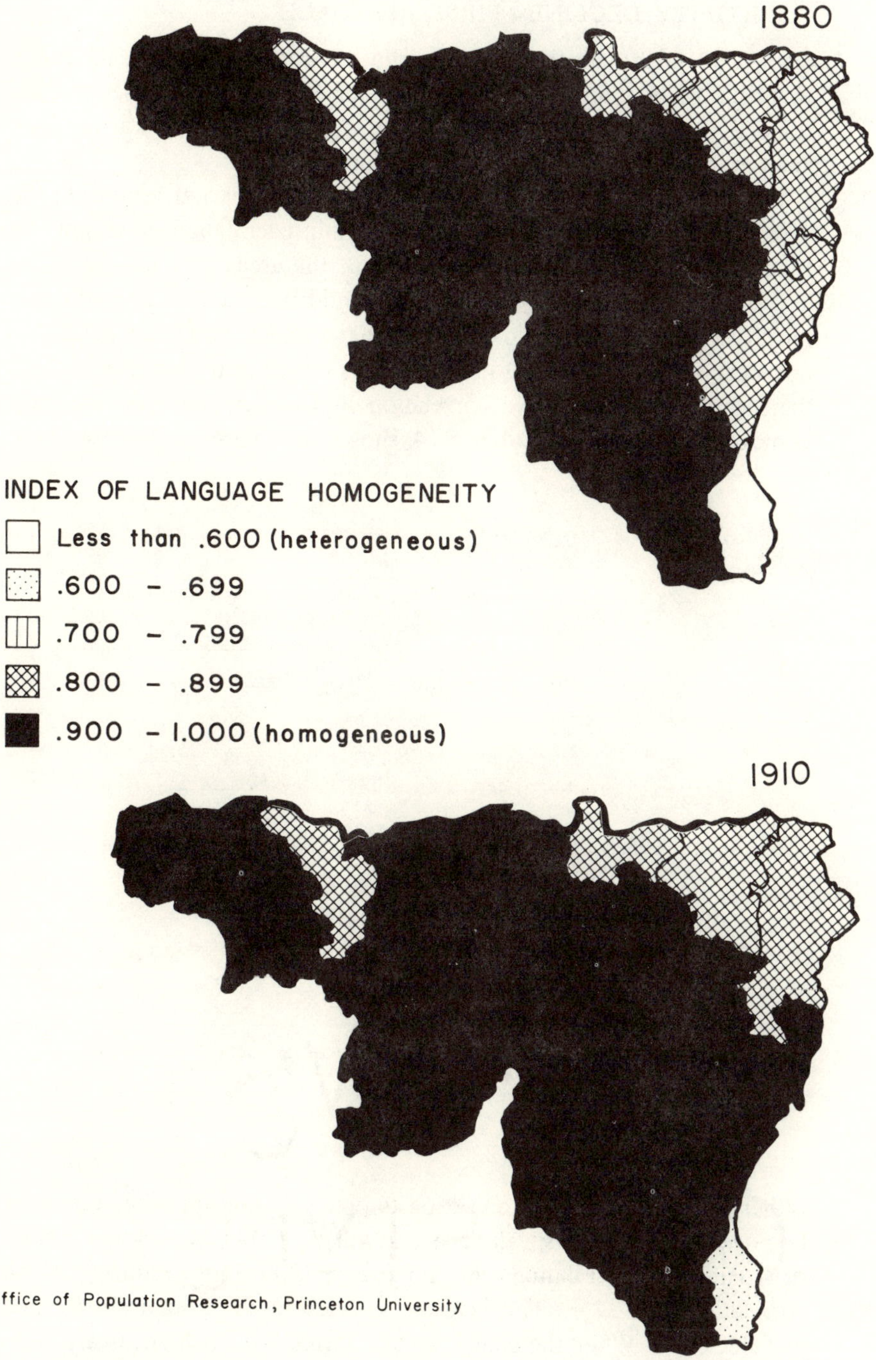

Map 5.7 Language Homogeneity, Percentage Speaking French, by Arrondissement, Wallonia: 1880 and 1910.

ment, a Flemish majority shows up, but, as can be expected, the index is substantially smaller than in any other Belgian arrondissement, irrespective of whether we define the index for the Brussels arrondissement in the way we did for Flanders or for Wallonia.

Let us now see whether the hypothesis linking marital fertility to the degree of language homogeneity holds within each language region. In Flanders we expect a positive association: the areas that are characterized by a high language homogeneity should maintain more traditional fertility values and behavior and thus have higher values of I_g. These areas can also be expected to experience a slower fertility transition, i.e., there should be a negative correlation in Flanders between language homogeneity and ΔI_g. Table 5.14 shows that these hypotheses hold

TABLE 5.14

MARITAL FERTILITY MEASURES (I_g AND ΔI_g), CORRELATION WITH LANGUAGE HOMOGENEITY, FLANDERS AND WALLONIA: 1880 TO 1910

		Correlation coefficients between index of language homogeneity and							
		I_g				ΔI_g			
Area	Date	1880	1890	1900	1910	1880-1900	1890-1900	1900-1910	1890-1910
Flanders (N = 22)	1880	+.735	--	--	--	-.430	--	--	--
	1890	--	+.784	--	--	--	-.552	--	-.526
	1900	--	--	+.738	--	--	--	-.553	--
	1910	--	--	--	+.653	--	--	--	--
Wallonia (N = 19)	1880	-.353	--	--	--	+.143	--	--	--
	1890	--	-.321	--	--	--	+.042	--	+.107
	1900	--	--	-.241	--	--	--	+.061	--
	1910	--	--	--	-.184	--	--	--	--

NOTES: The index of language homogeneity is defined as the ratio of the population aged 15 and older which speaks only the language of the area (Dutch in Flanders, French in Wallonia) to the total population aged 15 and older.

ΔI_g is defined as $\dfrac{I_{g1880} - I_{g1910}}{I_{g1880} - .200}$.

rather well. In Wallonia, one expects precisely the opposite: the more homogeneous French-speaking areas will probably have lower values of I_g (negative correlation) and a more rapid fertility decline (positive correlation with ΔI_g). This is also supported by the evidence presented in Table 5.14. When the magnitudes of correlation coefficients are compared between the two language regions, we find that a lack of homogeneity had a markedly greater influence on Flemish than on Walloon levels of I_g. This may reflect an important sociological feature. As indicated earlier, the linguistic minorities in Flanders were essentially the better-educated upper and middle classes who were generally setting the fashions and trends and whose life style was imitated or despised. In Flanders there may have been a polarization of different social groups along language and fertility dimensions simultaneously. In Wallonia the linguistic minorities were composed essentially of immigrant industrial workers or relatively small rural populations, i.e., a part of the lower echelons of the social-stratification scale. By changing languages and by reducing their family size, these groups could conceal their origin as much as possible and open up two possibilities for increasing intergenerational social mobility. Consequently when the minorities in Wallonia changed their fertility behavior almost as quickly as they switched languages, we should indeed find that their presence has only a small impact on the level of I_g in the Walloon arrondissements.

5.10 *Literacy and Marital Fertility*

We argue here that the increase in educational levels, observed in Belgium (see Table 5.15) especially in the second half of the nineteenth and in the first decade of the twentieth century must have affected the degree of fertility control through more than just one of the variables specified in the theoretical framework. One can argue first that a rise in educational level would have a favorable impact on the rationality factor. Education is then seen as an instrument with which a society combats traditional beliefs, social apathy, and economic backwardness. It replaces these by greater social and political awareness, by an expansion of the cultural horizons, and, above all, by awakening a sense for critical evaluation. Individuals discover that personal and social problems may have more than just one standard solution; they detect possibilities for choice and they learn how to calculate better ways of using their own training and skills to their social and economic advantage. In this way, an improvement of the educational level should have a positive impact upon the spreading of the knowledge and means of fertility control. Moreover, an increase in educational level generally reflects an acceleration of the mechanism of social capillarity and an increase in the demand for "higher quality children," thereby altering fertility behavior.

So far, we have identified the level of education as an agent of modernization, and in this perspective we should a priori expect a nega-

TABLE 5.15

LITERACY, BY ARRONDISSEMENT: 1880 TO 1910

Flanders	1880	1890	1900	1910
Aalst	63.6	70.1	78.0	85.0
Antwerp	75.2	82.1	87.6	92.0
Bruges	63.0	72.2	80.4	86.8
Brussels	75.9	81.3	87.8	91.9
Dendermonde	63.7	69.0	77.6	84.2
Diksmuide	68.1	71.4	82.4	88.3
Eeklo	62.0	63.8	73.4	85.4
Ghent	66.4	73.8	82.4	88.9
Hasselt	68.5	75.4	84.3	90.4
Kortrijk	59.4	65.0	76.6	85.5
Leuven	69.6	81.3	85.1	91.3
Maaseik	85.0	89.2	94.8	97.5
Mechelen	77.6	82.6	88.5	93.2
Ostend	71.6	74.7	84.4	90.3
Oudenaarde	64.7	68.2	81.2	87.1
Roeselare	72.0	72.4	81.9	91.0
St. Niklaas	63.3	66.2	74.7	83.1
Tielt	66.6	72.6	82.8	91.9
Tongeren	73.1	79.6	88.9	93.9
Turnhout	75.3	78.4	84.8	90.7
Veurne	80.8	86.6	91.9	96.0
Ypres	69.7	76.5	82.6	90.4
Wallonia				
Arlon	89.2	90.3	95.5	95.7
Ath	68.2	76.1	86.6	91.0
Bastogne	89.7	93.0	96.2	98.6
Charleroi	66.4	72.9	80.7	86.3
Dinant	88.5	93.3	96.7	98.1
Huy	80.5	88.7	94.4	96.2
Liège	74.2	81.5	87.9	92.7
Marche	87.6	90.6	96.8	98.2
Mons	63.4	69.3	77.7	84.9
Namur	84.0	88.6	93.5	96.0
Neufchâteau	93.1	95.8	97.1	98.7
Nivelles	72.8	81.3	88.0	91.9
Philippeville	89.1	93.8	96.6	98.1
Soignies	62.7	71.2	79.7	85.3
Thuin	74.8	80.7	87.2	89.8
Tournai	68.9	76.4	86.3	90.0
Verviers	82.1	88.9	93.5	96.6
Virton	94.1	96.7	98.2	98.9
Waremme	76.1	84.1	90.1	93.3

SOURCE: Population census of 1880, 1890, 1900, and 1910, Institut National de Statistique - Nationaal Instituut voor de Statistiek, Brussels.

NOTE: Level of literacy is defined as the percentage of the total population aged 15-55 that can read and write.

tive correlation between education and marital fertility levels, or, a positive correlation between education and the rate of fertility decline.

Since education is an element of the socialization system, however, it can also become a forceful agent of social control. Especially when education is organized along ideological, ethical, and religious lines, it can be used as an instrument for ensuring the continuity of the traditional moral and ethical codes, rather than as an instrument of modernization. Consequently, the education factor can have a dual impact, and its effect on the fertility decline will depend to some extent on the degree to which the prevailing school system stresses continuity or the alteration of the moral code.

When we turn to the Belgian scene of the late nineteenth century and operationalize educational level (either through the degree of literacy or through the proportion of the population with at least five years of primary-school education), we should expect this two-way impact of education to emerge. As indicated earlier, Belgium had a dual school system, one section controlled by the Catholic church, the other by the state or by communal authorities. Enrollment in the Catholic schools has always been larger than that in the state schools, particularly at the turn of the century. In fact, before 1900 many villages possessed only a Catholic parish school; and when, around 1880, non-Catholics were eager to establish an alternative school system in the countryside, a school war burst out. Ever since, this dual system has yielded an ample amount of tension among families, school associations, and partners in successive coalition governments. In short, the Belgian Catholic church occupied a leading role in organizing primary education during the nineteenth century, and thanks to some active religious orders, illiteracy had almost disappeared among adults under age 55 around 1910. At the same time, however, the church exercised a monopoly in education in the rural and semirural areas of the country.

This particular situation probably explains to a large degree a number of findings that are otherwise puzzling. First, there is a negative association between the level of literacy (age group 15-55) and the level of industrialization and urbanization. To bring this out, we have calculated the percentage literate in these age groups for 1890 and 1910, as shown in Map 5.8. There were not only important increases in adult literacy between the two dates, but also marked regional differences. In Flanders, there were only two arrondissements with literacy levels above 80 percent in 1880, and these arrondissements turn out to be two typically rural ones: Veurne and Maaseik. The arrondissement with the lowest level of literacy in 1880 was Kortrijk, with just over 40 percent illiterate adults. In addition to Kortrijk, the home of much of the Flemish textile industry, all other arrondissements with a substantial female employment had low literacy levels. We find a rather analogous situation in Wallonia in 1800. The entire Hainaut industrial belt had low literacy levels, whereas the rural arrondissements of the Ardennes had the high-

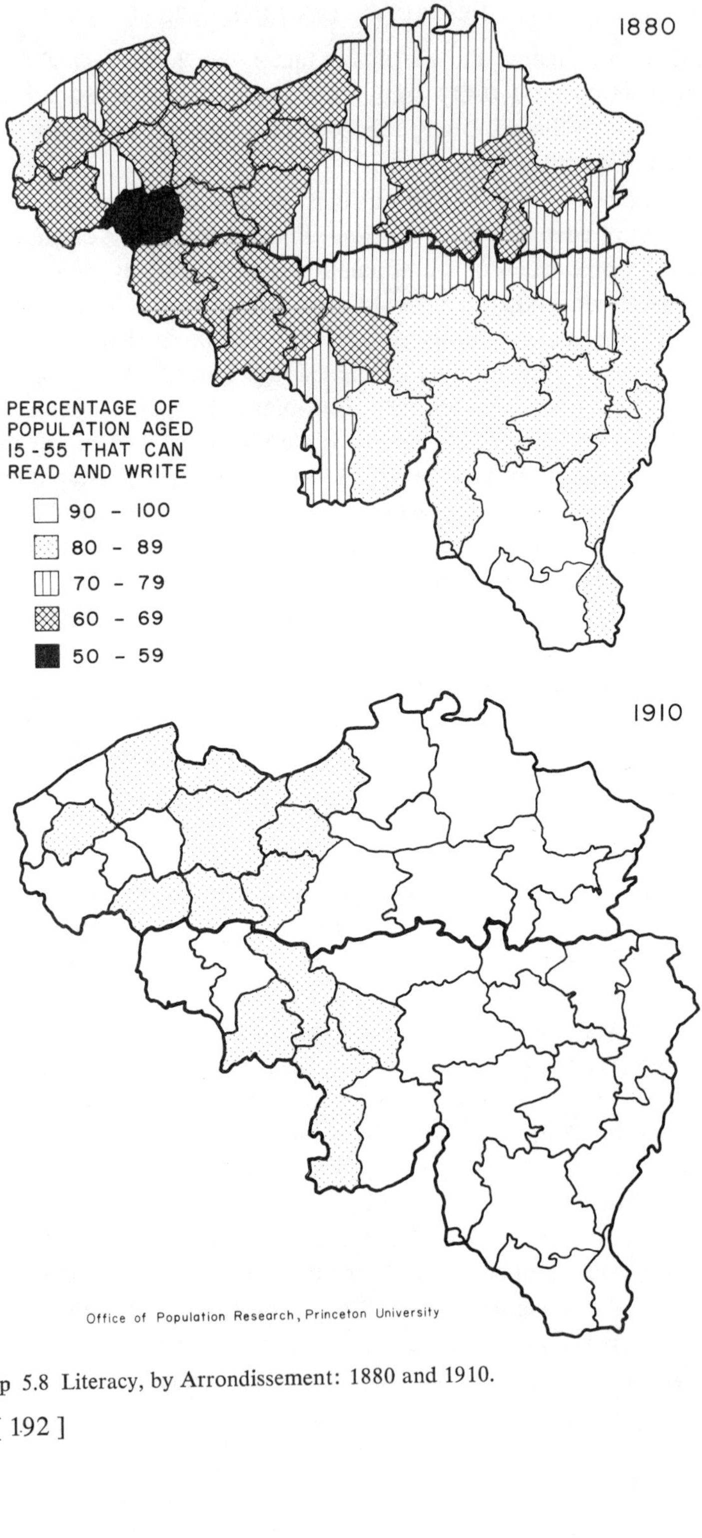

Map 5.8 Literacy, by Arrondissement: 1880 and 1910.

est levels in the country (less than 10 percent illiterate adults). In addition, the relationship between literacy level and the indicators of industrialization, urbanization, and secularization are much stronger in Wallonia than in Flanders. Thus, we find for Wallonia 1910 a correlation coefficient of −.684 between literacy level and the index of industrialization-urbanization, and −.793 between literacy and secularization. The corresponding coefficients for Flanders were only +.018 and −.100 respectively.

If we now turn to the degree of association between literacy and marital fertility, we again find a weak correlation in Flanders and a much stronger one in Wallonia. But the sign of the coefficient for Wallonia is opposite from that expected if the degree of literacy were interpreted as an indicator of modernization. The correlation coefficients are given in Table 5.16, and they show undeniably that high literacy levels in

TABLE 5.16

MARITAL FERTILITY MEASURES (I_g AND ΔI_g), CORRELATION WITH LITERACY, FLANDERS AND WALLONIA: 1880 TO 1910

		Correlation coefficients between level of literacy and							
		I_g				ΔI_g			
Area	Date	1880	1890	1900	1910	1880-1900	1890-1900	1900-1910	1890-1910
Flanders (N = 22)	1880	-.326	--	--	--	+.075	--	--	--
	1890	--	-.386	--	--	--	+.183	--	-.096
	1900	--	--	-.251	--	--	--	-.186	--
	1910	--	--	--	-.108	--	--	--	--
Wallonia (N = 19)	1880	+.412	--	--	--	-.737	--	--	--
	1890	--	+.431	--	--	--	-.784	--	-.786
	1900	--	--	+.590	--	--	--	-.707	--
	1910	--	--	--	+.677	--	--	--	--

NOTES: Level of literacy is defined as the percentage of the total population aged 15-55 that can read and write.

ΔI_g is defined as $\frac{I_{g1880} - I_{g1910}}{I_{g1880} - .200}$.

Wallonia are associated with higher marital fertility levels and with lower rates of fertility decline. In view of the negative correlation between literacy and the other exogenous variables, however, it may well be that the correlation coefficients in Table 5.16 for Wallonia are spurious to a considerable extent. Consequently, just as in the previous sections, a definite need emerges to study the entire correlation matrix and ultimately to take a multivariate approach.

As a tentative conclusion, it seems that the eradication of illiteracy through the development of primary-school education contributed more to the continuity of the existing moral norms than to their change. As a result, the degree of literacy in Belgium could be a better indicator of traditionalism than of modernization. The unexpected negative correlations with the measures of social change and with marital fertility point this out rather strikingly.

References—Chapter 5

Ariès, P. 1960. Interprétation pour une histoire des mentalités. In *La prévention des naissances dans la famille, ses origines dans les temps modernes,* by H. Bergues et al., pp. 311-327. Paris: INED, Presses Universitaires de France.

Demeny, P. 1968. Early fertility decline in Austria-Hungary: A lesson in demographic transition. *Daedalus* Spring:502-522.

De Smet, R., and Evalenko, R. 1956. *Les élections belges, explications de la répartition géographique des suffrages.* Brussels: Institut de Sociologie Solvay, Université Libre de Bruxelles.

De Smet, R., Evalenko, R., and Fraeys, W. 1958. *Atlas des élections belges, 1919–1954.* Brussels: Institut de Sociologie Solvay, Université Libre de Bruxelles.

Duchène, J., and Lesthaeghe, R. 1975. Essai de reconstitution de la population belge sous le régime francais: quelques caractéristiques démographiques de la population féminine. *Population et Famille* (Brussels).

Easterlin, R. 1972. The economics and sociology of fertility: a synthesis. Paper read at Seminar on Early Industrialization, Shifts in Fertility, and Changes in Family Structure, at Institute for Advanced Study, Princeton, N. J.

Habakkuk, H. 1972. *Population growth and economic development since 1750.* Leicester: Leicester University Press.

Henry, L. 1956. *Anciennes familles genevoises—étude démographique: XVIe-XXe siècle.* Paris: INED, Presses Universitaires de France.

Jacquart, C. 1907. *La mortalité infantile dans les Flandres: étude de démographie belge.* Brussels: Editions A. Dewit.

Landry, A. 1934. *La révolution démographique.* Paris: Recueil Sirey.

Leibenstein, H. 1957. *Economic backwardness and economic growth.* New York: J. Wiley and Sons.

Ohlin, G. 1973. Economic theory confronts population growth. Paper read at Conference of the International Economics Association, August 1973, at Valescure, France.

Peterson, W. 1960. The demographic transition in the Netherlands. *American Sociological Review* 25:334-347.

Pourbaix, C. 1973. La pratique pascale dans le diocèse de Namur. Unpublished thèse de licence at Faculté de Philosophie et Lettres, Université Catholique de Louvain.

Rombauts, W. 1971. *Het paasverzium in het Bisdon Brugge, 1840–1911*. Leuven: Editions Nauwelaerts.

Sauvy, A. 1960. Essai d'une vue d'ensemble. In *La prévention des naissances dans la famille, ses origines dans les temps modernes* by H. Bergues et al., pp. 375-391. Paris: INED, Presses Universitaires de France.

Schultz, T. P. 1973. Determinants of fertility: a micro-economic model of choice. Paper read at Conference of the International Economics Association, August 1973, at Valescure, France.

Spengler, J. J. 1938. *France faces depopulation*. Durham: University of North Carolina Press.

van der Wee, H. 1972. *Historische aspecten van de economische groei*. Antwerp-Utrecht: De Nederlandsche Boekhandel.

Chapter 6: Factors Associated with the Fertility Decline—Multivariate Analyses

In the previous chapter we described the various elements of socioeconomic change that might have been responsible for the fertility transition in Belgium, and developed a short theoretical framework. Then we translated some of this into a more readily testable set of simple propositions by operationalizing some concepts and by adding new variables that seemed relevant in the Belgian context. So far, each independent variable has been related to the fertility measures without introducing more than two variables at a time. This elementary approach is necessary in order to explore the nature of the independent variables in greater depth; but, when it comes to offering a more compact picture of all interrelations involved, this first approach is far from satisfactory. As already indicated at various points in chapter 5, a multivariate approach is indispensable: the correlation coefficients, measuring the overall strength of associations, have to be broken down into statistically measurable direct and indirect effects, and spurious relations have to be eliminated. In the subsequent sections, such a multivariate approach will be taken.

First, we shall reconsider the dichotomy between Flanders and Wallonia. Judging from the zero-order correlation coefficients presented so far, it seems that several relationships were different in the two language areas; now we shall examine whether or not the two subpopulations remain different with respect to marital fertility once we control for more than a single independent variable. An answer to this problem will be given in Section 6.1. In the other sections of the chapter we shall attempt to construct and to quantify a set of models. In these models, the demographic variables (nuptiality and marital and illegitimate fertility) will be treated as endogenous, or dependent, variables, and the other measures of social change will be taken as exogenous, or predetermined, variables.

Let us now see if the construction of these models should be done for the two subpopulations separately, or for the national population as a whole.

6.1 *Differences between the Marital Fertility Levels in the Two Language Regions after Control for the Effects of Exogenous Variables*

A classic explanation of the difference in marital fertility between Flanders and Wallonia states that it is simply the result of differences in literacy, urbanization, and especially the degree of industrialization. In other words, given that marital fertility levels are causally determined by industrialization levels, one should normally expect that the Walloon fertility decline would be different from the Flemish pattern. Translated into statistical terminology, this implies that the difference between the mean value of all I_gs in Wallonia and the mean value of all I_gs in Flanders should disappear, once we have eliminated the effect of a series of exogenous variables. In Table 6.1 we can see on the first line that the mean of 22 values of I_g for Flanders exceeded the mean of 19 values for Wallonia by .242 in 1880, by .274 in 1890, by .311 in 1900, and by .271 in 1910. Recalling that I_g takes the value of unity if Hutterite

TABLE 6.1

MARITAL FERTILITY (I_g), DIFFERENCE BETWEEN MEANS FOR FLANDERS AND WALLONIA, ADJUSTED FOR EFFECTS OF SELECTED VARIABLES BY COVARIANCE ANALYSIS: 1880 TO 1910

Difference	Covariate (X_J)	1880	1890	1900	1910
Original difference (no adjustments made for X_J)	--	.242	.274	.311	.271
Difference after adjustment for effects of X_J	Nuptiality (X_1)	.095 (.001)	.108 (.001)	.118 (.001)	.094 (.001)
	Industrialization (X_2)	.096 (.001)	.099 (.001)	.123 (.001)	.104 (.001)
	Literacy (X_3)	.127 (.001)	.142 (.001)	.167 (.001)	.155 (.001)
	Urbanization (X_4)	.132 (.001)	.153 (.001)	.177 (.001)	.159 (.001)
	Infant mortality (X_5)	.103 (.001)	.127 (.001)	.153 (.001)	.149 (.001)
	Covariates (X_1 - X_5)	.054 (.042)	.056 (N.S.)	.087 (.001)	.086 (.004)
	Secularization (X_6)	--	--	--	.011 (N.S.)
	Covariates (X_1 - X_6)	--	--	--	.025 (N.S.)

NOTE: The values in parentheses indicate the level of significance of adjusted mean differences; N.S. = not significant at .050 level.

fertility is reached, these differences mean that marital fertility levels in Flanders were on the average a quarter to a third of Hutterite fertility higher than in Wallonia.

We should like to find out whether or not these differences can be explained by differences between the Flemish and Walloon levels of (1) nuptiality, (2) industrialization, (3) literacy, (4) urbanization, (5) infant mortality, and (6) secularization.

An answer to this question can be obtained by applying the technique of analysis of covariance. In this type of analysis, we can test the null-hypothesis that the original regression lines linking I_g to any of the background variables (covariates) for each of the language regions (nominal factor) will coincide, after these lines have been adjusted to allow for differences between the two areas with respect to the background variables. If the adjusted regression lines fail to coincide, a significant difference will remain between the two means of the dependent variable I_g. Moreover, if we are dealing with samples rather than populations, and the adjusted regression lines in the samples remain parallel, then the probability that the adjusted regression lines in the populations are the same will be very small (depending, of course, on the number of degrees of freedom and the size of the two samples).

The results of such operations are presented in Table 6.1, using five covariates for 1880, 1890, and 1900, and adding a sixth for 1910, when we are able to introduce an operationalized proxy for secularization. Before we turn to the details of that table, we should specify that nuptiality is operationalized here as the index of proportion married (I_m), and that industrialization is measured by the percentage of the male active population engaged in agriculture. (Recalling Section 5.6, we note that the composite index of industrialization-urbanization cannot be used here, since it contains a variable that is measured in a different way for Flanders and Wallonia. Therefore, another variable, a nearly perfect correlate of the composite index, is chosen for our purposes here.) The remaining variables of Table 6.1 are operationalized in the same way as in chapter 5.

If we now turn to Table 6.1, we see that a very important proportion of the original difference between the means of I_g in Flanders and Wallonia persists after controlling for the separate effects of nuptiality, industrialization, literacy, urbanization, and infant mortality. Hence, if the two language regions had been identical with respect to any one of these five covariates, they would still have had an important difference in marital fertility at the four dates at the start of the fertility transition. Moreover, if Flemish and Walloon arrondissements had had the same means for all five covariates combined, the difference in their mean levels of I_g would still range between .054 and .087. These differences are again significant for 1880, 1900, and 1910 at the .05 level (and at the 0.65 level for 1890).

The results of Table 6.1 for the first five covariates indicate very clearly that the nominal factor (here the distinction between the two language regions) has an impact on the levels of marital fertility that is independent of the impact of the five covariates. The low marital fertility in Wallonia cannot be attributed solely to the more advanced position of this area with respect to nuptiality, industrialization, literacy, urbanization, and infant mortality. Clearly another variable, possibly a cultural dimension, must be responsible for explaining the Flemish-Walloon difference in I_g. Before we try to find this variable, let us assess what the impact would have been if we had pooled the data for the language regions into one national set, thereby failing to recognize that we should be dealing with two subpopulations.

Figure 6.1 shows the regression lines for 1910 data linking I_g to several background variables used as covariates in Table 6.1. These regression lines, together with the corresponding coefficients of determination (i.e., the correlation coefficient squared), are given for Belgium as a whole and for the language areas separately. When we inspect the figure linking I_g to the percentage of males engaged in agriculture, we can see clearly that the regression lines for the two regions are parallel and clearly distinct in that they have approximately the same slope but different intercepts. This indicates once more that the nominal factor has an impact of its own on I_g. If we compare the value of r^2 for Belgium with those values for the language regions, the differences are not very large. This means that by pooling the data for the subpopulations we would not have altered the estimated strength of the relationship in a significant way. Also, the slope of the regression line for Belgium as a whole would have been distorted only slightly. The only effect of the use of a national data set would have shown up in the calculation of the residuals: the Flemish arrondissements would systematically have had positive residuals and the Walloon arrondissements negative ones.

The picture is much more distorted when I_g is related to the index of urbanization. There, the regression lines are again almost parallel when the two language areas are considered, but the coefficients of determination indicate that 32 to 51 percent of the variance of I_g is explained when Wallonia and Flanders are taken separately, whereas only 4 percent of the variance is determined if the pooled data are considered. Also the slope of the regression line for the national set is distorted.

When we relate I_g to infant mortality, the use of a national data set is even more misleading. In the two language areas taken separately there is clearly no relation whatsoever between I_g and infant mortality. In fact, the observations for Wallonia form a round cluster in the lower left hand corner of the scattergram, while the observations for Flanders form a similar cluster in the upper right hand corner. The regression

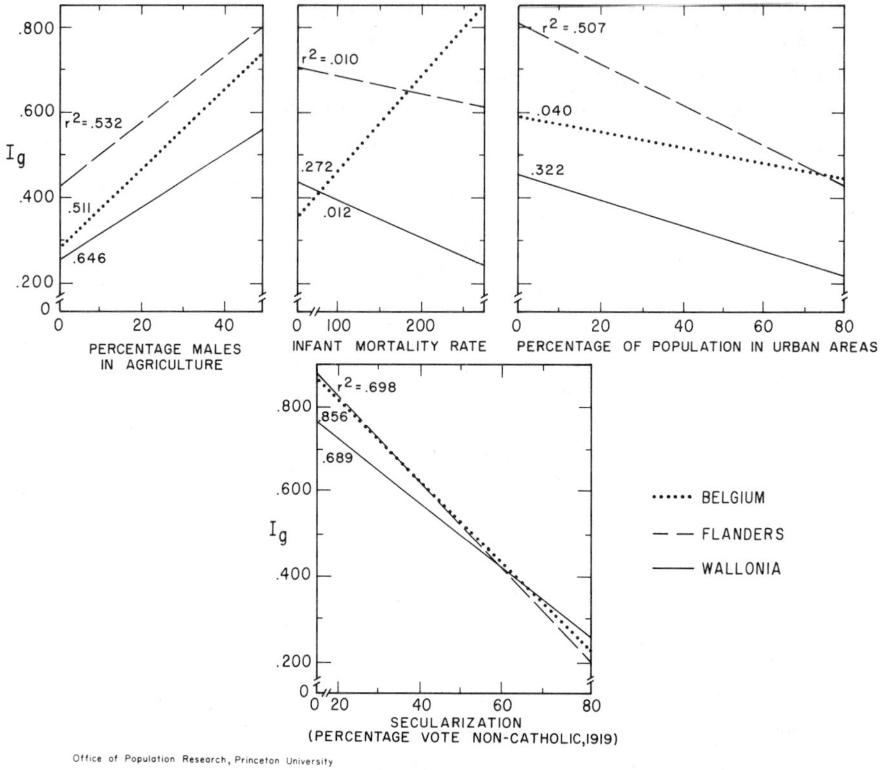

Figure 6.1 Marital Fertility (I_g), Relationship with Selected Variables as Shown by Regression Analysis, Flanders, Wallonia, and Belgium: 1910.

line for pooled data simply links these two clusters, thereby inflating r^2 to a considerable extent and totally misrepresenting the nature of the relationship. Put slightly differently, if we were working with only a national data set, a significant positive relationship would exist between I_g and infant mortality, whereas in reality we find that this positive association is an artifact produced by pooling two different subpopulations. In short, the evidence in Table 6.1 and Figure 6.1 shows clearly how misleading it would be to neglect the independent effect of the nominal factor.

As pointed out previously, however, there may be a variable other than the ones used so far that will give entirely different results when it is introduced in a covariance analysis. We have found such a variable: the difference between the mean levels of I_g in Flanders and Wallonia is reduced to zero when the difference in secularization is controlled for (see Table 6.1). In Figure 6.1, the regression lines between I_g and secularization for the two language areas are no longer parallel but intersect, and the difference in slopes and intercepts is no longer significant. This implies that the two subpopulations can be pooled and that a new meaningful, slightly curvilinear regression line is acceptable for the whole set of Belgian arrondissements.

The above supports the following conclusions: The first five covariates are essentially measures of the socioeconomic structure (occupational structure, urbanization, and literacy levels) or of the demographic structure (nuptiality and infant mortality). They do not reflect a cultural dimension or the difference in mentality between Flanders and Wallonia. The sixth covariate, secularization, measures this mentality difference much more closely, and the performance of this variable in the analysis of covariance procedure shows that the less-traditional outlook of the Walloon population is one of the prime factors responsible for the earlier transition of marital fertility in this region.

This particular view has been challenged by P. van Praag (1973, p. 370), who pointed out that the degree of secularization was a very strong correlate of industrialization in Belgium. Consequently, the prime cause of the fertility differential between the two language regions is industrialization, he believes, and secularization acted only as an intervening variable. Van Praag is undeniably correct in arguing that these variables were closely related. For 1910, we obtain correlation coefficients between them of +.620 in Flanders and +.873 in Wallonia. However, van Praag did not notice that the regression lines, which are at the basis of the correlation coefficients, are not identical but are parallel.

This means, more specifically, that for a given level of industrialization, the Walloon arrondissements had significantly higher levels of secularization than their Flemish counterparts. Obviously, if the regression lines linking secularization and industrialization levels for the two language regions were identical, the two variables would become nearly indistinguishable, and the industrialization variable would behave in very much the same way in the analysis of variance as the secularization variable. But the difference between the mean values of I_g in Flanders and Wallonia after the elimination of the effect of industrialization is far too large: industrialization and secularization do not measure the same phenomenon.

The fact that the Walloon arrondissements had a considerably higher level of secularization than the Flemish ones, after controlling for the level of industrialization, can be documented fairly easily. If we compare all the typical rural arrondissements with more than 30 percent of the male active population engaged in agriculture, the difference in levels of secularization is immediately evident. This is shown in Table 6.2, where the rural arrondissements are further subdivided into three groups, according to the size of the agricultural labor force. First, the most rural arrondissement of Wallonia, Bastogne, has no less than a 40 percent non-Catholic vote in 1919, compared with 27 percent in Diksmuide, the most rural arrondissement in Flanders. All the other Walloon arrondissements have a higher percentage of non-Catholic votes than Bastogne; in Flanders, 9 of the 12 rural arrondissements have substantially lower percentages with higher levels of industrialization than Bastogne. In total, only 8 Flemish arrondissements of the 22 have more than 40 percent non-Catholic votes. If we restrict ourselves again to the rural arrondissements only, this percentage ranges from 16.0 to 48.6 in Flanders, whereas in Wallonia percentages between 40.6 and 65.9 are found.

To summarize, the Walloon areas seem to have achieved lower levels of marital fertility partly because they were more urbanized and industrialized, but primarily because they coupled much higher levels of secularization to a given level of industrialization than was the case in Flanders. Without this secularization factor, which apparently has a meaning of its own independent of industrialization, the difference in marital fertility between Flanders and Wallonia cannot be explained.

TABLE 6.2

NON-CATHOLIC VOTE, 1919, AND MARITAL FERTILITY (Ig), 1910, BY PERCENTAGE MALE POPULATION OF 1910 IN AGRICULTURE, RURAL ARRONDISSEMENTS OF FLANDERS AND WALLONIA

Area	Percentage males in agriculture	Arrondissement	Percentage votes non-Catholic	I_g
Flanders	Over 50	Diksmuide	27.4	.705
	40-49	Eeklo	33.9	.629
		Hasselt	24.2	.791
		Maaseik	19.6	.953
		Oudenaarde	48.6	.658
		Tielt	16.0	.797
		Tongeren	33.5	.788
		Turnhout	22.6	.823
		Veurne	44.2	.595
	30-39	Aalst	38.2	.661
		Leuven	42.9	.610
		Ypres	29.0	.659
Wallonia	Over 50	Bastogne	40.6	.651
	40-49	Ath	64.4	.315
		Neufchâteau	46.8	.524
	30-39	Dinant	48.2	.423
		Marche	49.8	.523
		Virton	61.2	.457
		Waremme	65.9	.464

NOTE: Level of secularization is defined as the percentage votes non-Catholic in the 1919 election (the first election held under the system of universal male suffrage).

6.2 *The Development of a Regression Model*

From the analysis of covariance we learned that most of the independent variables related to marital fertility exercise their influence in different ways for the two language regions. Consequently, we are not justified in pooling the data for Flanders and Wallonia without allowing for their differences. This can be taken into account in two ways. First, we may introduce a dummy variable that would take the values of zero or unity, depending on the language region, and work with a national data set thereafter. A second procedure consists of quantifying a separate model for each of the language areas. The second procedure will be chosen here, primarily because we are not willing to lose an important variable whose definition is complementary in the two regions: the index of language homogeneity. In section 5.9 we indicated that this index correlates in a positive way with I_g in Flanders and in a negative way in Wallonia. Even if we used the complement of the index (an index of language heterogeneity) in one of the language regions, we would still fail to construct a meaningful variable for use in a national context. In fact, such an operation would result in a highly bimodal distribution, and the modes would be so far apart that the whole variable would take more or less the form of a nominal variable. In such circumstances, the effect of language homogeneity or heterogeneity *within* each language region could not be measured.

The model that will be considered for the two language regions takes the following form: first, as exogenous, or predetermined, variables we shall use the index of language homogeneity, the index of industrialization-urbanization, the infant mortality rate, the proportion literate, and the level of secularization (whenever possible). Then, the three demographic indices measuring nuptiality and marital and illegitimate fertility will be taken as endogenous, or dependent, variables. These endogenous variables will not only be related to the set of exogenous variables but also to each other. The format of the model is shown in Figure 6.2. There, the direction of the presumed asymmetric relationships is indicated by an arrow, and the expected sign belonging to each of the effects is also specified. Moreover, in order to express the model in the form of equations, the exogenous variables are abbreviated and numbered as Z-variables, whereas the endogenous variables are labeled as X-variables. With these conventions in mind, we shall now comment briefly on the model itself.

First, we assume that the level of and the change in I_g depends on the five exogenous variables simultaneously. The higher the degree of urbanization, industrialization, and secularization, the lower the level of marital fertility (I_g) or the greater its relative change (ΔI_g). According to the theories of Leibenstein, Ohlin, and Schultz, one would expect that a lower infant mortality rate would be associated with lower levels of I_g and larger relative changes, ΔI_g. We shall also maintain the original hypothesis with respect to the literacy variable: the higher the proportion literate, the lower the I_g and the faster the fertility decline. Finally, we expect that marital fertility drops faster in the Flemish arrondissements characterized by the presence of a substantial Francophone population and in the Walloon arrondissements with a negligible non-Franco-

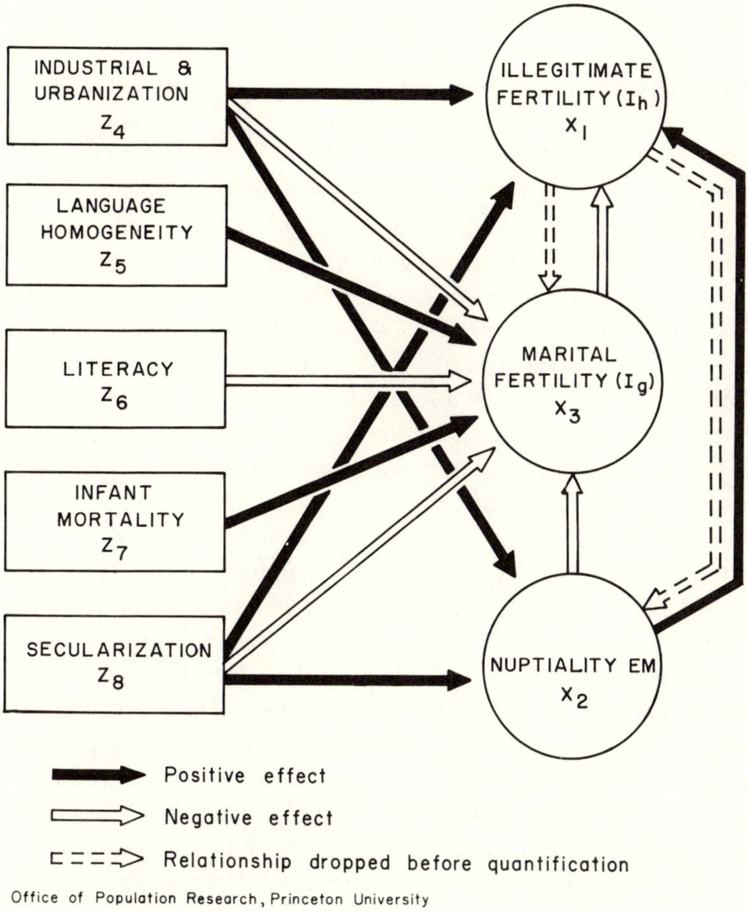

Figure 6.2 Causal Model, Basic Format Used to Relate Demographic Variables and Social Indicators.

phone population. In other words, a high degree of language homogeneity should be a reason for expecting a slower fertility decline in Flanders and a faster fertility decline in Wallonia.

Nuptiality and illegitimate fertility will be related to only two exogenous variables: industrialization-urbanization and secularization. We do not see any theoretical reason why these two demographic measures should depend on literacy, infant mortality, or language homogeneity. In all cases we expect positive associations: nuptiality and illegitimate fertility should be breaking away from the Malthusian principles, specified in Dupâquier's rules, especially in those areas increasingly more advanced with respect to their socioeconomic structure and level of secularization.

Between the endogenous variables themselves we have maintained the following effects: First, the decline in marital fertility has not influenced the change in nuptiality, as indicated in Section 5.8. Consequently, the arrow from I_g (ΔI_g) to EM (ΔEM) has been omitted. This leaves us with an asymmetric effect in the other direction, conforming with hypothesis A. The choice between hypothesis A ($EM \rightarrow I_g$) and hypothesis C (spurious relation) will be made when the structural parameters have been calculated for this particular asymmetric relationship. If it turns out that the structural parameter is not significantly different from zero, hypothesis C rather than A applies. Second, we introduce a two-way causation between I_g and I_h. From Section 4.6 we know that I_g and especially I_h are dependent on the degree to which extramarital conceptions are legitimized through pregnancy-precipitated marriages. When pregnancies fail to precipitate marriages, I_h will be inflated and I_g deflated; when the traditional pressures are applied, prenuptial conceptions will enter into the legitimate birth category and the opposite effect will appear. Whichever direction the births stemming from premarital conceptions may go, I_h and I_g will always be affected in opposite ways. A negative relationship is therefore expected. Third, nuptiality and illegitimate fertility are linked by direct paths in both directions. This two-way effect is justified on the basis that both variables are an integral part of the Malthusian pattern of family formation (see Dupâquier's rules). Therefore, the areas breaking away from this Malthusian pattern with respect to nuptiality should also depart from it with respect to illegitimate fertility.

As we shall see in the next section, the model of Figure 6.2 is nonrecursive, and it must fulfill certain conditions before it can be quantified. In applying these conditions, we shall see that two arrows will disappear: the effect of I_h on I_g and the effect of I_h on EM. The specific reasons for this elimination will now be discussed.

6.3 *The Quantification of the Model: Preliminary Problems*

Figure 6.2 contains in its original form two feedback relations or reciprocal causations: $I_g \rightleftarrows I_h$ and $EM \rightleftarrows I_h$ As a result, we are dealing with a nonrecursive system. This particular feature implies that we should not quantify the model via the ordinary least squares method (OLS), but that the two-stage least-squares technique (2SLS) is to be preferred. Since a knowledge of econometrics cannot be assumed for all readers, we shall come back to this issue further on. The second issue to be tackled is generally known as the identification problem. As usual, the arrow-diagram of Figure 6.2 will be translated into a set of linear equations. In working with such a set of equations, it is possible that there will be infinitely many sets of parameter values that can all generate the same empirical data. In other words, it may be impossible to obtain unique estimates of the true structural coefficients in the regression equations. To avoid this, certain a priori constraints must be placed on the theoretical model, and we must make sure that there is no excess of unknowns in the equations over the number of pieces of information that can be obtained empirically (H. Blalock, 1969, pp. 48-66). Therefore, the equations must meet the two identification conditions commonly used in econometrics. Having introduced the problems, we shall consider these two issues, identification and OLS bias in nonrecursive systems, in more detail.

As usually done in statistical work, the relationships specified in Figure 6.2 can be written in the form of the following linear equations:

$$X_1 = B_{14}Z_4 + B_{18}Z_8 + B_{12}X_2 + B_{13}X_3 + u_1$$

$$X_2 = B_{24}Z_4 + B_{28}Z_8 + B_{21}X_1 + u_2$$

$$X_3 = B_{34}Z_4 + B_{35}Z_5 + B_{36}Z_6 + B_{37}Z_7 + B_{38}Z_8 + B_{31}X_1 + B_{32}X_2 + u_3$$

In these equations, we predict each of the endogenous variables (X_i) in terms of a set of exogenous variables (Z_i) and other endogenous variables. Each of these predictors has a coefficient or "weight" (B), which we try to estimate. In addition, a u-term is specified. This is the disturbance or residual term, composed of two parts:

1. The residual component produced by all factors not explicitly considered in the equation, summarizing our ignorance about the other possible predictors of the dependent variable.
2. The measurement error component of the dependent variable.

Our basic problem is that these disturbance terms are generally correlated with the other endogenous variables when we are dealing with nonrecursive models. If this occurs, the OLS estimators of the structural parameters (B's) will be seriously biased (J. Johnston, 1972, pp. 277-279; C. F. Christ, 1966, pp. 453-464). Therefore, one must try to eliminate the effect of these u-terms as much as possible. This can be done by obtaining estimates of the endogenous variables, X_i on the basis of predetermined or "instrumental" variables that are good predictors of X_i. This operation is the first step in 2SLS, and it is performed through the following equations in our model:

$$\hat{X}_1 = B_{14}Z_4 + B_{18}Z_8$$

$$\hat{X}_2 = B_{13}Z_4 + B_{28}Z_8$$

$$\hat{X}_3 = B_{34}Z_4 + B_{35}Z_5 + B_{36}Z_6 + B_{37}Z_7 + B_{38}Z_8$$

The estimated values, X_i, are "purified" of their residuals, and in a second step of 2SLS, a particular endogenous variable will be regressed on the exogenous variables Z_i and on the previously calculated estimates of the remaining endogenous variables in the equation:

$$X_1 = B'_{12}\hat{X}_2 + B'_{13}\hat{X}_3 + B'_{14}Z_4 + B'_{18}Z_8 + u'_1$$

$$X_2 = B'_{21}\hat{X}_1 + B'_{24}Z_4 + B'_{28}Z_8 + u'_2$$

$$X_3 = B'_{31}\hat{X}_1 + B'_{32}\hat{X}_2 + B'_{34}Z_4 + B'_{35}Z_5 + B'_{36}Z_6 + B'_{37}Z_7 + B'_{38}Z_8 + u'_3$$

The new set of residuals (u') should now be negligible in comparison to the previous set (u) and the problem of correlation between residuals and endogenous variables, typical for a nonrecursive system, should be solved to a satisfactory degree.

This operation does not solve all our problems, however: we have not yet tested whether the equations satisfy the two identification conditions. The first and necessary condition requires the following: if K is the total number of exogenous variables, k is the number of exogenous variables included in equation i, and g the number of endogenous variables included in the same equation, then we must find for all equations that:

$$K - k \geq g - 1$$

If we apply this rule to our questions, we see that this necessary condition is not met in the equation predicting X_3. To achieve identification in this instance, we have to drop either an exogenous or an endogenous variable. In practice, we shall drop the relationship that is expected to be the least important in the model. In our case, we assume that the effect of I_h upon I_g is the closest to being negligible: the subtraction or the addition of a number of births and mothers involved in premarital conceptions to the numerator and denominator of I_g should have only a slight impact on the magnitude of I_g, especially since illegitimate fertility is not high in Belgium. As a consequence, we delete one of the reciprocal causations implied in the original model.

The second and sufficient condition to secure identification is of a strictly algebraic nature; in practical terms it requires that no pair of equations contain exactly the same combination of variables (C. F. Christ, 1966, pp. 314-331). In our example, this condition is met.

So far, we are left with one reciprocal causation in the model. This means that we should still apply the 2SLS procedure rather than OLS. But in doing so, another problem arises. When we executed the second step of 2SLS, serious multicollinearity problems appeared due to the high correlations between Z_4, Z_8, and the "purified" endogenous variables. In fact, all three endogenous variables, $\hat{X}_1$ through $\hat{X}_3$, are largely a function of the same two exogenous variables (Z_4 and Z_8). This leaves us with the following dilemma. We can maintain the reciprocal effects between I_h and *EM*, but then the basis of the model has to be changed, and different exogenous variables must be chosen as "instruments" to obtain $\hat{X}_1$, $\hat{X}_2$, and $\hat{X}_3$. Alternatively, we can maintain our relationships with the *Z* variables, but then we must eliminate the two-way causation linking I_h and *EM*. Of these alternatives, the latter solution seems preferable: the impact of I_h upon *EM* should not be important, and this relation is dropped.

If we inspect our model now, we see that it has become recursive: two feedback effects are assumed to be of minor importance, leaving us with a model involving only asymmetric relations. In a recursive system the reason for applying 2SLS no longer exists, and only the correlation between residuals or u-terms themselves must be negligible. If omitted factors assumed to affect X_i (incorporated with u_i) are uncorrelated with omitted factors producing variation in X_j (incorporated in u_j), there is no correlation between u_i and u_j, and OLS techniques will yield optimal estimations of the structural parameters (H. Blalock, 1969, p. 70; J. Johnston, 1972, pp. 377-380). Provided that the residuals are unrelated, the model can then be quantified via simple multiple regression techniques.

At first sight, it may appear that we have made a rather cumbersome statistical excursion to arrive at a situation where, after all, we will make use of one of the most classic types of multivariate analysis. If the model were immediately presented in its final form, however, a number of basic steps would have been hidden. We consider these steps of great importance in recasting relationships between social and demographic variables into a statistically quantifiable model. It is essential to show explicitly what logical weaknesses can be covered up by the verbal presentation of a set of propositions (identification problem) and what price we pay for quantification (multicollinearity in 2SLS).

6.4 *The Quantification of the Model: Results*

The model presented in Figure 6.2 will be quantified through multiple regression procedures. The structural coefficients are then obtained as the standardized regression coefficients (Beta-coefficients). As usual, the effect of the unspecified variables is obtained as $\sqrt{1-R^2}$, where R is the multiple correlation coefficient. The correlations between the residuals have been checked and found to be negligible. The calculations are performed for several subsamples: the levels of the endogenous variables are predicted for four dates and the relative changes are predicted for three periods. In this way, we are not only able to compare the relative weights of the predictors within a single period, but we can also inspect the degree of stability of a particular Beta-coefficient in the different time-specific subsamples. To facilitate reading, we have presented the results for one subsample on a diagram similar to the one shown in Figure 6.2. This gives Figure 6.3 when the levels of the endogenous variables are predicted, and Figure 6.4 when relative changes are determined. The Beta-coefficients for all subsamples are given in Tables 6.3 and 6.4. On the basis of this material, we can examine a number of the propositions made in Section 6.2 and in chapter 5.

Tables 6.3 and 6.4 support the proposition that industrialization-urbanization has a significant effect upon I_g in both language regions. The higher the degree of industrialization-urbanization, the lower the level of I_g and the higher the rate of the marital fertility decline, ΔI_g. The same holds between secularization and I_g. But, as secularization and industrialization-urbanization are significantly interrelated, their respective Beta-coefficients may be distorted. In other words, there is an important degree of multicollinearity between the predictors, which makes it difficult to state that the effect of secularization is larger than the effect of industrialization-urbanization by a specific amount. This problem can be lifted if we are willing to acknowledge that urbanization, industrialization, and secularization are different aspects of one syndrome. In this instance, we have certainly identified a set of interrelated variables that are responsible for a large part of the variance of I_g and

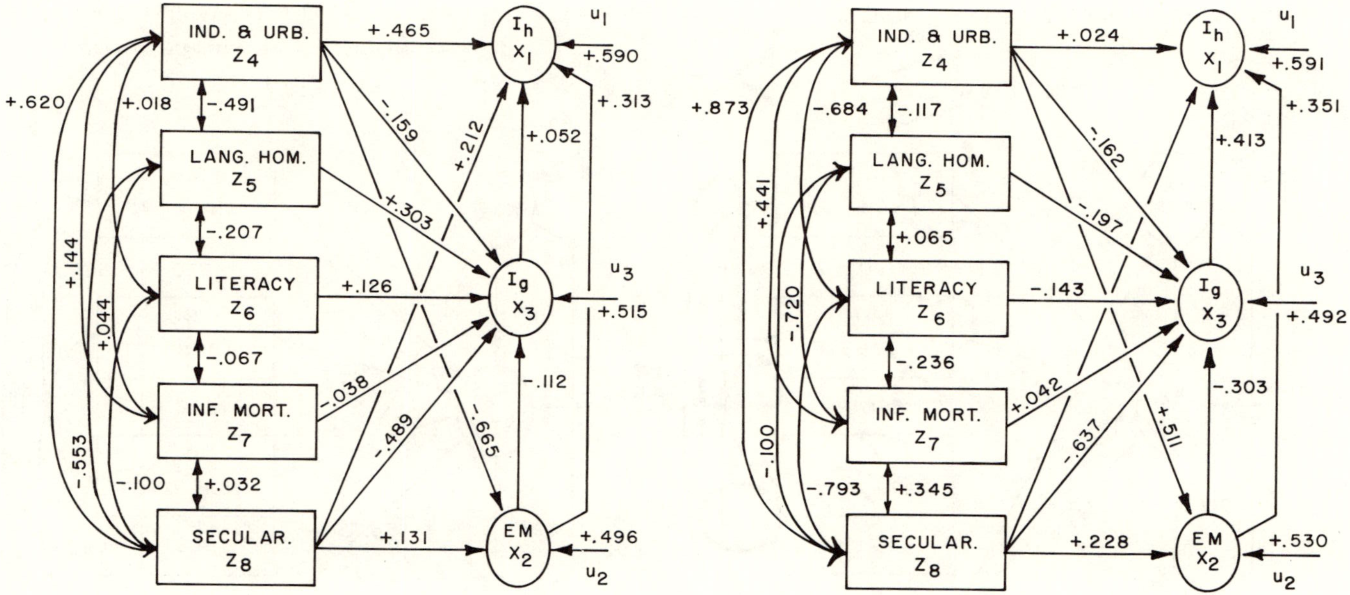

FLANDERS WALLONIA

Office of Population Research, Princeton University

Figure 6.3 Causal Model, Demographic Variables, 1910, as Related to Social Indicators, 1910, Flanders and Wallonia.

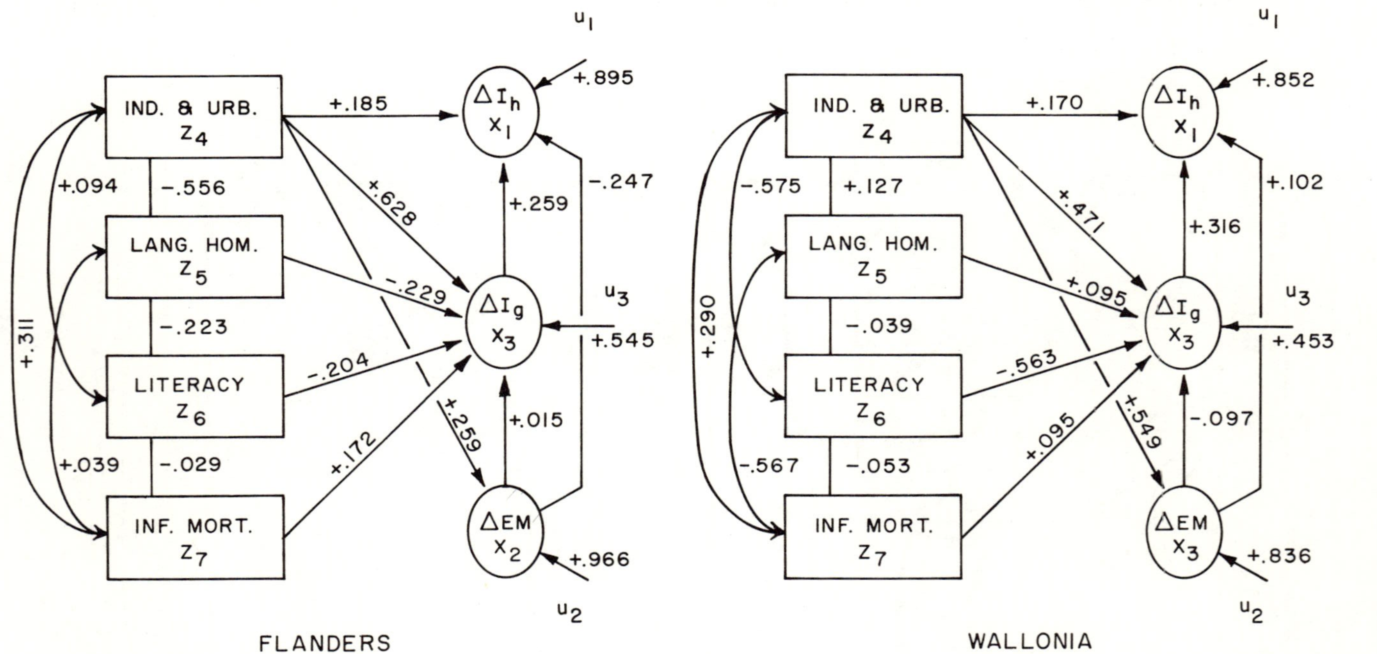

Office of Population Research, Princeton University

Figure 6.4 Causal Model, Change in Demographic Variables, 1890–1910, as Related to Social Indicators, 1890, Flanders and Wallonia.

TABLE 6.3

CAUSAL MODEL, DEMOGRAPHIC VARIABLES RELATED TO SOCIAL INDICATORS BY MULTIPLE REGRESSION ANALYSIS, FLANDERS AND WALLONIA: 1880 TO 1910

		Beta coefficients					
		Flanders			Wallonia		
		I_h	EM	I_g	I_h	EM	I_g
Variable	Date	(X_1)	(X_2)	(X_3)	(X_1)	(X_2)	(X_3)
Industrialization and urbanization (Z_4)	1880	+.446[a]	+.665[a]	-.241	+.544[a]	+.645[a]	-.245
	1890	+.435[a]	+.674[a]	-.312	+ 496[a]	+.721[a]	-.218
	1900	+.343	+.772[a]	-.322	+.465[a]	+.722[a]	-.388
	1910	+.465[a]	+.665[a]	-.159	+.024	+.511	-.162
Language homogeneity (Z_5)	1880	--	--	+.418[a]	--	--	-.113
	1890	--	--	+.527[a]	--	--	-.207
	1900	--	--	+.487[a]	--	--	+.071
	1910	--	--	+.303	--	--	-.197
Literacy (Z_6)	1880	--	--	-.161	--	--	-.050
	1890	--	--	-.207	--	--	-.133
	1900	--	--	-.067	--	--	+.015
	1910	--	--	+.126	--	--	-.143
Infant mortality (Z_7)	1880	--	--	+.428[a]	--	--	+.172
	1890	--	--	+.218	--	--	+.083
	1900	--	--	+.118	--	--	+.336
	1910	--	--	-.038	--	--	+.042
Secularization (Z_8)	1910	+.212	+.131	-.489[a]	+.889[a]	+.228	-.637[a]
EM (X_2)	1880	+.243[a]	--	-.348	+.342	--	-.524
	1890	+.251	--	-.120	+.473	--	-.637[a]
	1900	+.416	--	-.256	+.421	--	-.569[a]
	1910	+.313	--	-.112	+.351	--	-.303
I_g (X_3)	1880	-.409[a]	--	--	+.025	--	--
	1890	-.350[a]	--	--	+.144	--	--
	1900	-.230	--	--	+.058	--	--
	1910	+.052	--	--	+.413	--	--
		u_1	u_2	u_3	u_1	u_2	u_3
Unspecified variables	1880	+.371	+.756	+.507	+.648	+.764	+.744
	1890	+.490	+.739	+.548	+.632	+.693	+.697
	1900	+.482	+.636	+.539	+.670	+.692	+.532
	1910	+.590	+.496	+.515	+.591	+.530	+.492

NOTES: The causal model relates a set of dependent or endogenous variables (abbreviated as X-variables) to a set of independent or exogenous variables (abbreviated as Z-variables) and to each other. The influence of unspecified variables is embodied in the coefficients u_1 through u_3.

The results for 1910 are also presented in Figure 6.3.

The effects of the unspecified variables are obtained as $u = \sqrt{1-R^2}$ where R is the multiple correlation coefficient, corrected for the effect of n (number of predictors) approaching to N (number of observations). (See Q. McNemar, 1955, p.186.)

Measurement error is included in the concept of unspecified variables.

[a] Indicates significant values (B/Standard Error (B) ≥ 2.0).

ΔI_g. To this, however, we should add that it is meaningful to refer to this syndrome only when language regions are considered separately and not when we have the whole of Belgium in mind. We know from Section 6.1 that the Flemish and Walloon arrondissements have considerably different levels of secularization for a given level of industrialization-

TABLE 6.4

CAUSAL MODEL, CHANGE IN DEMOGRAPHIC VARIABLES RELATED TO SOCIAL INDICATORS BY MULTIPLE REGRESSION ANALYSIS, FLANDERS AND WALLONIA: 1880 TO 1910

			Beta coefficients					
			Flanders			Wallonia		
Variable	Date of Variable Z	X	ΔI_h (X_1)	ΔEM (X_2)	ΔI_g (X_3)	ΔI_h (X_1)	ΔEM (X_2)	ΔI_g (X_3)
Industrialization and urbanization (Z_4)	1890	Δ1890-1900	+.445	+.423	+.609[a]	+.387	+.600	+.333
	1890	Δ1890-1910	+.185	+.259	+.628[a]	+.170	+.549	+.471[a]
	1890	Δ1900-1910	-.164	-.169	+.602[a]	-.045	+.364	+.516[a]
	1900	Δ1900-1910	-.032	-.146	+.536[a]	-.180	+.439	+.682[a]
Language homogeneity (Z_5)	1890	Δ1890-1900	--	--	-.190	--	--	+.002
	1890	Δ1890-1910	--	--	-.229	--	--	+.095
	1890	Δ1900-1910	--	--	-.299	--	--	+.134
	1900	Δ1900-1910	--	--	-.395[a]	--	--	+.110
Literacy (Z_6)	1890	Δ1890-1900	--	--	+.093	--	--	-.609[a]
	1890	Δ1890-1910	--	--	-.204	--	--	-.563[a]
	1890	Δ1900-1910	--	--	-.354[a]	--	--	-.483[a]
	1900	Δ1900-1910	--	--	-.410[a]	--	--	-.341
Infant mortality (Z_7)	1890	Δ1890-1900	--	--	+.254	--	--	+.030
	1890	Δ1890-1910	--	--	+.172	--	--	+.095
	1890	Δ1900-1910	--	--	+.089	--	--	+.156
	1900	Δ1900-1910	--	--	+.054	--	--	+.00[illegible]
ΔEM (X_2)	--	Δ1890-1900	-.174	--	+.099	-.151	--	-.031
	--	Δ1890-1910	-.247	--	+.015	+.102	--	-.097
	--	Δ1900-1910	-.023	--	+.128	+.194	--	-.190
	--	Δ1900-1910	-.014	--	+.106	+.238	--	-.265
ΔI_g (X_3)	--	Δ1890-1900	+.017	--	--	-.006	--	--
	--	Δ1890-1910	+.259	--	--	+.316	--	--
	--	Δ1900-1910	+.316	--	--	+.483	--	--
	--	Δ1900-1910	+.217	--	--	+.578	--	--
			u_1	u_2	u_3	u_1	u_2	u_3
Unspecified variables	1890	Δ1890-1900	+.909	+.906	+.467	+.948	+.632	+.557
	1890	Δ1890-1910	+.895	+.966	+.545	+.852	+.836	+.453
	1890	Δ1900-1910	+.974	+.986	+.570	+.854	+.931	+.480
	1900	Δ1900-1910	+.980	+.989	+.566	+.849	+.898	+.547

NOTES: The causal model relates a set of dependent or endogenous variables (abbreviated as X-variables) to a set of independent or exogenous variables (abbreviated as Z-variables) and to each other. The influence of unspecified variables is embodied in the coefficients u_1 through u_3.

The results for Z variable 1890 and X variable Δ1890-1910 are also presented in Figure 6.4.

[a]Indicates significant values (B/Standard Error (B) ≥ 2.0).

urbanization. This also seems to be very meaningful when illegitimate fertility is predicted.

Our a priori proposition with respect to the relationship between language homogeneity and marital fertility holds as well. In Flanders, a high degree of homogeneity is definitely associated with higher levels of I_g and lower rates of fertility decline. In Wallonia, the signs are reversed, as expected, and the Beta-coefficients are much smaller than in Flanders. Hence, we find here some evidence in support of the thesis that the

Francophone minorities in Flanders may have been among the first social groups to have adopted forms of fertility regulation. Additional evidence should be obtained, however, from individual fertility records to complement these findings made on the basis of ecological data only.

The effect of literacy on level of marital fertility appears to be negligible in the two language regions, and when the rate of fertility decline is predicted, the sign of the Beta-weights is reversed. As a result, we reject the hypothesis that elementary education has been instrumental in reducing marital fertility. Infant mortality, too, obtains Beta-weights that are either small or fail to be in line with the hypothesis of Leibenstein et al. In fact, when ΔI_g is predicted in both language regions, the infant mortality variable obtains a positive Beta-coefficient, which would mean that higher infant mortality levels provoked higher rates of marital fertility decline. Furthermore, when we introduce a series of models, identical to those used here except for a time lag of 10 or 20 years between the exogenous and endogenous variables, the Beta-coefficients of infant mortality remain extremely low and fall just on the positive or negative side of the zero-value.

On the basis of the Beta-coefficients in Tables 6.3 and 6.4 we can also see the effect of nuptiality on marital fertility. If we restrict ourselves to the prediction of the level of marital fertility, the hypothesis formulated in Section 5.9 should be accepted. In Wallonia we find substantial negative values of the Beta-weights, which means that nuptiality has the expected effect on marital fertility according to hypothesis A. In Flanders, the Beta-weights also have the expected negative sign, but their values are smaller than those of the Beta-coefficients of industrialization-urbanization, secularization, and language homogeneity. If the rate of marital fertility decline (ΔI_g) is determined on the basis of the relative increase in *EM,* as is done in Table 6.4, the Beta-coefficients are small and fall just above or under the zero-value. For Flanders, this means that the effect of nuptiality on marital fertility is small and that, as a simplification, we may accept that the relation between *EM* and I_g is virtually spurious (hypothesis C). In Wallonia, however, we are left with a clear contradiction: on the basis of the results of Table 6.3, we should accept hypothesis A, but the Beta-weights of Table 6.4 indicate that hypothesis C holds. As a result, we are not able to discern which hypothesis should be accepted in Wallonia on the basis of the model we have introduced.

In the definition of the model in Figure 6.2 we stated that whenever the Malthusian rules break down with respect to nuptiality, they should also break down with respect to illegitimate fertility. The Beta-coefficients of *EM* in the regression with I_h in Table 6.3 seem to support this hypothesis in both language regions. This statement is only acceptable, however, if the Beta-coefficient is only partially affected by the "automatic" relationship between measures of nuptiality and the index of illegitimate fertility I_h (see Section 4.6). Consequently one should be on guard against interpreting the full weight of the Beta-coefficient from *EM* to I_h in strictly behavioral terms.

In Section 6.2, we expected a negative effect of I_g and I_h on the grounds that the exclusion of births stemming from prenuptial conceptions from the category of legitimate births must necessarily decrease I_g and inflate I_h. The Beta-coefficients in Table 6.3 show that this negative effect originally existed in Flanders, but, as time progresses, we observe that this effect becomes weaker and turns into a positive effect in 1910. Moreover, the Beta-coefficients for Wallonia are all positive and, in 1910, I_g obtains the second-highest coefficient in the regression predicting the level of I_h. Obviously, some other mechanism is at work, but before specifying it, we should see what characteristics the Beta-coefficients have when ΔI_h is predicted.

As we know from Section 4.6, the levels of illegitimate fertility reached a maximum in the last decade of the nineteenth century and steadily declined after 1900. This implies that ΔI_h 1880–1900 still measures a relative increase in illegitimate fertility in several areas, whereas ΔI_h 1900–1910 measures the rate of decline in all arrondissements . As a result, we see that the industrialization-urbanization factor causes an increase with respect to illegitimate fertility when the prediction is made for ΔI_h 1890–1900, while the effect of ΔI_g is virtually nil (see Table 6.4). When the relative decrease is measured by ΔI_h 1900–1910, the roles of the two predictors are reversed. A higher rate of marital fertility decline (ΔI_g) provokes a higher rate of decline in illegitimate fertility, while the effect of industrialization-urbanization is reduced. Very probably, the positive effect of ΔI_g on ΔI_h after 1900 indicates that the increase in control of marital fertility is matched by a similar increase in control of fertility outside wedlock.

Up to this point we have used regression analysis as a way of finding statistical evidence for the hypotheses that form the model in Figure 6.2. We do not know, however, exactly how successful we were in predicting the values of the endogenous variables. An idea of the degree of accuracy of the prediction can be obtained by inspecting the values of u_1 through u_3 in Tables 6.3 and 6.4. These values indicate the magnitude of the effect of the unspecified variables in each regression equation. As can be seen in the tables, the predictions of the levels of I_g, I_h, and ΔI_g are very satisfactory. In most cases the unspecified variables carry a weight varying between .400 and .600, and in only one instance (prediction of I_g 1880) is the .700 level exceeded. These levels correspond to multiple correlation coefficients of .800, .920, and .710 respectively for exogenous with endogenous variables, indicating that 64 to 84 percent of the variance of I_g, I_h, and ΔI_g is explained by the specified variables (51 percent of the variance of I_g 1880). The other variables are predicted with less accuracy. The unspecified factors influencing ΔI_h and ΔEM carry a weight higher than .850, which means that generally less than 28 percent of the variance of ΔI_h and ΔEM is explained by the variable explicitly introduced in the regression equations.

With excellent prediction results for ΔI_g, we can see which arrondissements were more advanced or more backward with respect to the rate of marital fertility decline, once we have controlled for the effects of industrialization-urbanization, language homogeneity, literacy, infant mortality, and ΔEM. This can be done by inspecting the standardized residuals (i.e., the differences between the predicted and observed values of ΔI_g divided by their own standard deviation). In addition to the four predictions of ΔI_g used in Table 6.4, we have also looked at the residuals of ΔI_g 1880–1900 and ΔI_g 1880–1910. These six series of residuals show such a high degree of conformity that their mean can easily be taken as representative for the whole period 1880–1910. These average standardized residuals are represented on Map 6.1. A comparison with Maps 5.2 and 5.4 reveals that, despite the introduction of more predictors, the two classic pockets still exist where the rate of the marital fertility decline was systematically too low for the given values of the independent variables. These pockets are the province of Limburg and the neighboring arrondissement of Turnhout in Flanders, and the four Ardennes arrondissements in Wallonia (Bastogne, Marche, Neufchâteau, and Virton). In addition to these pockets we also find negative residuals in several arrondissements of West Flanders and of Hainaut. On the basis of the darker shadings in southern West Flanders (arrondissements of Ypres and Kortrijk) we can now rule out that fertility regulation was imported from France. Rather, the central part of Flanders, incorporating the three large urban areas of Antwerp, Brussels, and

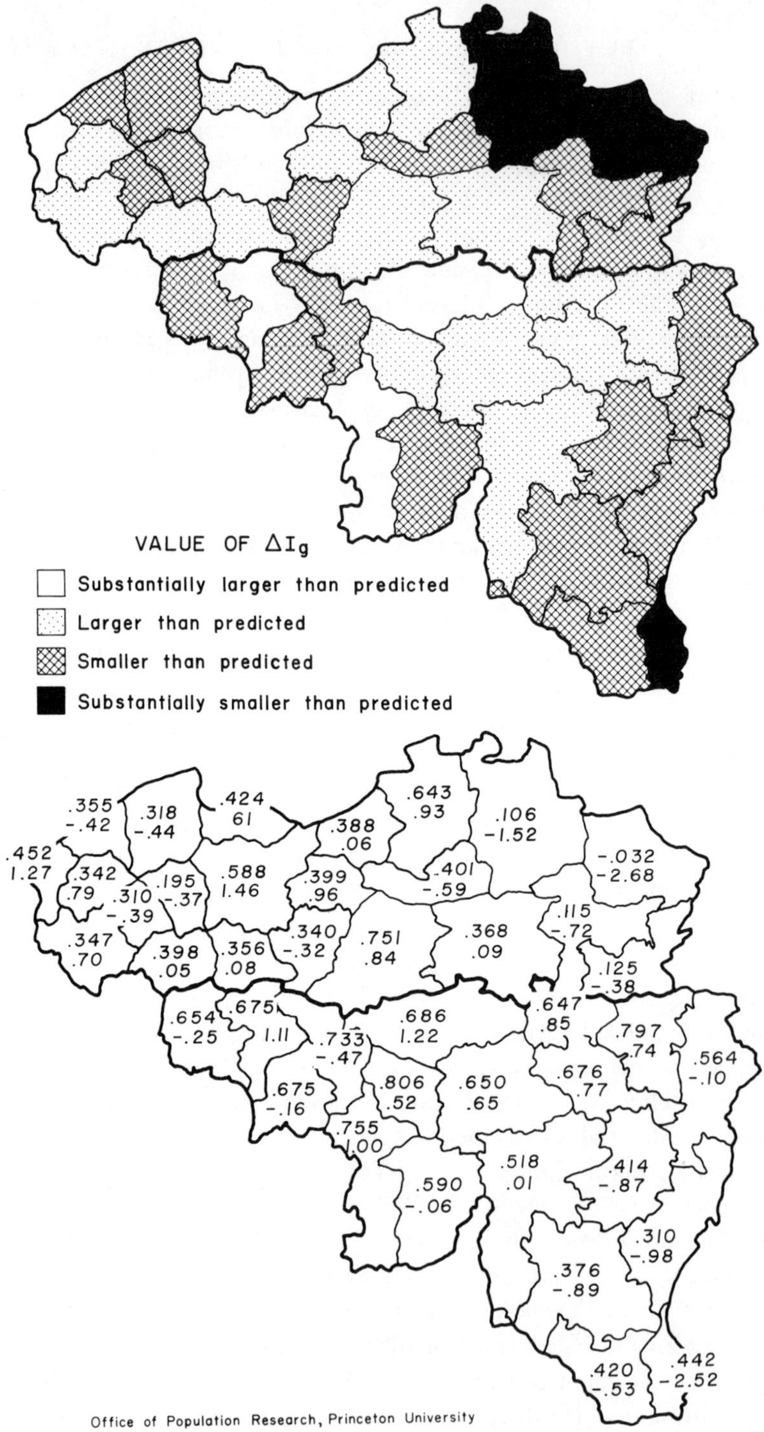

Map 6.1 Change in Marital Fertility (ΔI_g), Deviations from Predicted Value (prediction based on variables in causal model) by Arrondissement: 1880–1910.

NOTE: Separate regressions for each language area.

Ghent, was more advanced, and the extreme eastern and western parts (with the exception of the Polder arrondissements of Veurne and Diksmuide) stayed behind.

At first sight, the geographical dispersion pattern referred to in Section 5.6 for Wallonia seems difficult to accept, given the darker shadings in the Hainaut arrondissements of Charleroi, Mons, and Soignies. But, as was already indicated in Section 5.6, these three arrondissements have by far the highest rates of marital fertility decline in Belgium, and they could hardly be expected to have the still higher values of ΔI_g that were predicted in the linear regressions. Stated in a simplified way, if the conditions are twice as favorable in the leading arrondissements compared to any other arrondissement, it is much harder for the trend setter to reduce its marital fertility at twice the rate observed in the other place. The sheer fact of being in a leading position implies a built-in braking effect, and this particular effect is probably responsible for the negative residuals in Charleroi, Mons, and Soignies. In this case, we are still willing to accept the existence of the geographical dispersion pattern in Wallonia described in Section 5.6.

6.5 *Conclusion*

In chapters 5 and 6 we tried to offer a short verification of some mechanisms described in the theoretical framework. In addition to such variables as industrialization, urbanization, infant mortality, and secularization, two others were introduced: literacy and language homogeneity. This was done because of their presumed importance for the Belgian experience. As a result, several specific hypotheses could be examined empirically and accepted or altered, depending on the outcome of the multivariate procedure.

From this we learned that a statistical account of the regional variation in fertility decline in Belgium must be based on two factors: the industrialization-urbanization factor and the secularization factor. The former gives us an idea of the impact of the degree of modernization on the socioeconomic structure, whereas the latter enables us to bring out a cultural component, i.e., the more traditional outlook of the Flemish and the more flexible or more modern mentality of the Walloon and Francophone subpopulations. If these two factors are introduced simultaneously, two-thirds to three-quarters of the regional variation in marital fertility can be explained. All the other factors seem to be of a rather subsidiary nature: the literacy, infant mortality, and nuptiality variables had at most a very small impact on the ecological pattern of the marital fertility decline, and in several instances they manifested their smaller influence in the opposite direction of what was expected. Only language homogeneity can be singled out as an additional important variable in Flanders, but there, this variable points at the difference between the Francophone and the Dutch-speaking subpopulations, i.e., a dimension that is already partially taken into account in the urbanization component and in the secularization variable.

When it comes to explaining the regional variance in illegitimate fertility, our predictions are less powerful. Nevertheless, it seems that increasing industrialization, urbanization, and secularization, and the gradual breakdown of the Malthusian marriage pattern provoked a weakening of the restrictions vis-à-vis illegitimate fertility. After an initial increase of I_h, however, illegitimate fertlity dropped again after 1890. The emerging relationship between ΔI_g and ΔI_h indicates that this decline was primarily a result of the introduction of contraception.

References—Chapter 6

Blalock, H. M. 1969. *Theory construction, from verbal to mathematical formulations.* Englewood Cliffs, N. J.: Prentice Hall.

Christ, C. F. 1966. *Econometric models and methods.* New York: John Wiley.

Johnston, J. 1972. *Econometric methods.* 2nd ed. Tokyo: Kogakusha.

McNemar, Q. 1955. *Psychological statistics.* New York: John Wiley and Sons.

van Praag, P. 1973. Kanttekeningen bij vruchtbaarheidscontrole, nuptialiteit en sociaal-economische veranderingen in België, 1846–1910. *Bevolking en Gezin* 2:369-373.

CHAPTER 7: Final Considerations

The statistical and qualitative evidence presented in the preceding chapters calls for a final reappraisal of the findings. In such an appraisal we will consider the features of the Belgian experience more cohesively.

In the middle of the nineteenth century the Belgian demographic situation showed the following characteristics: high mortality and non-controlled marital fertility, late and nonuniversal marriage, and negligible illegitimate fertility.. There is some evidence that mortality was considerably lower in certain parts of Wallonia, that nuptiality restrictions were more severe in Flanders, and also that marital fertility may have been sligthly higher in Flanders than in Wallonia. It is also likely that there were fluctuations in the levels of mortality, nuptiality, and marital fertility over time. In the census of 1846, which was the first fully reliable measurement of these phenomena, the Flemish part of the country was in the middle of a severe economic crisis; it is likely that the nuptiality restrictions and marital fertility levels recorded then were not completely typical of the first half of the nineteenth century as a whole. The upward trend in I_g and I_m observable for the subsequent decades probably contains an element of restoration to the situation existing before the crises of the 1840s and 1850s.

Despite the heterogeneity in space and fluctuations over time, we can apply the term "Malthusian" to the demographic characteristics existing before 1870. In this Malthusian situation, one particular feature stands out quite distinctly: given the pattern of late nuptiality, high levels of both fertility and mortality, and the young age composition, the average family size was fairly small. In fact, it was far too small to accept the hypothesis that Belgian families of the early nineteenth century were of the extended type. Instead, family structures were quite modern. Without doubt, the foundations were already laid for the emergence of an almost exclusively nuclear family structure. This structure could develop fully only in the twentieth century, however, when fertility had declined to low levels.

After 1870, the signs of a genuine transition appeared: nuptiality broke away from its restrictions, illegitimate fertility rose, and marital fertility was brought under greater control. As hypothesized by Hofstee, the change in nuptiality seems, at least partially, the result of a proletarization. To this we should add, however, that the rural and semi-agricultural proletariat changed its nuptiality pattern much later than the population of the industrial centers. Geographical imbalances between eligible male and female populations also seem to be a factor. In this way, urbanization and industrialization exercised a double but opposite influence. In general, it gave people the chance to marry earlier; but, wherever new economic activities attracted a labor force in which one sex was more numerous than the other, the local sex balance could be upset and the marriage intensity among the overrepresented sex reduced. Lower levels of I_m, quite independent of the intensity of nuptiality in adjacent areas, have also been found for urban centers in Germany (J. Knodel, 1974). We suspect that an explanation similar to the one offered for Belgium may hold for other urban areas of Western Europe as well.

The increase in illegitimate fertility between 1870 and 1890 also fits the image of a fundamental demographic change. As Dupâquier indicates, the western European Malthusian system discouraged not only early marriage but also conceptions of births outside wedlock. Since we find that the levels of I_h tripled between 1860 and 1890 in some Belgian provinces, it is clear that both Malthusian principles were under attack.

Which factors were responsible for this increase? First, it is highly unlikely that the lower levels of I_h prior to 1860 were due to a high incidence of contraceptive practice. This would imply that the application of contraception was less effective in 1890 than it was in 1860 and would contradict the basic trend toward increasing contraceptive practice and effectiveness. Alternatively, it could be that the increase in I_h reflected a form of moral decadence and that adultery and concubinage became more frequent. Certainly, the *fin de siècle* period may have been less Victorian, but the level of I_h, even taken at its maximal value, is still far too small to justify the use of the term moral decadence. Rather, we see the increase in I_h as being primarily related to the change in nuptiality behavior. There is some evidence that changes in the incidence and outcome of premarital conceptions may have been responsible for a substantial part of the rise of I_h.

Several factors could have influenced the incidence of premarital conceptions. We can assume that the effectiveness of contraception was not high among young single adults in the nineteenth century. We can also assume that young people engaged more freely in premarital relations towards the end of the century than they did near the middle of the century, as the chances of marrying earlier were becoming less and less hampered by enforcement of the restrictive Malthusian marriage code.

Moreover, we are dealing with a situation in which parentally arranged marriage were not the rule and where only the choice of a particular partner could possibly be obstructed by parents. As a result, a modern form of partner choice emerged, characterized by a relatively high degree of freedom within fairly broad boundaries of social classes. In this context an increase in premarital conceptions would be normal as long as contraception among the younger adults was not widespread or was largely ineffective.

At the same time, the range of possible outcomes of an unmarried woman's pregnancy presumably widened. First, the man would be under less pressure to marry the mothers of his child as the effectiveness of village opinions and social sanctions declined. Second, even if he did plan to marry her, there may have been a decrease in the social pressure to marry before the confinement. In this instance, the child would be legitimized later. The statistics on legitimations show that such marriages occurred fairly soon after the birth and that the number of legitimations increased rapidly. One would expect that all these alterations in premarital behavior and in the arrangement of marriages, leading to higher values of I_h, would be most typical of more industrialized, urbanized, or secularized areas. Our multivariate analysis supports this last hypothesis; it shows that these three variables affect the level of I_h not only directly, but presumably to some extent also indirectly via the nuptiality variable. This last element is subject to caution, since we do not know exactly to what degree our measure of illegitimate fertility I_h is by definition affected by the changes in the mean age at marriage.

After 1900, there emerged a growing link between the rates of decline in illegitimate and marital fertility. This indicates that more effective contraceptive practices were being used in premarital (and extramarital) relations. As a result, the values of I_h fell back to levels observed before 1860. In the more industrialized, urbanized, and secularized areas, this upward and downward movement of I_h was completed in 1930. In the more traditionally oriented as rural areas, this illegitimate fertility hump was considerably less marked. In these areas the proportions married at young ages did not rise ar rapidly as they did elsewhere. Most probably, by the time dating and marriage behavior had become modernized to the same degree as in the more advanced areas, the emergence of more effective contraception had intervened, and this was enough to suppress the hump in the evolution of I_h that might otherwise have occurred.

The dates of the appearance of marital fertility control in the 41

Belgian arrondissements are scattered over a period of about half a century. From 1866 marital fertility followed an uninterrupted downward movement in several arrondissements of Hainaut and in the adjacent arrondissement of Philippeville; it was not until after World War I that such a trend appeared in the arrondissement of Maaseik. These dates set the stage: we can say that the marital fertility decline occurred in a period characterized by a substantial and unprecedented transformation of the economic and social structure. The fact, however, that two areas in Belgium, which are not even 100 miles apart, experienced their fertility declines with a time lag of 60 years between them, shows very clearly that such a general statement is far from satisfactory.

There is no shortage of questions that can be posed. Let us consider the following:

1. Given a general link between the modernization of the socioeconomic structure and the decline of marital fertility, what are the mechanisms through which these social changes affect a decline in marital fertility?
2. Given the detection of these mechanisms, can they be sufficiently universal to repeat themselves in other regions? Put slightly differently, is there a threshold of modernization (or a checklist of essential characteristics measured along some multidimensional socioeconomic scale) that will identify a population in which marital fertility is ready to fall? (see A. J. Coale, 1973, p. 64).

On the basis of this study, the first question can be answered only partially. We have only a limited set of variables to work with, and they are not measured on the basis of individual units of observation; thus, it is impossible to test a fairly intricate model in all details. As discussed, we have had to restrict ourselves to those elements for which an operationalization was possible.

The strong relationship between the rate of the marital fertility decline and the index of industrialization-urbanization indicates that modernization of the occupational structure was indeed a forceful agent in the process of fertility reduction. The mechanism of social capillarity, directly linked to the expansion of the occupational structure and the social-stratification system, was probably at work. It is equally likely that the modification of the socioeconomic structure resulted in a pronounced desire for "high quality children" and in a reduced economic utility of children. One could also argue, however, that an increase in real incomes could more easily meet the demand for "high quality children" and that, as a consequence, there would have been no need to curb fertility. This conjecture is not in line with the empirical findings: the more urbanized and industrialized areas in Belgium were definitely those where real income rose more rapidly and where, on the whole, fertility declined earlier and at a faster pace. As a result, it seems more likely that an increased preference for "high quality children" was reinforced rather than satisfied by increasing real income. In other words, the income factor probably acted as an intensifier that magnified the desire to give children more chances to succeed in life and that reduced their prospective economic utility as well.

Given that the situation is characterized at the outset by natural fertility and that the socioeconomic development acted in the direction of a decline in the desired number of children, excess fertility should develop (see R. Easterlin, 1972, pp. 33, 42). In other words, the desired family size would fall short of the fertility level implied by the traditionally prevailing level of natural fertility. This excess could be reinforced further by a decline in infant mortality and by an increase in the number of reproductive years added by a decrease in the age at marriage. From the evidence gathered in Belgium, however, it seems that these two factors were of secondary importance. The decline in infant mortality came too late in several areas and was unrelated to the initial decline in marital fertility. A similar observation has been made for Germany (J. Knodel, 1974). There, the national trends of infant mortality and marital fertility were remarkably parallel; but once the national population is broken down into provincial populations, it is clear that the infant-mortality decline came after the drop in I_g in about half the provinces. As a result, it is sometimes difficult to maintain a view of the infant-mortality decline as one of the initial causes of the marital fertility decline. Very much the same can be said about nuptiality. In Flanders, the high inverse correlation found between nuptiality intensity and marital fertility seems to be spurious to a considerable degree; and in Wallonia, the relationship breaks down when the rate of fertility decline is predicted on the basis of the rate of nuptiality increase.

If excess fertility did indeed emerge in Belgium, it was not sufficient to provoke on its own such a steep drop in marital fertility as that witnessed after 1870 or 1880. Knowledge about effective forms of contraception must have been available, the couples must also have been willing to pay a psychological "price" for adopting sexually less satisfying practices such as abstinence or coitus interruptus, and the ethical or religious restrictions on contraception must have been overcome. These constraints were important in Belgium because of the rather militant position of Catholic officials, the restrictive legal system, the presumed heavy use of coitus interruptus, and the late modernization of contraceptive technology. If we add to these restrictions the observation that the eradication of illiteracy, the decline of infant mortality, and the change in nuptiality were not important as incentives, then it becomes clear that the metamorphosis of the economic basis and of the occupational structure must have accounted for a substantial part of the increasing motivation to limit fertility.

Up to this point, the modernization of the occupational structure and related factors have received ample credit. It is possible that we may have overlooked other factors characteristic of the modernization of the socioeconomic structure that deserve a share of the credit as well. All these socioeconomic elements combined may be able to indicate the direction of the fertility trends, but it is nevertheless unlikely that they fully account for the regional differences with respect to the date and pace of the marital fertility decline. It is difficult to define a socioeconomic threshold that will identify a population in which marital fertility is ready to fall. Van de Walle and Knodel (1967, pp. 47-55) were willing to look for such a threshold in a larger western European context. Rather than revealing a socioeconomic threshold, however, their analysis showed instead how heterogeneous the socioeconomic characteristics of the various national popultions were at the time of their marital fertility decline. At one end of the scale they found that most of France had engineered its fertility transition entirely within the preindustrial era. At the other end came nations like Germany where substantial socioeconomic transformation occurred before marital fertility decreased steadily. The examples of England and Wallonia are equally interesting in this respect: the two industrial pioneers of Western Europe failed to reduce their marital fertility levels until 1870, whereas rural Normandy succeeded in doing so 70 years earlier.

Within the limits of a small country such as Belgium, we are equally unsuccessful in identifying a socioeconomic threshold, despite the fact that the modernization of the occupational structure accounts for a large part of the regional variation in I_g. First, as long as we introduce only socioeconomic characteristics, a substantial difference between Walloon and Flemish marital fertility remains unexplained. Second, this difference is particularly sharp, and a real demarcation line between high and low fertility can be found over the entire length of the language border, i.e., even within pairs of Walloon and Flemish villages that are, on the average, only 4 miles away from each other. Third, similar indications of earlier fertility control are found among the Francophone populations of Brussels and of the Flemish cities. Fourth, the three arrondissements of Limburg and the adjacent arrondissement of Turnhout remained behind in the evolution of marital fertility, even when a series of socioeconomic variables are controlled for. As late as the 1950s and early 1960s, these Limburg arrondissements recorded values of I_g considerably higher than those found in most of the country after World War I.

Obviously, a second set of factors, other than strictly socioeconomic ones, are at work. In this respect the impact of language and secularization is far from negligible. These two variables cannot be taken as entirely dependent. In other words, there is a partial, but no complete, overlap between the socioeconomic variables and these two cultural dimensions. Let us document this more specifically.

The index of language homogeneity in Flanders largely reflects the size of the socially, economically, and culturally distinct groups of Francophone Flemings. As these groups were found essentially in urban areas and belonged to the more educated middle and upper classes, the index must correlate with the degree of urbanization and with measures that reflect the existence of a more diversified social stratification system and a more modernized occupational structure. In this way, a more complex syndrome emerges in which socioeconomic and cultural features are reflected simultaneously. It is in this particular sense that language differences are partly related to socioeconomic ones.

The language factors has a meaning of its own, however, independent of socioeconomic characteristics. Language acts as a communication barrier, as an obstacle in the process of diffusion. In this respect, the early adoption of fertility control, emerging in Hainaut and spreading to the rest of Wallonia, stopped at the language border. Not only did Flemings and Walloons who lived as neighbors in this very narrow strip along the language border fail to intermarry to a considerable extent, but they also did not take each other's attitude toward fertility. As a result, two separate diffusion patterns developed in Flanders and Wallonia and at no point did we find traces of a spill-over across the language border.

The effect of secularization upon marital fertility is also partly linked to socioeconomic factors and partly independent of them. In both language regions, a higher degree of secularization developed in areas characterized by higher levels of industrialization and urbanization. As a result, we again find the emergence of a complex syndrome that incorporates socioeconomic and cultural features. Despite this, we find that Walloon arrondissements had reached much higher levels of secularization than the Flemish ones for a given level of socioeconomic development. Hence, secularization reflects dimensions other than socioeconomic ones. The most obvious of these dimensions is the less traditionally oriented mentality of the Walloon population. The fact that this is highly associated with earlier and a more rapid fertility decline leads us to the conclusion that, on the average, Walloons were bringing their fertility within the calculus of conscious choice earlier than the Flemish. In Flanders, this new, more rational mode of thought remained longer in conflict with deeply rooted religious and traditional ethics, and as a result, marital fertility declined later. To summarize, the secularization factor seems to have influenced marital fertility—

1. by helping to bring the fertility of couples within the frame of conscious choice and rational calculation;
2. by reducing the tradtiional religious and ethical constraints toward contraception in general and toward specific contraceptive practices in particular;
3. by intensifying the effect of the socioeconomic elements of modernization.

Given that the secularization variable contains a large amount of information about both socioeconomic and cultural determinants of fertility, and considering that it was the only variable able to explain the fertility differentials between Walloon and Flemish arrondissements, we should not be surprised that a threshold can be established on the basis of this "contextual" variable. To establish this, it suffices to plot the proportion of the total decline of marital fertility occurring between 1880 and 1910 (ΔI_g 1880–1910) against the level of secularization. As the latter variable cannot be measured for this period, we have to establish a retrospective threshold, and predict ΔI_g 1880–1910 on the basis of secularization 1919. The resulting relationship can then be interpreted as follows: from the knowledge that a specific arrondissement has evolved to a particular level of secularization, we should be able to infer how far it has come with respect to the marital fertility decline. The scattergram relating ΔI_g 1880–1900 to the level of secularization in 1919 is given in Figure 7.1. It shows a remarkable feature: the percentage change in I_g is almost exactly equal to the percentage of the vote non-Catholic. When one-third of the votes goes to non-Catholic parties in

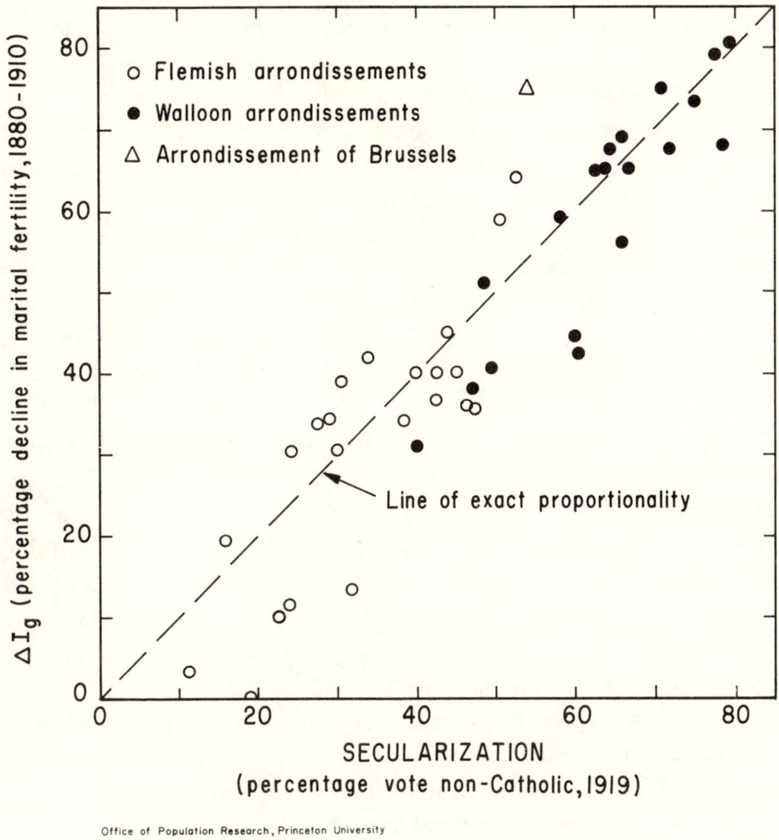

Figure 7.1 Secularization and Fertility, Scattergram Relating Non-Catholic Vote, 1919, with Change in Marital Fertility (ΔI_g), 1880–1910, by Arrondissement.

1919, about one-third of the fertility transition has been completed by 1910. Hence, if we know that a particular arrondissement reported more than 40 percent of its votes as non-Catholic in 1919, we know that its level of marital fertility must have dropped during the preceding decades to around .600 or lower, i.e., below the level that was accepted as a definite indication of the appearance of conscious fertility control in Belgium. For example, to take an extreme case, even if I_g was as high as .900 or .950 in 1880, ΔI_g of 40 percent would bring I_g down to .620 by 1910.

The impact of secularization or its complement, religiosity, did not disappear during the subsequent decades. In fact, it continued to influence general fertility (I_f) through both the nuptiality (I_m) and marital fertility (I_g) components. C. Wattelar and G. Wunsch (1967, p. 108) analyzed the mean age at marriage and the proportion never marrying in the Belgian arrondissements for the early 1960s. They found that no indicator performed better in their predictions than the percentage of votes Catholic or Socialist. Moreover, a higher non-Catholic vote was associated with earlier and more universal marriage in the 1960s in just the same way as it was at the turn of the century. The fertility of individual couples in the 1950s and 1960s has been the subject of several studies: here, too, the degree of religiosity has been shown to be a crucial factor (K. Dobbelaere, 1967, pp. 360-367; J. Morsa and G. Julémont, 1972, pp. 42-55).

In the 1950s and 1960s, the distribution of parity-specific fertility varied far less than it did in 1910. Since 1965, this variance has been even further reduced to an unprecedented minimum. Even in these circumstances, R. van Malderghem (1974) has found on the basis of data of the National Fertility Survey of 1971 that two variables stand out in predicting the current and expected parity of women aged 30-34 years and married for five years or more: religiosity and female labor force participation. Other variables, such as education, individual income, social mobility, degree of urbanization, and language, have either a secondary effect or none at all. Of all the variables that have emerged as indicators of fertility reduction in late nineteenth century Belgium, secularization seems to be the one that can be singled out, both as the most powerful variable at the outset of the fertility decline and as the one with the longest lasting effect or the highest degree of persistence.

The Belgian example is not an isolated case in Europe. France was a European leader with respect to fertility control and probably also with respect to secularization; in Italy and Portugal, fertility declined precipitously among populations and in regions renowned for their lack of sympathy toward religion (M. Livi Bacci, 1965; 1971); and the Dutch experience shows that not only Catholic subpopulations, but also more traditional Protestant groups were more resistant to the spread of fertility control (F. van Heek, 1963, pp. 81-103; S. van Poppel, 1974).

As a conclusion, it appears to us that it is difficult to establish a strictly socioeconomic threshold to predict the appearance of conscious fertility regulation, even if relatively homogeneous cultural regions are considered. Flanders and Wallonia are often taken as culturally homogeneous areas; yet we can assert that a relatively precise socioeconomic threshold is absent within their boundaries. Too many areas remained essentially rural or economically less advanced but nevertheless had a relatively early fertility decline. Conversely, too many areas failed to experience a particularly early fertility decline despite their rapid socioeconomic development. Rather, the effect of socioeconomic modernization is partially channelled through the increase in secularization. This variable absorbs several cultural traits, and it reflects better the degree to which traditional moral and religious barriers are overcome. As a result, such a contextual variable emerges as the most powerful predictor of the fertility decline in the whole of Belgium and reduces to a secondary exercise the search for a regional socioeconomic threshold. This analysis contains a classic lesson: traditional ethical and religious constraints had to yield to a more rational outlook before fertility was brought within the calculus of conscious choice, and before the direct impact of socioeconomic development could be felt . The main reasons for Belgium's second place in the chronological list of countries that experienced a fertility transition can then be stated succinctly as follows: fairly early economic and social transformations coincided with and were partly responsible for an early breach in ethical and religious barriers; a relatively low level of secularization was sufficient to release the mechanisms that would bring fertility down; and once the process was set in motion, most of the country experienced a fast evolution to higher levels of secularization and, simultaneously, to lower levels of marital fertility.

The diagnosis of C. Jacquart, Father Vermeersch, and Cardinal Mercier in 1908 was in essence correct: fertility control and securlarization were an interacting set of phenomena. Their pleas and action against onanism came too late, however. By 1900, a large number of Belgians had already chosen in favor of smaller families; they had decided that the church could maintain its authority in strictly religious matters but that fertility regulation was their own private affair.

References—Chapter 7

Coale, A. J. 1973. The demographic transition. In *Proceedings of the International Population Conference,* pp. 53-71. Liège: International Union for the Scientific Study of Population.

Dobbelaere, K. 1967. Ideal number of children in marriage in Belgium and the USA. *Journal of Marriage and the Family* 29:360-367.

Easterlin, R. 1972. The economics and sociology of fertility: a synthesis. Paper read at Seminar on Early Industrialization, Shifts in Fertility, and Changes in Family Structure, at Institute for Advanced Study, Princeton, N. J.

Knodel, J. 1974. *The decline of fertility in Germany, 1871–1939.* Princeton: Princeton University Press.

Livi Bacci, M. 1965. Il declino della fecondità della popolazione Italiana nell'ultimo secolo. *Statistica.*

———. 1971. A century of Portuguese fertility. Princeton: Princeton University Press.

Morsa, J., and Julémont, G. 1972. Une enquê nationale sur la fécondité—attentes et souhaîts (1966). *Population et Famille,* pp. 15-68.

van de Walle, E., and Knodel, J. 1967. Demographic transition and fertility decline: the European case. In *Proceedings of the International Population Conference,* pp. 47-55. Sydney: International Union for the Scientific Study of Population.

van Heek, F. 1963. Het Nederlands geboortepatroon en de godsdienstfactor gedurende de laatste halve eeuw. *Mens en Maatschappij* 38:81-103.

van Malderghem, R. 1974. Evolutie van de gezinsgrootte in de Nederlandse Kultuurgemeenschap van België tussen 1966 en 1971. Mimeographic report at Vrije Universiteit Brussel.

van Poppel, S. 1974. De differentiële vruchtbaarheid in Nederland in historisch perspectief: de invloed van de religie. *Bevolking en Gezin.*

Wattelar, C., and Wunsch, G. 1967. *Etude démographique de la nuptialité en Belgique.* Louvain: Institut de Recherches Economiques, Sociales et Politiques, Université Catholique de Louvain.

APPENDIX: The Quality of the Demographic Data

A.1 *Introduction*

The measurements of nuptiality and fertility used in this monograph are based mainly on censuses and records of vital registration. The former source yields information relative to the female population by age and marital status, and the latter provides the number of births by legitimacy. Both sources existed prior to 1846, the date of Belgium's first census as an independent nation, but they were not always complete in terms of geographic or demographic coverage. The census of 1846 was preceded by six others: the census of 1784 conducted under the Austrian regime; the censuses of 1801, 1806, 1811, and 1816 ordered by the French Republic; and the census of 1829 taken in the last year of the Dutch occupation. Two of these enumerations (1811 and 1816) contain merely a count of the total population and are consequently not suitable for further demographic use. While the other censuses are more detailed, a systematic publication of their data does not yet exist. It is still a task for historians and demographers to gather the scattered information buried mainly in the French and local Belgian archives (see A. Quételet, 1847, X. Heuschling, 1875).

Our series of nuptiality and fertility indices starts in 1846 with the first national census. Ever since independence, the government had felt a need for more detailed information on the Belgian population. An important workgroup was installed, the *Commission centrale de Statistique,* under the presidency of A. Quételet. This leading scientist not only established the first life tables for Belgium, but was also familiar with the modern demographic notions of stationary and stable population models; as the director of the National Observatory he started the first series of meteorological statistics and won admiration in the French-speaking world with his sociological treatise (A. Quételet, 1848). Under the leadership of this capable man, the *Commission* prepared and conducted the census of 1846 with great care. In 1842 and again in 1845 tests were held in the Brussels urban area and the system of enumeration on the basis of household questionnaires was set up. These questionnaires were filled out by the head of each household in the presence of a census agent, or, in the case of insufficient literacy, by the census agent himself at the dwelling of the subjects. The whole operation of 1846 was strongly decentralized: controls were performed at the level of each community by a commission of local notables, and again on the provincial level by a commission of better-qualified scientists. Defective household questionnaires were sent back for re-enumeration or completion. It should be noted that the data gathered in this way were relative to the de facto population; it was only from 1866 that the household questionnaires were filled out on the basis of the de jure population.

The system of vital registration also underwent considerable reorganization during this period. Beginning in 1792, parish records of baptisms, burials, and marriages kept by the clergy were deposited in town halls and administered by the municipal authorities. In 1834, the first regular publication of the vital registration started; this incorporated more-detailed information (data on migration, age at death, and births and deaths by month). In 1841, the statistical tables were further expanded and standardized and remained the basis for vital registration in the following decades. In this reorganization, the hand of Quételet and his colleague, X. Heuschling, is clearly visible. Both men undertook regular inspection trips all over the country, sometimes severely reprimanding the local authorities and clerks for the slightest deficiency in the vital statistics records.

As a result, both the census and the vital registration are believed to be of excellent quality. In 1890, a member of the French Academy, E. Levasseur, considered the enumeration of 1846 as "the first really scientific census ever taken." Whether or not this compliment was merited is the question posed in this appendix.

A.2 *The Age Distribution and the Mortality Experience*

It is a common feature in partially illiterate populations that when ages are recorded, a pattern of age-heaping emerges. This results from the reporting of ages in multiples of five or ten years. Other age misstatement also frequently occurs. The best-known example of this is the phenomenon where young married women report older ages, closer to the generally accepted average age at marriage, whereas older single women report younger ages. This systematic age misstatement is not as readily detected by visual inspection of the age pyramid as the phenomenon of age heaping.

The age pyramids for Belgium for the first four censuses have been constructed in Figure A.1. They reveal immediately that age-heaping occurred very clearly from age 30 onward at multiples of 10 years. Of these first four enumerations, the census of 1846 is most affected, but

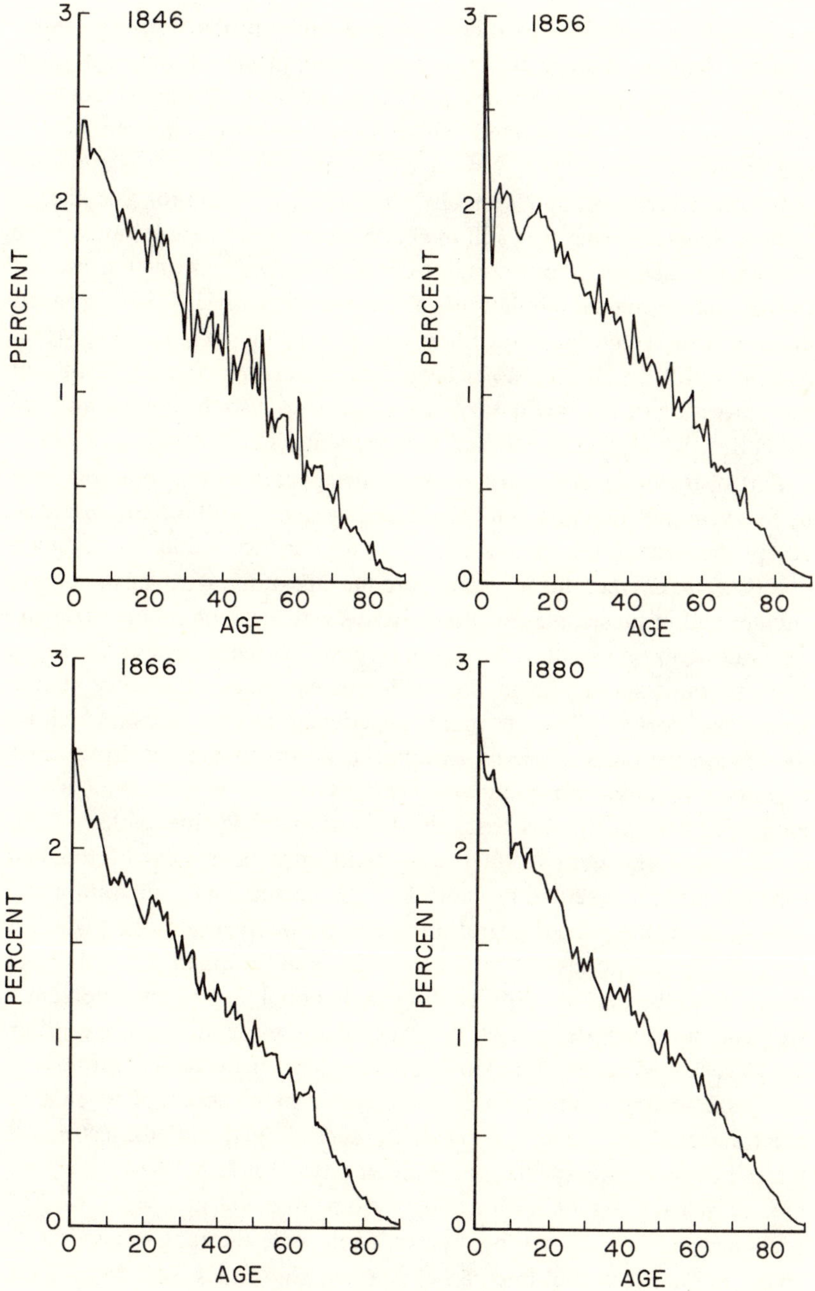

Office of Population Research, Princeton University

Figure A.1 Age distribution by Single Years of Age: 1846, 1856, 1866, and 1880.

age-heaping diminishes gradually to negligible proportions in 1880. Another striking feature is the drastic misreporting of the first three years of life in the census of 1856. The number of infants between 0 and 1 year is clearly inflated, whereas the number of children from 2 to 3 years is undercounted. No trace of such a misstatement is apparent in the other censuses, and we really have no explanation for this phenomenon. Quételet, who was still in charge of the 1856 census, must have noticed this deficiency but remains conspicuously silent on that matter. In fact, the summary tabulations of the age structure in 1856 grouped the first three single ages together, concealing this irregularity. Moreover, it would be difficult to believe that the error occurred mainly in the processing of the raw data, since it shows up also in the regional age structures, which were compiled independently of each other.

Part of the error in the first censuses disappears by grouping the data by five-year age intervals, but the remaining error is still too important to accept the age structures of 1846 and 1856 at face value. A common procedure to correct this is to compare the size of five-year birth cohorts enumerated in successive censuses. In this way, a set of cohort survivorship rates can be calculated from one census to the next and the series of these rates should be in line with the mortality experience in the intercensal period. This mortality experience can be measured either directly on the basis of the registration of deaths by age, or, in the case of suspect or unknown quality of mortality registration, on the basis of model life tables. In this case, the Princeton model life tables (A. J. Coale and P. Demeny, 1966) were used and the results of the first calculations are presented in Table A.1. No correction for migration was applied, since the annual migration rate in the intercensal period was less than -2.0 per thousand in 1846–1856 and dropped to -0.3 per thousand in the period 1866–1880 (female population). The intercensal survivorship rates, defined as the ratio of the population in age group $x+10$ to $x+15$ to the population 10 years earlier in the age group x to $x+5$, shows important fluctuations. This is more apparent when they are translated into levels of mortality according to the Princeton life tables in which the expectation of life at birth (for females) is 2.5 years greater at each higher level, ranging from 20 years at level 1 to 77.5 years at level 24. As can be seen in Table A.1, the range of mortality levels implied by the intercensal survivorship rates for 1846–1856 exceeds 7.00 levels, which indicates the existence of important irregularities in the enumeration of the female population by age at both dates.

APPENDIX

TABLE A.1

INTERCENSAL SURVIVORSHIP RATE AND IMPLIED LEVELS OF MORTALITY: 1846-1856 AND 1856-1866

Age	1846-1856		1856-1866	
	Survivorship rate	Level of mortality (West)	Survivorship rate	Level of mortality (West)
0-4 /10-14	.8616	7.47	.9050	10.89
5-9 /15-19	.9009	3.72	.9463	10.08
10-14/20-24	.9244	8.06	.9414	10.61
15-19/25-29	.8989	7.04	.8862	5.47
20-24/30-34	.8446	3.64	.8866	7.29
25-29/35-39	.9094	10.87	.8582	6.00
30-34/40-44	.9080	11.81	.8563	6.88
35-39/45-49	.8836	10.39	.8429	6.77
40-44/50-54	.8716	11.04	.8494	8.98
45-49/55-59	.8057	8.47	.8126	8.97
50-54/60-64	.7509	8.81	.7821	10.90
55-59/65-69	.7160	11.73	.7309	12.66
60-64/70-74	.5736	9.69	.5949	10.88
65-69/75-79	.4542	10.46	.4658	11.08

NOTE: Intercensal survivorship rate is defined as:

$$\frac{\text{population aged } x+10 \text{ to } x+15 \text{ at time } t}{\text{population aged } x \text{ to } x+5 \text{ at time } t+10}$$

The levels of mortality implied by the intercensal survivorship rates for the period 1856–1866 are slightly more consistent, but the implied life expectancy still varies from 32.5 years (level 6) to 47.5 years (level 12). The ups and downs of the survivorship rates can also be followed in Figure A.2, where they are compared to survivorship rates of two model life tables. The sequence of rates for the period 1866–1880 was also calculated for a 14-year interval, and they were considerably more regular as could be expected from the limited amount of age misstatement apparent in the censuses of 1866 and 1880. Hence, only the census results of 1856, and, to a larger degree, those of 1846 have to be corrected, whereas the figures for 1866 and 1880 can be accepted.

A classic way of estimating the appropriate level of mortality is offered by projecting the initial age distribution over the next 10 years by means of the model life table survivorship rates corresponding to various levels of mortality. Each resulting projected age structure can then be cumulated starting at the highest age, and the result can be compared with the enumerated age distribution at time t+10, cumulated in the same way. In this manner, cumulation has an important dampening

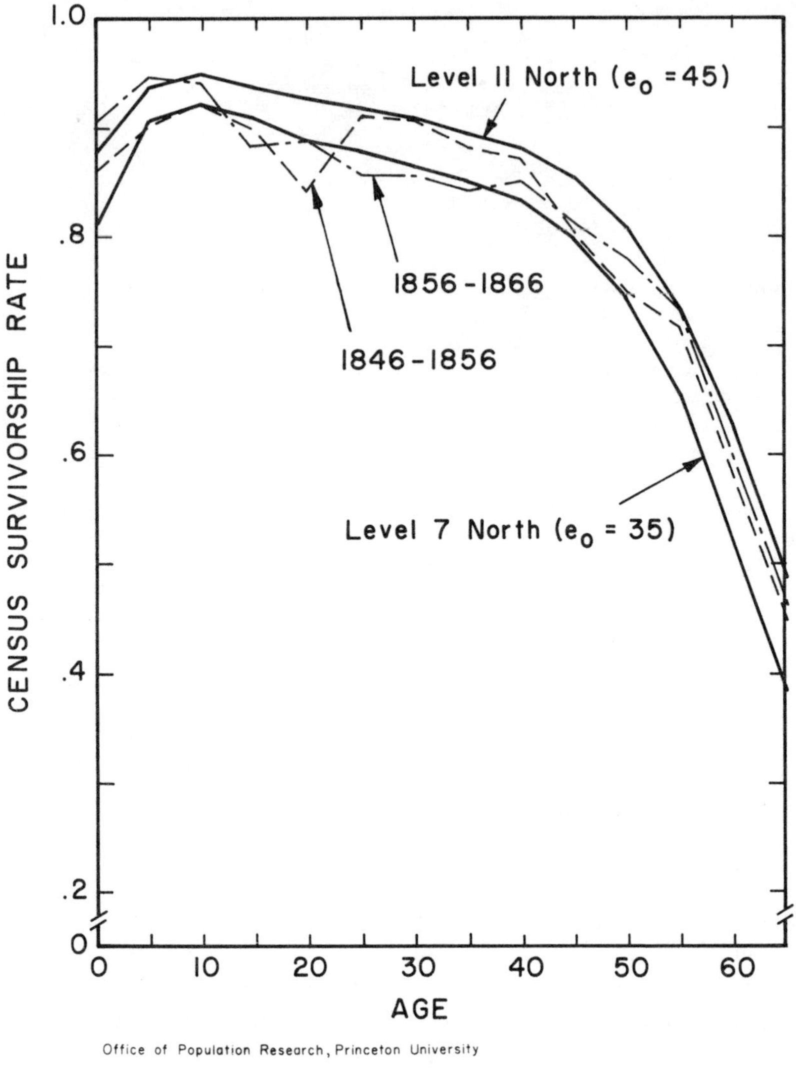

Figure A.2 Intercensal Survivorship Rate and Implied Levels of Mortality: 1846–1856 and 1856–1866.

effect on the irregularities shown on Figure A.2, and the revealed levels of mortality are considerably more consistent than those implied by the intercensal survivorship rates. On the basis of this sequence of mortality levels, one single level can be chosen, representing the mortality experience of the intercensal period. Here, the initial population was projected with West and North model life tables, and the results of the calculations are presented in Table A.2. Since we are basically interested in the correction of the younger sections of the age distribution, we have also compared the range of levels implied by the first nine age categories. In both 1846–1856 and 1856–1866, the North models yield more consistent results: they imply a variation in life expectancy at birth of 3.83 and 2.75 years respectively, compared to 7.25 and 5.78 years for the West models. The North models of the Princeton life tables have a higher mortality among young adults for a given mortality intensity among older adults (above age 40 or 45), and hence a smaller discrepancy exsits between mortality intensities of infants and children on one hand and intensities among young adults on the other hand. These North schedules represent more fully the prevalence of mortality from tuberculosis than the West family. Since tuberculosis was the major

TABLE A.2

IMPLIED LEVELS OF MORTALITY, WEST AND NORTH MODEL LIFE TABLES: 1846-1856 AND 1856-1866

	1846-1856		1856-1866	
Age	West	North	West	North
0-4 /10-14	7.57	8.35	8.99	8.78
5-9 /15-19	7.95	7.96	8.75	8.08
10-14/20-24	9.20	8.16	8.67	7.76
15-19/25-29	9.30	8.20	8.53	7.57
20-24/30-34	9.55	8.49	8.83	7.91
25-29/35-39	10.47	9.49	9.28	8.35
30-34/40-44	10.42	9.42	9.77	8.78
35-39/45-49	10.23	9.17	10.24	9.16
40-44/50-54	10.20	9.06	10.84	9.67
45-49/55-59	10.02	8.92	11.19	9.98
50-54/60-64	10.46	9.37	11.75	10.47
55-59/65-69	11.01	9.99	12.02	10.81
60-64/70-74	10.71	9.90	11.69	10.70
Median of first 9 levels:	9.55	8.46	9.28	8.78
Range of first 9 levels:	2.90	1.53	2.31	1.10
Variation in life expectancy at birth corresponding to the range of first 9 levels (in years):	7.25	3.83	5.78	2.75

disease in Belgium at this time, it is not surprising to find a smaller range among North levels.

Taking the median of the first nine levels as representative for the intercensal mortality experience, one can compare the functions of the most appropriate North models with those calculated directly on the basis of the registration of deaths and census data. Again, it was A. Quételet who compiled the first trustworthy life table for Belgium for the period 1841–1850, using registered deaths by age centered on the age structure given in the 1846 census (A. Quételet, 1853). The comparison of Quételet's results and ours, given in Figure A.3, is based on the l_x-function, or the number of surviving women at an exact age x, stemming from an initial cohort of 10,000 female live births. The agreement between the l_x-functions is nearly complete from age 25 on. Before that age, Quételet finds a slightly smaller infant mortality of 150 per thousand live births, compared to 164 (1846–1856) and 166 (1856–1866) in the North models. This initial difference between Quételet's results and ours remains the same up to age 20, as shown in Table A.3.

TABLE A.3

LIFE TABLE POPULATIONS BY FIVE-YEAR INTERVALS TO AGE 35: QUETELET FOR 1841-1850 AND NORTH FOR 1846-1856 AND 1856-1866

Age	Quételet, 1841-1850	North, 1846-1856	North, 1856-1866	Differences (1)-(2)	(1)-(3)
0	10,000	10,000	10,000	--	--
1	8,497	8,358	8,337	139	160
5	7,253	7,147	7,114	106	139
10	6,886	6,704	6,664	182	222
15	6,626	6,482	6,440	144	186
20	6,350	6,256	6,214	94	136
25	6,036	6,006	5,962	30	74
30	5,730	5,728	5,683	2	47
35	5,427	5,420	5,373	7	44

SOURCE: A. Quételet [1853, p. 20].

NOTE: North levels are 8.49 in 1846-1856 and 8.35 in 1856-1866.

If all series were adjusted for the same intensity of infant mortality, the discrepancy would hardly be noticeable in Figure A.3. Several factors can explain this difference: (1) Infant mortality could have been underregistered by 10 percent; (2) the link between infant and adolescent mortality postulated in the North models, is not fully applicable to the

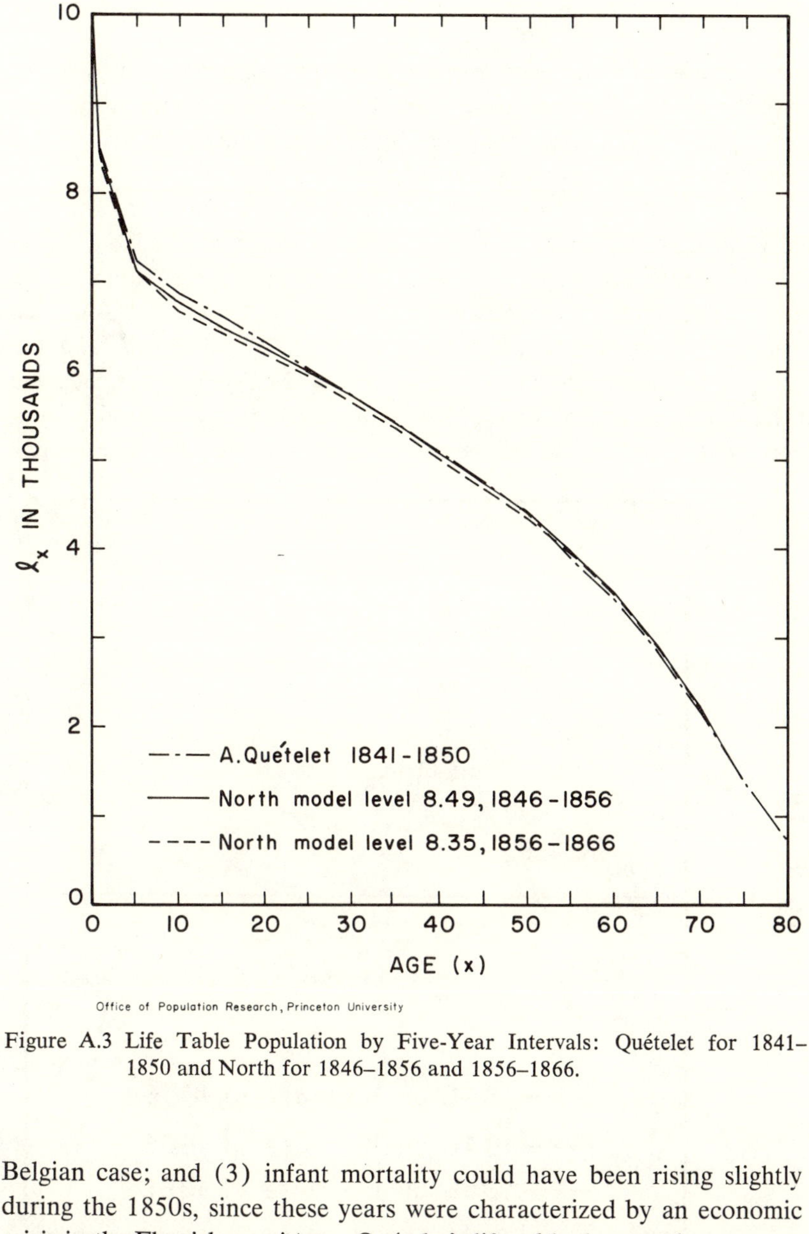

Figure A.3 Life Table Population by Five-Year Intervals: Quételet for 1841–1850 and North for 1846–1856 and 1856–1866.

Belgian case; and (3) infant mortality could have been rising slightly during the 1850s, since these years were characterized by an economic crisis in the Flemish provinces. Quételet's life table does not incorporate data after 1850, which partly explains his lower figure for infant mortality. On the whole, one should not push the importance of such small differences in l_x-values to the extreme, and the close agreement found in Figure A.3 supports the usefulness of the Princeton models and the completeness of infant and overall mortality registration in Belgium since the 1850s. Consequently, when this matter is taken up in the next section, we will not accept estimates of infant mortality rates that exceed the reported ones by more than 10 percent.

The close agreement between the mortality experiences according to the vital registration and according to the North models enables us to reconstitute the age distribution for 1846 with confidence, either on the basis of the figures for 1856 or on the basis of those for 1866. The results of the backward projections are given in Table A.4 and the ratios of enumerated to calculated quantities (E/C-ratios) for each age interval are reported in Figure A.4. The ratios for 1846 reveal a common pattern of age mistatement, but the ratios for the age groups

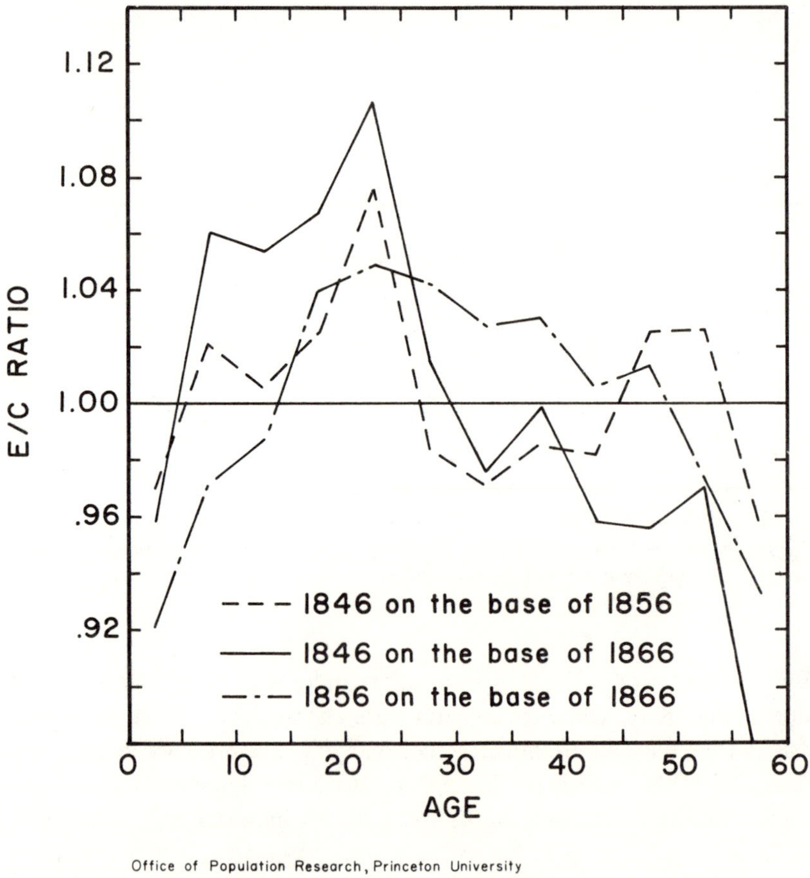

Figure A.4 Ratio of Enumerated to Calculated Population: 1846 and 1856.

TABLE A.4

CORRECTION OF FEMALE AGE DISTRIBUTIONS OF 1846 AND 1856 BY BACKWARD PROJECTION WITH NORTH MODEL LIFE TABLES

Age	Enumerated 1866 (1)	Calculated 1856 (2)	Calculated 1846 (3)	Enumerated 1856 (4)	Calculated 1846 (5)	Enumerated 1846 (6)	E/C-ratios (6)/(3)	(6)/(5)	(2)/(4)
0-4	---	264,482	261,810	243,679	258,438	250,755	.958	.970	.921
5-9	--	228,104	220,352	221,385	228,822	233,544	1.060	1.021	.971
10-14	220,530	218,905	196,674	216,085	206,073	207,324	1.054	1.006	.987
15-19	209,500	202,623	180,331	210,411	187,840	192,516	1.068	1.025	1.038
20-24	233,387	182,902	177,232	191,642	182,217	196,121	1.106	1.076	1.048
25-29	186,474	166,127	159,645	173,045	164,611	162,052	1.015	.984	1.042
30-34	166,078	161,120	153,383	165,652	154,262	149,806	.976	.971	1.028
35-39	148,513	142,923	140,901	145,369	142,823	140,707	.999	.985	1.031
40-44	141,856	135,246	132,849	136,022	129,694	127,344	.950	.982	1.006
45-49	124,216	122,661	128,339	124,335	119,779	122,725	.954	1.025	1.013
50-54	115,536	113,692	103,277	110,992	97,681	100,221	.970	1.026	.973
55-59	101,039	105,943	95,918	98,877	86,495	82,721	.862	.956	.933
60-64	86,808	79,566	--	75,255	--	--	--	--	--
65-69	72,262	65,684	--	59,231	--	--	--	--	--
70-74	44,768	--	--	--	--	--	--	--	--
75-79	27,588	--	--	--	--	--	--	--	--

NOTE: The backward projection from 1866 to 1856 is performed with North model life table, level 8.35, whereas the backward projection for 1856 to 1846 was level 8.49.

between 5 and 35 years are larger in the case of a backward projection starting in 1866 than those calculated in a reconstitution from 1856. This is caused by the general overenumeration of women in childbearing ages in 1856, and these larger quantities are then shifted 10 years backward. In 1846, the number of children between 0 and 5 years of age is probably underreported by some 3 to 4 percent; the figure is probably larger in 1856.

Hence, in addition to heaping around ages that are multiples of 10 years, there are also other forms of distortion. On the whole, if the reported female age structure is represented in five-year age intervals, it can be assumed that the maximum magnitude of error in most age groups does not exceed 4 to 5 percent. However, the age intervals of 0-5 years and 20-25 years are exceptional, and the magnitude of distortion may increase to 8 percent.

A.3 *The Registration of Live Births*

The second element needed in the calculation of the basic demographic measures of fertility is the number of live births given by the vital registration. The method for verifying the completeness of birth registration is based on the comparison of the reported number of live births in the five-year period prior to a census, deflated by infant and early childhood deaths, to the reported number of children under age 5 in the census. Before the results of such calculations will be considered, a few remarks have to be made. First, this system works only in the case of properly registered infant and childhood mortality and accurately enumerated population size in the youngest age interval. Equality of the child population estimated from the registered births and enumerated in the census can hence be obtained in a setting where all three pieces of information—births, deaths, and population size—are underestimated. Hence, the remarks made in the previous section relative to infant mortality and population size in the age group from 0 to 5 years should be kept in mind.

The E/C ratios of enumerated to calculated population under age 5 (E/C-ratios) for 1846 are given in Table A.5, where the information is also broken down by province and level of urbanization. The overall picture shows good agreement between the calculated and the enumerated quantities. Focusing on the E/C-ratios for the entire age interval of 5 years, one observes that no province other than Brabant has an error exceeding 2 percent. The explanation for Brabant can be found in the disparity between the E/C-ratios for urban and rural areas: the

TABLE A.5

RATIO OF ENUMERATED TO CALCULATED NUMBER OF CHILDREN BY SINGLE YEARS OF AGE FROM 0 TO 5, BY PROVINCE AND DEGREE OF URBANIZATION: 1846

Area		0-1	1-2	2-3	3-4	4-5	0-5
Province:	Antwerp	.972	1.046	1.081	.951	1.007	1.006
	Brabant	.925	.929	.963	.950	.999	.952
	East Flanders	1.015	.985	.999	.980	1.016	.998
	West Flanders	1.069	1.000	1.062	.933	1.028	1.017
	Hainaut	.935	.984	.976	.999	1.023	.983
	Liège	.956	.972	.966	.995	1.026	.982
	Limburg	.983	.926	1.131	1.030	1.039	1.021
	Luxemburg	.982	.957	1.048	1.026	1.048	1.005
	Namur	.963	.979	1.050	.980	1.013	.998
Urban areas		.912	.949	.976	.928	.948	.943
Rural communities		1.002	.986	1.019	.992	1.043	1.007
Belgium		.978	.977	1.008	.976	1.019	.991

former have a deficit in the enumerated number of children, whereas the latter have a surplus. There is a fair possibility that this is caused by the migration of infants from the cities and mainly from Brussels (province of Brabant) to wet nurses in the countryside. The custom of sending off nurslings to the rural areas was practiced in Belgium, but to a considerably smaller extent than in certain French areas (E. van de Walle, 1974).

Following the E/C-ratios over the censuses of the previous century, one notices that the ratios for the 1846 census were very close to unity (Table A.6). The ratios for 1856 reveal large errors in the first three years of age, a feature already shown in the analysis of the census results for that year.

On the surface, the ratios suggest an accurate registration of births

TABLE A.6

RATIO OF ENUMERATED TO CALCULATED NUMBER OF CHILDREN BY SINGLE YEARS OF AGE FROM 0 TO 5: 1846 TO 1900

Date	0-1	1-2	2-3	3-4	4-5	0-5
1846	.978	.977	1.008	.976	1.019	.991
1856	1.229	.938	.754	.974	.964	.977
1866	.960	.982	.959	.966	1.002	.973
1880	.999	.950	.991	.986	.989	.982
1900	1.005	.991	.993	1.004	1.009	1.000

and an underenumeration of infants and young children of no more than 3 percent. In the previous section, however, we accepted a higher figure of 4 percent for 1846 and 7 to 8 percent for 1856. If mortality would be accurately measured in the register, and the higher set of figures for census underenumeration would hold, how large would the consequent error in birth registration be? Corrected for underenumeration by 4 percent, the size of the female population between 0-5 years in 1846 becomes 523,244 instead of 505,042. The calculated population on the basis of registered births and assuming correct death registration is 509,412. The E/C-ratio is consequently equal to 1.031, so that the calculated population becomes too small by 3.1 percent, attributable to underregistration of live births. Assuming a 7 percent underenumeration of infants and young children in 1856, one would obtain a 4.5 percent birth underregistration. If, in addition, mortality were slightly in error—10 percent in the first year of life and 1 percent in the other four years—the amount of birth underregistration would increase by another percent. The maximum figures are 4.1 percent for 1846 and 5.5 percent of 1856. Hence, accepting the reported numbers of live births at face value may lead to an error, but not to a serious one.

A.4 *The Distribution According to Marital Status*

The third element needed to establish the basic demographic measures is the distribution of the female population according to marital status. Here we have been working with a procedure suggested by A. J. Coale. This procedure was first tested using Swedish material from 1750 to 1900, and the excellent results justify the use of it in the Belgian case. The calculations are performed as an iteration process yielding an appropriate distribution of ever-married women and widows on the basis of two model functions.

Coale has shown that first-marriage frequencies observed in a number of diverse societies can be scaled in such a way that a single pattern of nuptiality emerges (1971, pp. 193-214; Coale and McNeil, 1972, pp. 743-749). On a standardized age scale this pattern is represented by the following function:

$$r(x) = 0.174 \exp(-4.411 e^{0.309x})$$

where $r(x)$ represents the risk of first marriage at different ages on a standard time schedule. Three parameters and this standard nuptiality distribution suffice to fit observed patterns. The parameters are:

a_0, the lowest age at which a noticeable proportion in the population first enters marriage;

k, a measure of the time scale at which the first marriages occur;

C, the final proportion ever-married at the age at which first marriages become negligible.

The values of a_o and k relate the observed time schedule of first marriages to the time schedule used in defining the standard pattern in the equation above. A k of 0.5, for instance, means that as many first marriages occur in 0.5 years in the actual case as in 1.0 year in the standard distribution; and a C equal to unity implies that, eventually, every woman gets married. Given values for a_o and k, and setting C equal to unity, the first-marriage frequencies can be calculated in a specific case by the following equation:

$$r(x) = (0.174/k)\exp(-4.411)\exp(-0{,}309/k)(x-a_o)$$

From these first-marriage frequencies an entire nuptiality table can be derived and on the basis of the number of person-years lived as ever-married in a cohort not subject to mortality, the proportions of women ever-married in each given age group can be compiled. These proportions applied to the age distribution, corrected in Section 2, yield the number of ever-married women by age group in the case of $C = 1.0$. The sum of these numbers divided by the total number of ever-married women in the actual population gives an estimate of C and adjusts the entire distribution for a C smaller than 1.0. So far, an infinite number of distributions of ever-married women can be calculated, but only one specific combination of C and k, given a fixed a_0, will yield a distribution satisfying the recorded total number of deaths to ever-married women. Hence, the deaths by age of all women are introduced and death rates to ever-married women are calculated on the basis of a standard set of ratios of death rates by age among ever-married women to death rates by age among single women. This set of ratios is obtained in a period for which it can be assumed that the registration of deaths by age and by marital status was accurate. In the Belgian case, they were taken from the data on mortality for the period 1890 to 1900. The program starts its iteration of the appropriate function of ever-married women with a schedule characterized by too low a value of k, and consequently a low value of C. In this schedule, the number of ever-married women in the lower age groups is too high and the number in the higher age groups too low. Since the bulk of mortality occurs among the higher ages, the calculated number of deaths to ever-married women is too low in comparison with the corresponding number taken from the register. The program increases the value of k, and hence also of C, until the total calculated number of deaths to ever-married women exceeds the actual number, and the appropriate distribution of ever-married women is then interpolated. Hence, a set of weights characterizing differential mortality by marital status and age, the number of overall deaths by age, the total number of ever-married women and the total number of deaths to them specify a unique distribution of single and ever-married women by age.

A similar procedure was adopted for the calculation of the age distribution of widows (and a negligible number of divorced women). A standard distribution of widows was taken from the 1900 census together with a series of weights (death rates among nonwidows to death rates among widows) from the 1890–1900 mortality experience. Two parameters adjusted this standard by iteration, so as to yield a distribution of widows by age conforming to both quantities, the total number of widows and the total number of deaths among them.

As the preliminary calculations on the Swedish material covering the experience of more than a century had shown, this system is extremely sensitive. A small discrepancy between the actual marital status distribution and the registered total number of deaths by marital status is revealed immediately by the comparison between the reported and calculated proportions single or ever-married. The results for Belgium 1846 are given in Figure A.5. The agreement between the enumerated- and calculated-proportions single and currently married is certainly very close but nevertheless not complete. The iterated value of C remained, in fact, nearly 2 percent higher than the actual value, accounting for a slightly higher value of k and consequently causing a difference of 2 to 3 percent between observed and calculated percentages currently married in the age groups of 25-29 and 30-34 years. Hence, a slight discrepancy existed between the deaths by marital status recorded in the period 1844–1848 and the marital status distribution given in the census of 1846, or the assumptions incorporated in the calculations do not hold perfectly. At any rate, this discrepancy is too small to affect our measure of nuptiality, as we will show in the section below.

A.5 *Final Remarks*

As the calculations in the previous section have revealed, the basic data taken from the register and the census are clearly imperfect in 1846

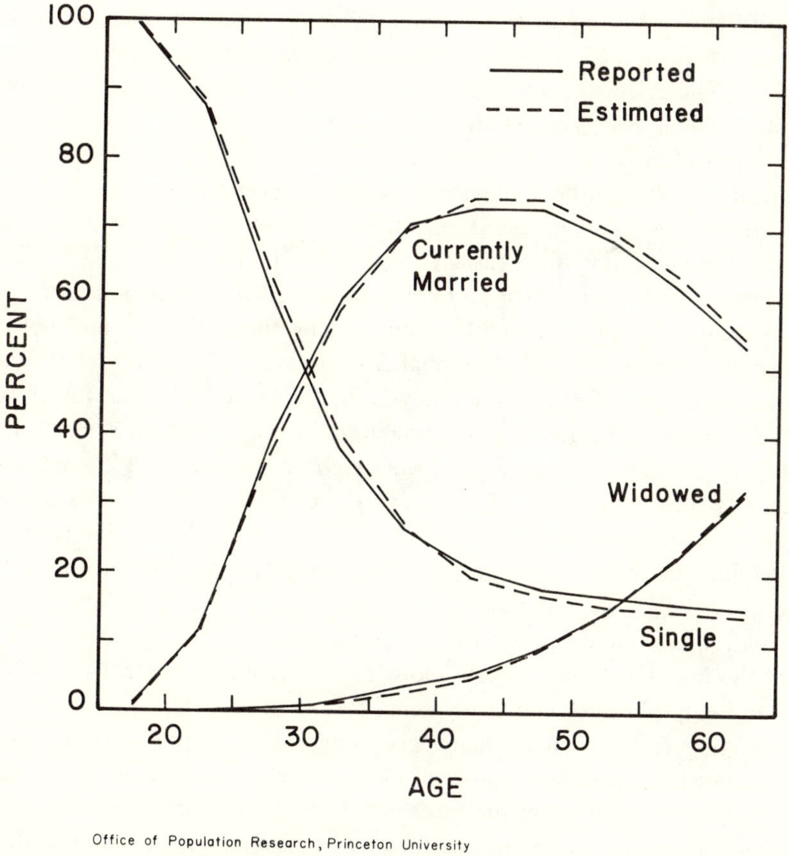

Figure A.5 Reported and Estimated Marital Status Distribution by Age: 1846

and 1856. However, our family of demographic indices is not quickly affected by certain types of census errors. The weights F_i are relatively similar for the age groups between 20 and 35 years, and shifts across boundaries within this interval will not have a marked effect. Age or marital status misstatement affecting the age group 15-19 or the age groups above 40, provoke a more important bias, together with under-registration of births. If one accepts the hypothesis concerning under-registration of infant mortality made in Section 2 and a consequent undercount of live births by 4 percent in 1846, together with the calculated age structure (Section A.3) and marital status distribution (Section A.4), a value of I_g equal to .822 is obtained. Compared to the reported value of .764 on the basis of the data taken at face value, this represents a maximum error of 7.5 percent. Similarly, the calculated value of I_m is .367, which is 3 percent lower than the reported one of .375. The calculated and reported values of I_f are respectively .325 and .302, which leaves a difference of 5 percent. Given these possible margins of error, it would be an overstatement to regard the quality of the data in the middle of the previous century as excellent.

So far, we have discussed only the nature of the data necessary for calculation of the four basic demographic indices. There are some questions, however, whose solution requires other information based on different types of demographic data. Using the indices I_m and I_g, for instance, one is able to link nuptiality to marital fertility through the use of correlation and regression analysis, but as these indices are based on the average behavior of the population in each arrondissement, the fallacy of ecological correlation runs high. Tables where the nuptiality and fertility experience of individuals are directly related (individual rather than ecological information) are, therefore, of great interest. In Belgium the first attempt to produce such data was made in the 1910 census, but then the number of surviving (rather than ever-born) children was tabulated against age and duration of the current marriage of the father (rather than the mother). Moreover, the census question was badly phrased, and many remarried men reported the number of surviving children to all marriages combined. Later on, tables were produced showing the number of children ever-born related to age and duration of marriage of the mother, which is, at least for demographic analysis, a much more meaningful way of relating fertility to nuptiality. Regrettably, these data were not available until 1930, by which time the demographic transition was nearing its end.

Hence, the quality of our analysis is more impaired by the absence of tables describing relations on an individual basis than by existence of deficiencies in enumeration and registration in the earlier periods.

References-Appendix

Coale, A. J. 1971. Age patterns of marriage. *Population Studies* 25:193-214.

Coale, A. J., and Demeny, P. 1966. *Regional model life tables and stable populations.* Princeton: Princeton University Press.

Coale, A. J., and McNeil, D. R. 1972. Distribution by age of frequency of first marriage in a female cohort. *Journal of the American Statistical Association* 67:743-749.

Heuschling, X. 1875. *Notice sur la statistique ancienne en Belgique.* Liège: Verhoven-Debeur Imprimeurs.

———. Situation territoriale et population des provinces belges sous le gouvernement autrichien. *Athénée historique.* Recueil de Memoires et Traités, pp. 18-27.

Quételet, A. 1847. Sur les anciens recensements de la population belge. *Bulletin de la Commission Centrale de Statistique* (Brussels) 3:1-26.

———. 1848. *Du système social et des lois qui le régissent.* Paris: Guillamin et Cie.

———. 1849. Nouvelles tables de mortalité pour la Belgique. *Bulletin de la Commission Centrale de Statistique* (Brussels) 4:1-16.

———. 1853. Sur les tables de mortalité et de population. Ibid., 5:1-24.

van de Walle, E. 1974. *The female population of France in the nineteenth century.* Princeton: Princeton University Press.

Index

LIBRARY OF CONGRESS CATALOGING IN PUBLICATION DATA

Lesthaeghe, Ron J. 1945-
The decline of Belgian fertility, 1800-1970.

"A publication of the Office of Population Research, Princeton University."

Includes bibliographical references and index.

1. Fertility, Human—Belgium—History.
I. Princeton University. Office of Population Research. II. Title.
HB1013.L47 301.32'1'09493 77-71991
ISBN 0-691-05253-0

ERRATUM

Page 50, figure 3.1

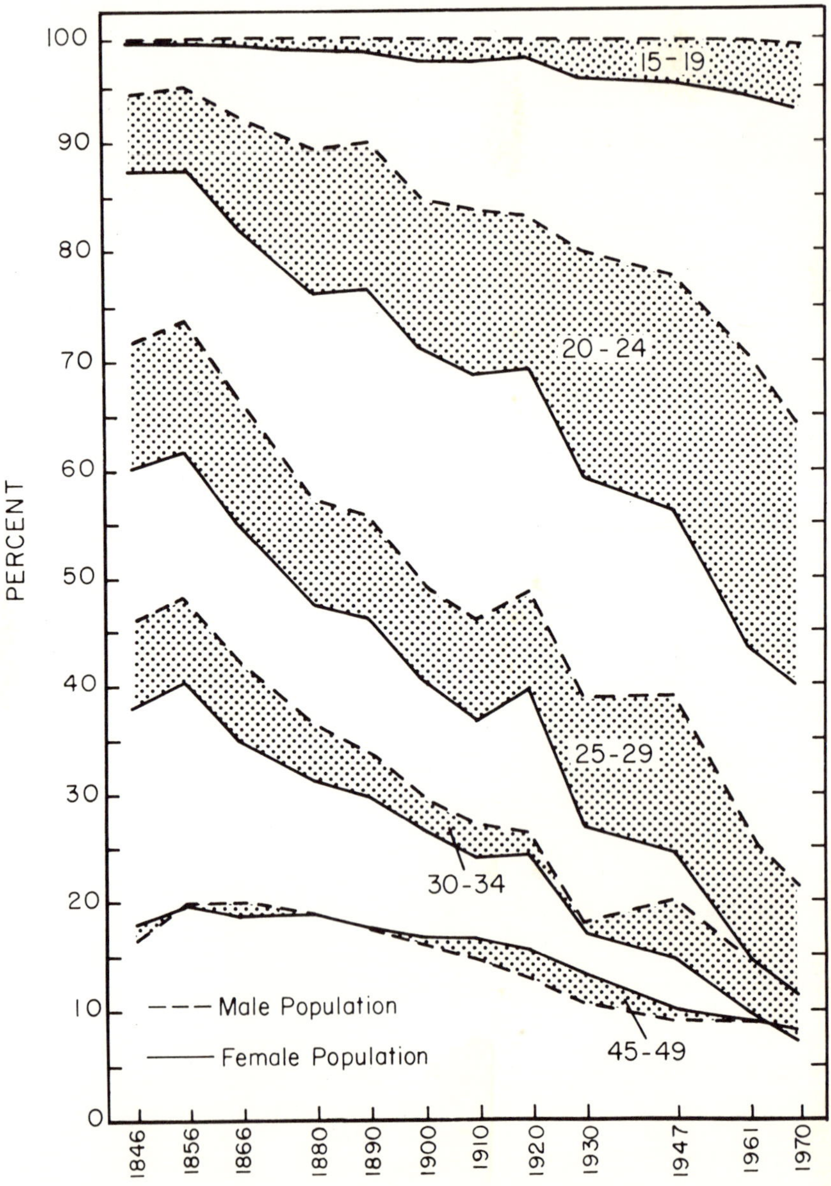

Figure 3.1 Percentage Single, by Sex and Age Group: 1846 to 1970.